Introduction to
Clinical Neurology

Introduction to Clinical Neurology

Fourth Edition

Douglas J. Gelb, MD, PhD
Department of Neurology
University of Michigan Medical School
Ann Arbor, Michigan

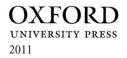
OXFORD
UNIVERSITY PRESS
2011

OXFORD
UNIVERSITY PRESS

Oxford University Press, Inc., publishes works that further
Oxford University's objective of excellence
in research, scholarship, and education.

Oxford New York
Auckland   Cape Town   Dar es Salaam   Hong Kong   Karachi
Kuala Lumpur   Madrid   Melbourne   Mexico City   Nairobi
New Delhi   Shanghai   Taipei   Toronto

With offices in
Argentina   Austria   Brazil   Chile   Czech Republic   France   Greece
Guatemala   Hungary   Italy   Japan   Poland   Portugal   Singapore
South Korea   Switzerland   Thailand   Turkey   Ukraine   Vietnam

Published by Oxford University Press, Inc.
198 Madison Avenue, New York, New York 10016
www.oup.com

Oxford is a registered trademark of Oxford University Press

Library of Congress Cataloging-in-Publication Data

Gelb, Douglas James, 1957–
    Introduction to clinical neurology / Douglas J. Gelb. – 4th ed.
       p.; cm.
    Includes bibliographical references and index.
    ISBN 978-0-19-973484-9
1. Neurology.   2. Nervous system—Diseases.   I. Title.
    [DNLM: 1. Nervous System Diseases. WL 140 G314i 2011]
    RC346.G45 2011
    616.8–dc22
                                                        2010011749

The science of medicine is a rapidly changing field. As new research and clinical experience broaden
our knowledge, changes in treatment and drug therapy occur. The author and publisher of this
work have checked with sources believed to be reliable in their efforts to provide information that is
accurate and complete, and in accordance with the standards accepted at the time of publication. In
light of the possibility of human error or changes in the practice of medicine, however, neither the
author, nor the publisher, nor any other party who has been involved in the preparation or
publication of this work warrants that the information contained herein is in every respect accurate
or complete. Readers are encouraged to confirm the information contained herein with other
reliable sources, and are strongly advised to check the product information sheet provided by the
pharmaceutical company for each drug they plan to administer.

9 8 7 6 5 4 3 2 1
Printed in the United States of America
on acid-free paper

To my father, the best teacher I know

Preface

In the five years since the publication of the third edition of this book, controlled trials and systematic reviews have helped to resolve or clarify many longstanding clinical debates. The current edition incorporates recent evidence regarding such topics as the role of steroids in treating Bell's palsy, surgical vs. non-surgical treatment of lumbar disc herniation, the relative value of clopidogrel and aspirin/extended-release dipyridamole in stroke prevention, the comparative effectiveness of glatiramer and interferons in treating multiple sclerosis, and the relative risks and benefits of carotid endarterectomy and angioplasty/stenting. In the same time period, the FDA has approved four new anti-epileptic drugs, a drug for Huntington's disease, and a new symptomatic medication for multiple sclerosis. There have also been recent revisions to the definitions of some fundamental neurologic conditions, notably "transient ischemic attack" and "epilepsy." The current edition includes all of these developments.

Although the details have been thoroughly updated, the overall organization and focus of the book remain unchanged. As before, the emphasis is on diagnosis and management, stressing general principles and a systematic approach. I have tried to maintain a consistent tone throughout the book, but to make sure that the discussion did not become too tainted by my personal biases and idiosyncrasies, I asked some of my colleagues to review chapters in their areas of expertise. I am grateful to Jim Burke, Ron Chervin, Kelvin Chou, Praveen Dayalu, Simon Glynn, Kevin Kerber, Steve Leber, Dan Leventhal, Linda Selwa, Jonathan Trobe, and Darin Zahuranec for many helpful comments. Of course, I was too stubborn to follow all of their advice, so any flaws that remain in the book are my fault, not theirs. As with all three previous editions of the book, I want to thank my wife, Karen, and my daughters, Elizabeth and Molly, for helping me avoid distractions when deadlines loomed and for providing the best possible distractions at other times.

D.J.G.

Preface to the First Edition

Is neurology obsolete? Two current trends prompt this question. First, dramatic biologic and technologic advances have resulted in increasingly accurate diagnostic tests. It is hard to believe that CT scans have only been widely available since the 1970s; MRI scans, PET scans, and SPECT scans are even more recent, and they are constantly being refined. While chess-playing computers have not quite reached world champion status yet, neurodiagnostic imaging studies have long since achieved a degree of sensitivity that neurologists cannot hope to match. There is more than a little truth to the joke that "one MRI scan is worth a roomful of neurologists." Moreover, advances in molecular genetics and immunochemistry now permit more accurate diagnosis of many conditions than could have been imagined 25 years ago. Some conditions can even be diagnosed before any clinical manifestations are evident. With tests this good, what is the point of learning the traditional approach to neurologic diagnosis, in which lesion localization is deduced from patients' symptoms and signs?

The second major trend challenging the current status of neurology is health care reform. As of this writing, the first great national legislative debate concerning health care reform has ended, not with a bang but a whimper. Yet the problem itself has not disappeared. The already unacceptable costs of health care will continue to escalate if the current system remains unchanged. While the various reform plans that have been proposed differ in many fundamental respects, there appears to be a consensus that there should be more primary care physicians and fewer specialists. Indeed, several forces are already pushing the medical profession in that direction even in the absence of a comprehensive national legislative plan. As a concrete example, it is anticipated that the number of residency training positions in neurology will drop, perhaps to only half of the current level. With so much nationwide emphasis on primary care, what is the point of studying neurology?

Ironically, these two trends together provide a compelling reason to study neurology. In coming years, there will be increasing pressures on primary care physicians to avoid referring patients to specialists (and there will be fewer specialists in the first place). One response of primary care physicians might be to order more diagnostic tests. Unfortunately, the only thing more impressive than the sensitivity of the new tests is their price tag. Just at the time when diagnostic tests are reaching unprecedented levels of accuracy, the funds to pay for the tests are disappearing. Rather than replacing neurologists with MRI scans and genetic testing, primary care physicians will have to become neurologists (to some degree) themselves.

In short, the role currently played by neurologists may well be obsolete, but neurology itself is not. All physicians, regardless of specialty, must become familiar with the general principles of neurologic diagnosis and management. That is the rationale for this book.

The purpose of this book is to present a systematic approach to the neurologic problems likely to be encountered in general medical practice. The focus throughout the book is on practical issues of patient management. This is a departure from the traditional view of neurologic diseases as fascinating but untreatable. Neurologists are often caricatured as pedants who will pontificate interminably on the precise localization of a lesion, produce an obscure diagnosis with an unpronounceable eponym, and smugly declare the case closed. In years past, this stereotype was not wholly inaccurate. Even when therapeutic options existed, there were few controlled studies of efficacy, so it was easy to take a nihilistic approach to therapy. "First do no harm" could often be legitimately interpreted to mean "Do nothing." This was obviously a frustrating position for physicians, and even more so for patients, but at least it kept things simple. All this has changed. Controlled trials of both new and traditional therapies are being conducted with increasing frequency. In the two years since the original versions of some of the current chapters were first prepared, sumatriptan has been approved for treatment of headache, beta interferon for use in multiple sclerosis, ticlopidine for stroke, and tacrine for Alzheimer's disease. Felbamate has appeared and (practically) disappeared. Gabapentin and lamotrigine have been approved for use in epilepsy. The long-term results of a large cooperative study of optic neuritis have challenged traditional practices involving the use of steroids for that condition and for multiple sclerosis. Preliminary reports have appeared concerning the value of endarterectomy for asymptomatic carotid stenosis, a new preparation of beta interferon for MS, and Copolymer I for MS. These are exciting developments, but many of the studies raise as many questions as they answer. They certainly change the way physicians have traditionally approached many neurologic diseases. This book reflects that change. Esoteric diagnostic distinctions with little practical relevance are avoided. Distinctions that affect treatment are emphasized. In most chapters, the available treatment options and general approach to management are presented first, to clarify which diagnostic distinctions are important and why.

For many physicians and medical students, the most difficult aspect of neurology is deciding where to start. It is relatively straightforward to manage a patient who has had a stroke; it is often harder to determine whether the patient had a stroke in the first place. When does hand weakness indicate carpal tunnel syndrome, and when is it a manifestation of multiple sclerosis? When does back pain signify metastatic cancer or a herniated disk? These general issues are addressed in the three chapters of Part I. In Part II, common neurologic disease categories are discussed. Part III concerns common symptoms and issues that cross disease categories. Features that distinguish neurologic problems in the pediatric and geriatric populations are discussed in Part IV.

This book is not meant to be comprehensive. Certain topics are omitted, notably specialized management issues that primary care physicians will probably not need to address and other conditions for which treatment is a matter of standard medical care. For example, most patients with primary brain cancer will probably be referred to specialists even in an age of health care reform, so the different types of brain cancer and their treatment are not addressed in this book. Diabetes, chronic alcohol abuse, vitamin B12 deficiency, and other metabolic disturbances can affect many parts of the nervous system. These conditions are mentioned in the relevant sections of this book, but there is no chapter devoted specifically to metabolic problems and their management because these topics are covered in standard medical textbooks. Even for the topics that are included in the book, much detail has been omitted. Again, detailed discussions are available in standard reference books. Use of those books requires some sophistication about neurology, however. A physician trying to figure out why a patient's hand is weak may be overwhelmed by a one or two thousand page textbook. Even when the patient's diagnosis is known, the standard references often fail to distinguish the forest from the trees, making it difficult to glean the main principles governing patient management. Those principles are the focus of this book.

Each chapter in this book begins with a set of clinical vignettes and associated questions. These are intended to help the reader focus on practical clinical questions while reading the chapter. Readers should try to answer the questions before reading the rest of the chapter. After finishing the chapter (but before reading the discussion of the clinical vignettes) readers should return to the questions and revise their answers as necessary. Readers can then compare their answers with those given in the discussion at the end of the chapter.

The vignettes are also intended to convey the message that neurology is fun. Many students who used the original version of this book reported that they enjoyed working through the vignettes, and they even suggested that more be included. This response is gratifying. Still, the best "clinical vignettes" come from patients themselves, not from books. Ideally, readers of this book will be inspired to seek out patients with neurologic problems, and will approach them not only with confidence, but with enthusiasm.

Contents

PART III: Common Symptoms

Contributors

James W. Albers, MD, PhD
Professor Emeritus
Director, Electromyography Laboratory
Department of Neurology
University of Michigan Medical School
Ann Arbor, Michigan

Mark B. Bromberg, MD, PhD
Professor of Neurology
Department of Neurology
University of Utah School of Medicine
Salt Lake City, Utah

Linda M. Selwa, MD
Professor of Neurology
Medical Director, Outpatient Services
Department of Neurology
University of Michigan Medical School
Ann Arbor, Michigan

Introduction to
Clinical Neurology

I

The Basic Approach

Chapter 1

Where's the Lesion?

I. Sample Localization Problems

Example 1. A patient is found to have neurologic deficits that include the following:

1. weakness of abduction of the little finger on the right hand, and

2. reduced pinprick sensation on the palmar surface of the little finger of the right hand.

   Where's the lesion?

Example 2. A patient is found to have neurologic deficits that include the following:

1. reduced pinprick sensation on the left forehead, and

2. reduced pinprick sensation on the palmar surface of the little finger of the right hand.

   Where's the lesion?

Example 3. A patient is found to have neurologic deficits that include the following:

1. reduced joint position sense in the left foot, and

2. reduced pinprick sensation on the palmar surface of the little finger of the right hand.

   Where's the lesion?

Example 4. A patient is found to have neurologic deficits that include the following:

1. reduced joint position sense in the left foot,

2. reduced pinprick sensation on the palmar surface of the little finger of the right hand,

3. weakness of left ankle dorsiflexion, and

4. hyperreflexia at the left knee.

Where's the lesion?

Example 5. A patient is found to have neurologic deficits that include the following:

1. reduced joint position sense in the left foot,

2. reduced joint position sense in the right foot,

3. reduced joint position sense in the left hand, and

4. reduced joint position sense in the right hand.

Where's the lesion?

Example 6. A patient is found to have neurologic deficits that include the following:

1. reduced joint position sense in the left foot,

2. reduced pinprick sensation on the palmar surface of the little finger of the right hand, and

3. reduced visual acuity in the left eye.

Where's the lesion?

Example 7. The findings on a patient's neurologic examination include the following:

1. reduced joint position and pinprick sensation in the left foot,

2. reduced joint position and pinprick sensation in the right foot,

3. reduced joint position and pinprick sensation in the left hand,

4. reduced joint position and pinprick sensation in the right hand, and

5. normal strength and sensation proximally in all four limbs.

Where's the lesion?

II. The Game

The key to neurologic diagnosis is localization. By identifying the site—or sites—of nervous system dysfunction, the clinician can refine the list of likely disease processes. This approach is not unique to neurology. For example, hematemesis suggests a problem in the upper gastrointestinal tract, so the evaluation should be directed at diseases that typically strike there, rather than diseases that usually affect the jejunum or below (let alone diseases that primarily affect the heart or lungs).

The main reason neurologic localization is distinctive is that the nervous system has so many different functions, each one mediated by anatomic structures that overlap or abut structures responsible for many other functions. Moreover, most of the anatomic structures are inaccessible to direct examination. The nervous system is, in effect, a black box—we can observe what goes in (sensory input) and what comes out (a person's movements, language output, and behaviors), but not what happens inside the box. Fortunately, we know enough about the structure and function of the nervous system that by observing the "output" that results from a known sensory "input," we can typically deduce the site of nervous system dysfunction.

As an analogy, suppose you are trying to find a broken track in an urban subway system, but the only information available to you is a map of the subway lines and continuous satellite video footage (see Figure 1.1).

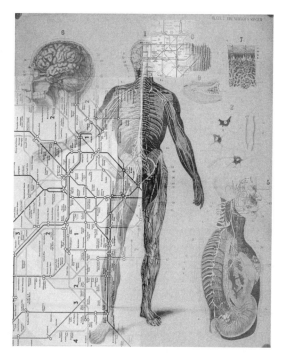

Fig. 1.1 Superposition of the human nervous system and a subway system.

Having monitored the video footage every day, you recognize certain people who routinely enter a particular station at the same time each day and always exit the system at some other station. Reviewing today's video, you see that some of those people have maintained their routine, which means that the tracks connecting their entry and exit stations are intact. Other people have revised their routine, indicating a disruption somewhere on the track between their entry and exit stations. By analyzing which people had to alter their routines and which did not, and referring to your map of the subway system, you should be able to pinpoint the damage.

Over the years, astute clinicians, anatomists, and physiologists have provided us with a detailed "subway map" of the nervous system. We also have plenty of "previous days' video footage"—patients can tell us how they functioned at baseline, and we know what to expect on a normal neurologic examination. We can determine which functions of the nervous system remain intact and which are disrupted, and use this information to deduce the site (or sites) of disease. Neurologic localization is essentially an exercise in logic—a game, but hardly a frivolous one. Once you learn to play the game, you can approach patients with neurologic symptoms and signs in a systematic manner rather than relying on pattern recognition (an overwhelming prospect given how many diseases affect the nervous system) or even worse, a shotgun approach, testing for every possible disease.

The rules of the game are presented in the following part of this chapter. For practicing neurologists, the reasoning involved in localization is so instinctive that explicit rules are unnecessary, but most would agree that localization ultimately depends on the kind of logical, stepwise approach summarized in these rules.

III. The Rules

1. Each symptom or abnormal physical finding can be thought of as a line segment connecting the central nervous system to the periphery (a muscle or sensory receptor). (In terms of the subway analogy in Part II, *each symptom or physical finding represents a different subway line.*)

2. If all of these line segments intersect at a single point, that point is the site of the lesion (i.e., *a station that is on every one of the damaged subway lines.*)

3. There may be two or more points where all the line segments intersect, and hence, two or more potential lesion sites. If so, each potential site must be evaluated further by determining whether the patient has the other symptoms or signs that would be expected with a lesion in that location. (*For every station common to all the damaged subway lines, check to see whether any additional subway lines travel through that station, then look to see if trains are running normally along those lines.*)

4. There may be no points that fall on all of the line segments. If so, the goal is to explain all of the patient's symptoms and physical findings on the basis of just two lesions (i.e., to find two points such that every line segment passes through one or the other point; or, in our analogy, to find **two** *stations that together account for all the damaged subway lines*).

5. If even two lesion sites are not sufficient to explain all the symptoms and findings, the process is likely to be either multifocal or diffuse. The goal then becomes one of detecting a unifying property that applies to all the lesion sites. For example, they may all be located at the neuromuscular junction, or they may all be in the white matter of the central nervous system (*all the stations that are above ground, say, or all the stations that are in suburbs*).

When stated in this way, the rules appear abstract and somewhat obscure, but they are actually quite straightforward to apply. This is demonstrated in the following three parts of this chapter by considering specific examples. It might seem that detailed knowledge of neuroanatomy would be required. Certainly, more precise neuroanatomic knowledge permits more refined localization, but for most purposes, some fairly rough neuroanatomic approximations are adequate. To show this, several examples of careful neuroanatomic analysis are presented in Part IV, and simpler analyses of the same clinical scenarios are presented in Part V. In Part VI, the kind of reasoning applied in Parts IV and V is used to derive some general principles that can expedite localization.

IV. The Play: The Long Version

Note: If the following discussion seems too complicated, you might want to proceed directly to Part V. In fact, you could skip even further ahead and focus on the simple rules presented in Part VI, which can be used to localize the majority of neurologic lesions. At some point, however, you should return to Part IV to understand the detailed reasoning process that underlies the more simplified approaches.

Example 1. A patient is found to have neurologic deficits that include the following:

1. weakness of abduction of the little finger on the right hand, and
2. reduced pinprick sensation on the palmar surface of the little finger of the right hand.

Where's the lesion?

Item 1 in Example 1 could be caused by a lesion anywhere in the line segment shown in Figure 1.2. The pathway begins in the precentral gyrus of the left cerebral cortex (i.e., the motor strip). The representation of the hand in this strip is midway between the leg representation medially and the face representation laterally. From this point of origin, the segment descends in order through the corona radiata, the internal capsule, the cerebral peduncle (in the midbrain), and the basis pontis, until it reaches the pyramid in the medulla. At this point, the pathway crosses to the right side, and proceeds downward in the lateral white matter of the spinal cord. At the C8 and T1 levels of the spinal cord, the pathway enters the anterior aspect of the gray matter (where the cortical neuron synapses on a motor neuron whose cell body is in the anterior horn), then exits the spinal cord via the right C8 and T1 roots, proceeds through the lower trunk and then the medial cord of the brachial plexus, exits in the ulnar nerve, passes through the neuromuscular junction, and terminates in the abductor digiti minimi muscle.

The line segment corresponding to item 2 is shown in Figure 1.3. It starts in sensory receptors in the little finger of the right hand, continues in the ulnar nerve, proceeds proximally through the medial cord and lower trunk of the brachial plexus, and enters the spinal cord via the right C8 nerve root. It ascends one or two segments in the cord, and then crosses to the left spinothalamic tract, ascending in this tract through the medulla, pons, and midbrain. After synapsing in the ventral posterolateral nucleus of the thalamus, the pathway continues through the internal capsule and corona radiata, terminating in the parietal cortex (just posterior to the region of the motor strip where the line segment for item 1 originates).

Figure 1.4 illustrates both of these line segments together. One obvious point of intersection is in the frontoparietal cortex, where one segment lies directly behind the other. In addition, there is a whole set of possible intersection sites falling between the ulnar nerve distally and the C8/T1 nerve roots proximally. To decide which of these potential localization sites is the true focus of pathology, the next step is to consider what other signs and

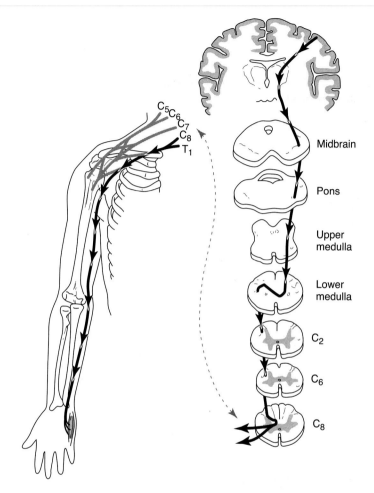

Fig. 1.2 The solid black arrows show the pathway corresponding to weakness of abduction of the little finger on the right hand.

symptoms might be expected from a lesion at each site. For example, a lesion in the C8/T1 nerve roots or the lower trunk of the brachial plexus would be likely to affect fibers destined for the median nerve, affecting muscles innervated by that nerve, whereas these muscles would clearly be spared by a lesion in the ulnar nerve itself. In contrast, a cortical lesion affecting the arm could extend far enough laterally or medially to affect the

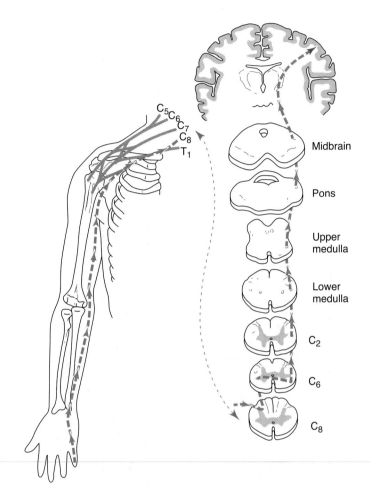

Fig. 1.3 The dashed gray arrows depict the pathway corresponding to reduced pinprick sensation on the palmar surface of the little finger on the right hand.

cortical representation of the right face or leg, whereas a nerve, plexus, or root lesion clearly would not affect anything outside the right upper extremity. Abnormalities of vision or language function would also imply a cortical localization and would be inconsistent with a lesion in the peripheral nervous system.

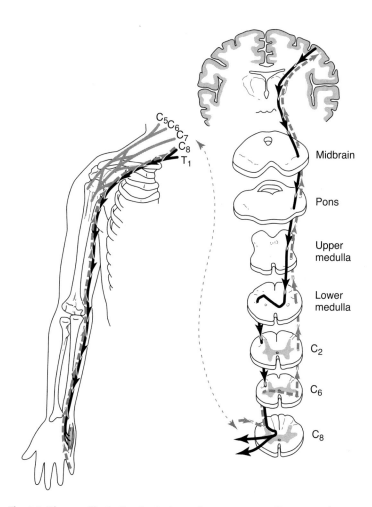

Fig. 1.4 Diagram illustrating both the pathway corresponding to weak abduction of the right little finger (black, descending arrows) and reduced pinprick sensation (gray, ascending arrows) in that finger (i.e., the pathways of both Figure 1.2 and Figure 1.3). The regions common to both pathways are in the left frontoparietal cortex and in the peripheral nervous system (from the right C8/T1 nerve roots to the right ulnar nerve).

Example 2. A patient is found to have neurologic deficits that include the following:

1. reduced pinprick sensation on the left forehead, and

2. reduced pinprick sensation on the palmar surface of the little finger of the right hand.

Where's the lesion?

The line segment corresponding to item 2 in Example 2 was already discussed in the previous example (see Figure 1.3). The pathway for item 1 is shown in Figure 1.5. It starts in sensory receptors in the left forehead and continues in the first division (the ophthalmic division) of the trigeminal nerve (cranial nerve V). This nerve travels through the superior orbital fissure and enters the lateral wall of the cavernous sinus. It then emerges to join the other two divisions of the trigeminal nerve in the trigeminal (gasserian) ganglion. From here, the pathway enters the pons, descends in the left spinal tract of the trigeminal nucleus, and synapses in the nucleus of that tract at about the C2 spinal level. At this point, the pathway crosses to the right side of the spinal cord and ascends in the ventral trigeminotha-lamic tract to synapse in the ventral posteromedial nucleus of the right thalamus. The final section of the line segment runs from the ventral pos-teromedial nucleus through the internal capsule and corona radiata to ter-minate in the lateral aspect of the postcentral gyrus of the parietal lobe.

Figure 1.6 combines Figures 1.3 and 1.5. Potential intersection sites lie between the mid-pons and the high spinal cord (C2) on the left. At all other points, the line segments are nowhere near each other. In fact, they are generally on opposite sides of the nervous system! Again, the localiza-tion can be made even more precise by determining whether the patient has other abnormalities that might result from a lesion at each potential site. For example, facial nerve involvement could occur with a lesion in the mid-pons, but not at any of the lower sites, whereas hypoglossal nerve involvement would indicate a lesion at the level of the medulla.

Although Figures 1.2 through 1.6 may seem excessively detailed, they are still relatively simplified versions of the underlying anatomy. For example, Figure 1.2 reflects a tacit assumption that the lateral corticospinal tract is the principal descending pathway affecting limb muscles. The ventral corticospinal tract and other descending motor pathways (such as the vestibulospinal, tectospinal, rubrospinal, reticulospinal, and ceruleus-spinal projections) are not included in the figure. The importance of these other descending pathways is best appreciated by recognizing that a

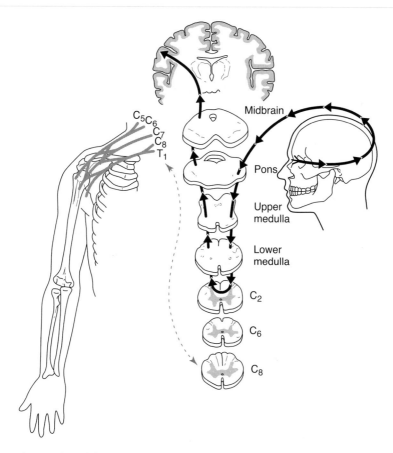

Fig. 1.5 The solid black arrows show the pathway corresponding to reduced pinprick sensation on the left forehead.

selective lesion of the corticospinal tract (e.g., in the medullary pyramid, one of the few locations where it is physically isolated from other descending tracts) results in minimal long-term weakness. Even so, the pathway presented in Figure 1.2 proves to be very useful in clinical localization. Presumably, the contributions of all the descending tracts sum up in such a way that the net effect is something similar to the pathway shown in the figure. This is just one example of how approximations and simplifications that we know are inaccurate can nonetheless lead to conclusions that are

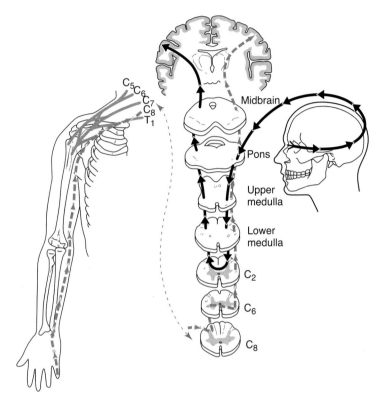

Fig. 1.6 Diagram illustrating both the pathway corresponding to (gray arrows) reduced pinprick sensation in the right little finger and (black arrows) reduced pinprick sensation on the left forehead (i.e., the pathways of both Figure 1.3 and Figure 1.5). The regions common to both pathways lie between the mid-pons and the C2 level of the spinal cord on the left.

clinically useful. In fact, we can ignore many anatomical details and still localize most lesions fairly reliably. Part V illustrates this.

V. The Play: The Abbreviated Version

The best way to identify all plausible lesion localization sites (and only those sites) is to follow the approach outlined in Part IV. In many cases, however, much coarser analysis of the symptoms and signs will give nearly the same results. In particular, the lesion can often be localized with surprising precision simply by considering where the relevant nervous system pathways cross the midline.

Example 1 Revisited. Figure 1.7 shows a schematic diagram of the pathway portrayed in Figure 1.2, corresponding to weakness of the right abductor digiti minimi muscle. Much of the detail has been eliminated. In fact, the same diagram would apply to any muscle in the right upper extremity. Figure 1.8 shows a schematic diagram for the right hand numbness represented in Figure 1.3. Figure 1.9 combines Figures 1.7 and 1.8. It is clear even from this simplified diagram that within the spinal cord the two pathways are on opposite sides, so the lesion could not possibly be located there. Instead, it must either be in the periphery (i.e., at the level of nerve roots, plexus, or peripheral nerves) or rostral to the level at which the motor pathway crosses in the medulla. Although the more detailed analysis presented in Part IV results in a more refined final localization (ruling out all of the rostral structures except the cortex), this additional refinement may not be that important in practice. The entire region from the medulla to the cortex is visualized on magnetic resonance imaging (MRI) of the brain, so as long as the lesion can be localized to somewhere within this region the appropriate diagnostic study will be obtained. In contrast, elimination of the cervical spinal cord from consideration does have a significant practical result, because it makes an MRI scan of the cervical spine unnecessary.

Example 2 Revisited. Figure 1.10 presents a schematic diagram for the pathway shown in Figure 1.5, representing left forehead numbness. Again, Figure 1.8 represents a schematic diagram for right hand numbness. Both pathways are shown together in Figure 1.11. It is clear from the diagram that the only potential intersection points lie in the region extending from the left mid-pons down to the left side of the spinal cord at the C2 level. This is exactly the same localization deduced earlier from the more detailed analysis.

Because the level at which a pathway crosses the midline is the most important feature for localizing central nervous system lesions, many different symptoms can be portrayed by the same schematic diagram. For example, Figure 1.7 represents weakness in any muscle of the right upper extremity, and an analogous figure can be drawn for weakness in any other limb. Figure 1.8 portrays a deficit in pain or temperature sensation anywhere in the right upper extremity, and analogous figures apply to pain/temperature deficits in other limbs.

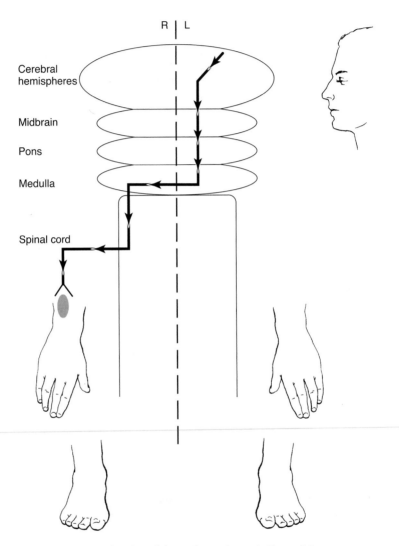

Fig. 1.7 Schematic drawing of the pathway shown in Figure 1.2, representing weakness of right little finger abduction. The same diagram would be used to represent weakness in any muscle of the right upper extremity.

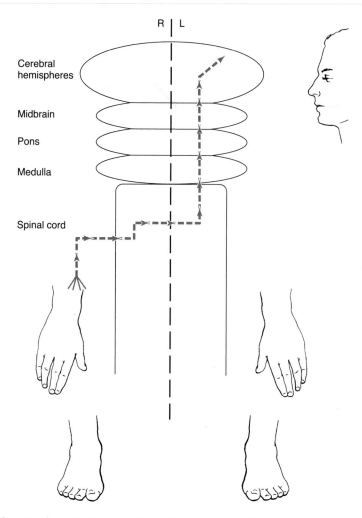

Fig. 1.8 Schematic drawing of the pathway shown in Figure 1.3, representing reduced pinprick sensation in the right upper extremity.

A deficit in proprioception or vibration sense is represented by Figure 1.12 (or something analogous in another limb). Figure 1.10 portrays the pathway for impaired pain and temperature sensation in the face. The pathway for facial weakness is represented in Figure 1.13, and analogous figures can be drawn for the motor components of other cranial nerves. These pathways

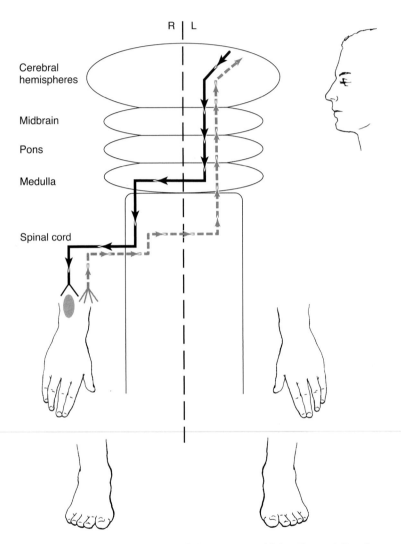

Fig. 1.9 Schematic representation of Figure 1.4, combining Figures 1.7 and 1.8. The only regions common to both pathways are at the level of the mid-medulla or above on the left, or in the peripheral nervous system on the right.

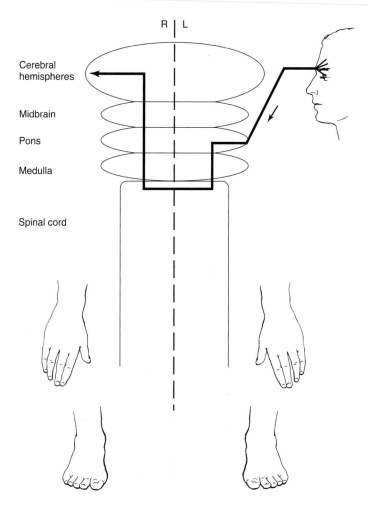

Fig. 1.10 Schematic drawing of the pathway shown in Figure 1.5, representing left facial numbness.

are complicated because there is bilateral cortical input to many of these cranial nerve nuclei, making interpretation difficult at times. Analogously, the auditory and vestibular pathways project bilaterally once they enter the central nervous system, making peripheral lesions much more straightforward to localize than central lesions. For example, unilateral hearing loss

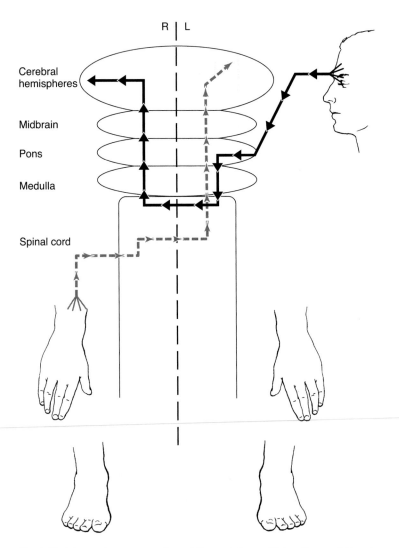

Fig. 1.11 Schematic representation of Figure 1.6, combining Figures 1.8 and 1.10. The only regions common to both pathways lie between the midpons and the C2 level of the spinal cord on the left.

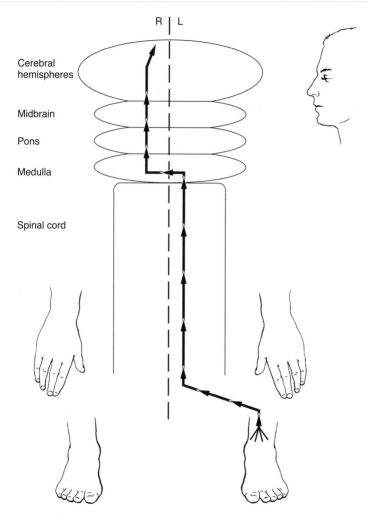

Fig. 1.12 Schematic drawing of the pathway corresponding to reduced position or vibration sense in the left lower extremity.

implies a lesion in the ipsilateral eighth nerve, cochlea, or inner ear. Bilateral hearing loss is of much less localizing value.

The distinction between the central and peripheral portions of a pathway is often very powerful. When considered schematically, the peripheral portion of a pathway (extending from a muscle or sensory receptor organ

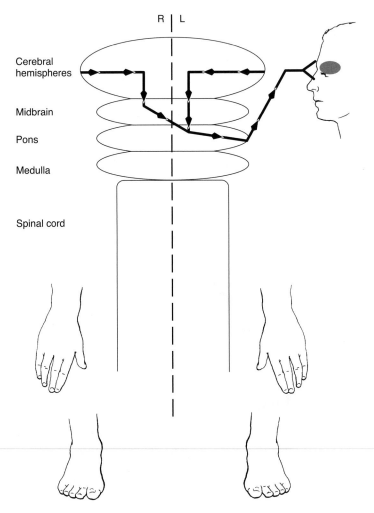

Fig. 1.13 Schematic drawing of the pathway corresponding to left facial weakness.

to the spinal cord or brainstem) is perpendicular to the "long axis" of the nervous system (the neuraxis), which runs from the cortex to the base of the spinal cord. A lesion that can be localized to the peripheral limb of one pathway (pathway X in Figure 1.14) and the central limb of another (pathway Y) is thus "caught in the cross-hairs," permitting very precise

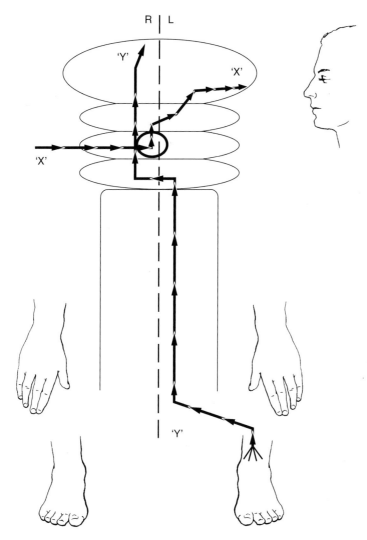

Fig. 1.14 Schematic drawing to illustrate the localizing value of identifying dysfunction in the peripheral portion of one pathway ('X') and the central portion of another pathway ('Y'), thereby localizing the lesion "in the cross-hairs" (small circle).

localization (the subway equivalent would be involvement of both a north-south line and an east-west line).

For example, a patient who has a lesion compressing the spinal cord typically has hypoactive deep tendon reflexes at the level of the lesion and hyperactive reflexes below that level. *Hypoactive reflexes indicate dysfunction in the peripheral portion of the reflex pathway, the reflex arc.* The reflex arc begins in a sensory receptor located inside a muscle, travels along sensory nerve fibers to the spinal cord, then synapses with a motor neuron in the anterior horn at the same level, and proceeds out along motor nerve fibers to the original muscle. In essence, the pathway combines the peripheral components of Figures 1.7 and 1.12. In normal individuals, the deep tendon reflexes are continually suppressed by descending motor tracts. These tracts constitute the central, or "upper motor neuron," portion of the reflex pathway. *When there is a lesion in this central pathway, the peripheral reflex arc is no longer suppressed, and a hyperactive reflex results.* Several different descending tracts are involved, but, as already discussed with regard to weakness, the central limb of the pathway shown in Figure 1.7 approximates the net effect. Both the peripheral and the central portions of the pathway for the right biceps reflex are represented schematically in Figure 1.15. A compressive lesion at the C5 level of the spinal cord interrupts the peripheral portion of the biceps reflex pathway and at the same time interrupts the central portion of the pathways mediating the triceps and lower extremity reflexes. Other examination findings useful in distinguishing central (e.g., upper motor neuron or supranuclear) from peripheral (e.g., lower motor neuron or nuclear) lesions are discussed in Chapter 2.

Visual information is transmitted from the eyes to the brain by another pathway that is perpendicular to the neuraxis (Figure 1.16). Detailed understanding of this pathway can lead to elegant and precise localization, but at the most basic level it suffices to know that the optic nerves from each eye merge at the optic chiasm. Anterior to the chiasm, a structural lesion will affect vision from only one eye, whereas a lesion at the chiasm or posterior to it will produce visual problems in both eyes. Moreover, when the fibers merge at the chiasm, they sort themselves so that all the fibers on one side of the brain correspond to visual input from the opposite side of the visual world. To be specific, stimuli in the right half of the visual world are focused by the lens system of each eye onto the left side of the retina. This is the temporal half of the left retina and the nasal half of the right retina. The ganglion cells in the left half of each retina send information to the left occipital cortex. Thus, the left occipital cortex processes visual input from the right half of the visual world. To accomplish this, the fibers

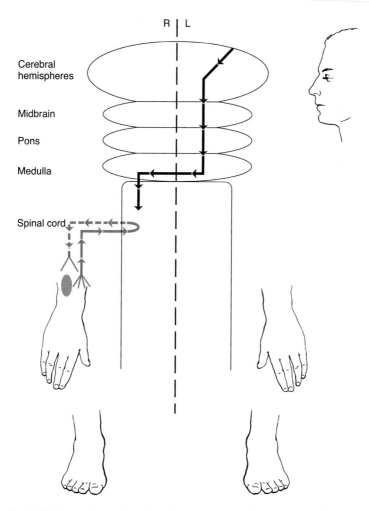

Fig. 1.15 Schematic drawing of a reflex arc in the right upper extremity, together with the central pathway providing descending inhibitory input to the reflex arc.

from the nasal half of the right retina must cross the midline. Analogously, the fibers from the nasal half of the left retina cross the midline to send information to the right visual cortex. This crossing occurs in the optic chiasm. A single large lesion at the chiasm can damage all the crossing and uncrossing fibers, resulting in total blindness. A smaller, centrally placed

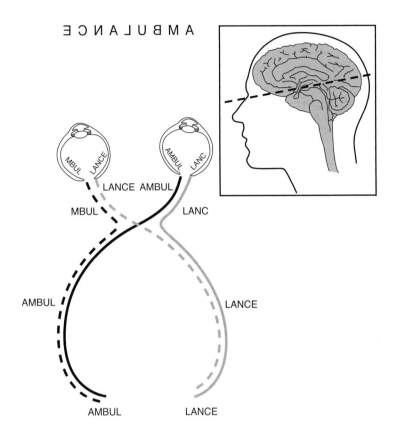

Fig. 1.16 Schematic drawing representing the visual pathways.

lesion may damage only the crossing fibers. Since these fibers originate in the nasal retina of each eye, the result is impaired vision in the temporal field of each eye (a bitemporal hemianopia).

The pupillary light reflex is mediated by another pathway that is perpendicular to the neuraxis (Figure 1.17). The pathway runs from the eye through the optic chiasm, just as in Figure 1.16, but soon after leaving the chiasm some fibers diverge from the rest of the visual fibers to synapse in the dorsal midbrain on parasympathetic nerve fibers that run with the oculomotor nerve (cranial nerve III) and terminate in the pupillary constrictor muscles. Note that even with input to just one eye, the bilateral

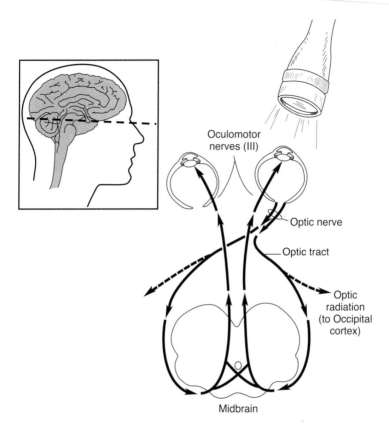

Fig. 1.17 Schematic drawing of the pathway mediating bilateral pupillary constriction in response to light in one eye.

projections in the optic chiasm and again in the midbrain result in bilateral output—that is, both pupils constrict. The net output is actually a function of the input to both eyes. In most natural circumstances, the overall illumination is the same in both eyes, so the input to each eye is the same. When the input to each eye is different (e.g., when an examiner holds a bright flashlight up to one eye, or when one optic nerve is defective), the midbrain essentially averages the illumination from the two eyes to produce a single net output signal that is the same for the two pupils.

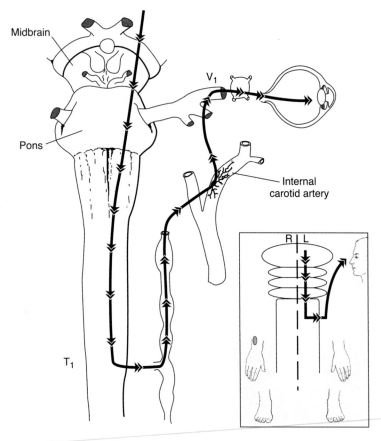

Fig. 1.18 Schematic drawing illustrating the pathway for sympathetic innervation of the left pupil.

Pupillary size is determined not only by the parasympathetic pathway but also by the sympathetic pathway, represented in Figure 1.18. This pathway begins in the hypothalamus, descends through the brainstem to the spinal cord at about the T1 level, then exits the spinal cord to enter the sympathetic chain and synapse in the superior cervical ganglion. From here, the pathway follows first the internal carotid artery and then the ophthalmic division of the trigeminal nerve (cranial nerve V), ultimately terminating in the pupil. Unlike most other pathways, the sympathetic pathway controlling the pupil remains on one side of the nervous system throughout its course. This is often extremely helpful in pinning down the site of a lesion.

Several neurologic deficits with localizing value do not readily lend themselves to a formulation in terms of line segments. For example, coordinated movements involve the interplay of motor cortex, basal ganglia, cerebellum, and brainstem nuclei. The interconnections between these structures result in "double-crossing" and "triple-crossing" pathways that sometimes resemble a tangled ball of yarn. It is often simplest to localize a lesion on the basis of other clinical features, and then check to see that the resulting localization is consistent with the patient's coordination problem, rather than trying to reason through all the potential sites that could cause the coordination abnormality.

Cognitive processing is another example of neural circuitry that is so complicated that it does not lend itself to simple diagrams based on isolated line segments. Language function is a partial exception. The neurophysiologic mechanisms involved in linguistic processing remain obscure, and undoubtedly involve intricate connections between many different brain regions. Despite this complexity, a very crude and simplistic model of language processing is surprisingly useful for clinical localization (Figure 1.19A and B). According to this model, Wernicke's area in the posterior temporal cortex is involved in recognizing the linguistic structures incorporated in a string of sounds. Areas of "higher" association cortex process these linguistic structures to extract meaning. Broca's area in the inferior lateral frontal lobe (just anterior to the region of the motor strip representing the face) translates linguistic structures into the motor programs necessary for producing speech. Thus, the comprehension of spoken language is represented in Figure 1.19B by pathway 1 from the ear to auditory cortex to Wernicke's area and thence to association areas. The ability to repeat a string of words is represented by pathway 3 from the ear to auditory cortex to Wernicke's area, and from there through the arcuate fasciculus to Broca's area to the motor strip and thence to the cranial nerves innervating the appropriate muscles of the face, tongue, pharynx, larynx, and diaphragm. This model is a gross oversimplification and fails to explain many clinical observations. For example, many patients with lesions in the arcuate fasciculus are able to repeat normally. Nonetheless, the model has some clinical utility—at least in giving an indication of whether a lesion is likely to be located anteriorly or posteriorly. In fact, an extension of the model that includes coding of written symbols in the angular gyrus (just above and behind Wernicke's area at the junction of the occipital, parietal, and temporal lobes) is also useful clinically.

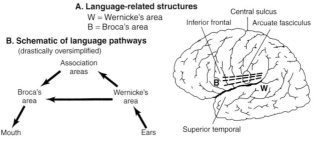

A. Language-related structures
W = Wernicke's area
B = Broca's area

B. Schematic of language pathways
(drastically oversimplified)

Pathways

1. Comprehension: ears -→ Wernicke's -→ association areas
2. Fluency: association areas -→ Broca's -→ mouth
3. Repetition: ears -→Wernicke's -→(via arcuate fasciculus) -→ Broca's -→ mouth

Note: Repetition pathway is peri-Sylvian (i.e., involves only structures adjacent to Sylvian fissure). Global hypoperfusion tends to spare this area, disconnecting it from association areas and producing transcortical aphasias (see Panel C).

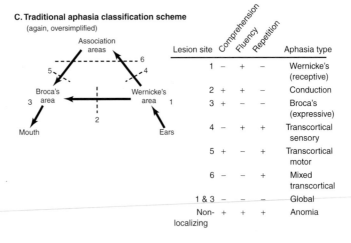

C. Traditional aphasia classification scheme
(again, oversimplified)

Lesion site	Comprehension	Fluency	Repetition	Aphasia type
1	–	+	–	Wernicke's (receptive)
2	+	+	–	Conduction
3	+	–	–	Broca's (expressive)
4	–	+	+	Transcortical sensory
5	+	–	+	Transcortical motor
6	–	–	+	Mixed transcortical
1 & 3	–	–	–	Global
Non-localizing	+	+	+	Anomia

Fig. 1.19 Schematic diagram representing language processing in the brain.

Example 3. A patient is found to have neurologic deficits that include the following:

1. reduced joint position sense in the left foot, and
2. reduced pinprick sensation on the palmar surface of the little finger of the right hand.

Where's the lesion?

The line segment corresponding to item 2 in Example 3 has already been discussed (see Figure 1.8). The line segment corresponding to item 1 is shown in Figure 1.12. Both line segments are shown together in Figure 1.20. The two line segments are on opposite sides of the nervous system except for a short segment running from the lower medulla on the left to about the C6/7 level of the spinal cord on the left. This region is the only potential localization site.

Example 4. A patient is found to have neurologic deficits that include the following:

1. reduced joint position sense in the left foot,
2. reduced pinprick sensation on the palmar surface of the little finger of the right hand,
3. weakness of left ankle dorsiflexion, and
4. hyperreflexia at the left knee.

Where's the lesion?

The first two items are the same as in Example 3 and imply a lesion localization somewhere between the low medulla and the C6/7 level of the spinal cord on the left (see Figure 1.20). Within this region, the line segments corresponding to the third and fourth items essentially coincide with the line segment for item 1. Thus, the additional deficits help to confirm the region of potential localization, but they do not help to refine it. One way to narrow the region would be to examine the left biceps reflex. This would be represented by a mirror image of the pathway shown in Figure 1.15. A depressed biceps reflex would imply a lesion in the reflex arc at the C5 or C6 level of the spinal cord. In contrast, a hyperactive biceps reflex would imply a lesion above the level of C5.

Example 5. A patient is found to have neurologic deficits that include the following:

1. reduced joint position sense in the left foot,
2. reduced joint position sense in the right foot,
3. reduced joint position sense in the left hand, and
4. reduced joint position sense in the right hand.

Where's the lesion?

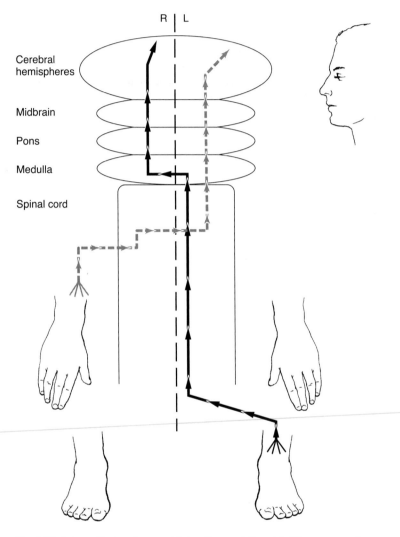

Fig. 1.20 Schematic drawing combining Figures 1.8 and 1.12, corresponding to reduced pinprick sensation in the right upper extremity and reduced joint position sense in the left lower extremity. The only regions common to both pathways lie between the low medulla and the C6/7 level of the spinal cord on the left.

Figure 1.12 shows the line segment corresponding to item 1 in Example 5. Figure 1.21 includes this line segment together with analogous line segments from each of the other three limbs representing items 2, 3, and 4. At first glance, it appears that there is only one level at which all these segments intersect: in the medulla, where they all cross. At every other level, two of the segments are on one side of the nervous system and two are on the other. On closer scrutiny, however, additional localization sites are evident. Even though the segments lie on both sides of the nervous system, there are two places where they are contiguous across the midline. Thus, whereas a unilateral lesion could not affect all four line segments, a bilateral lesion centered in the midline and extending out to each side could explain the pattern of deficits. The sites where this is possible are in the cervical spinal cord (at the level of C7 and above) and the postcentral gyrus of the cortex. The presence or absence of additional deficits (corresponding to additional line segments) would help to distinguish between these three potential lesion sites (medulla, cervical cord, and cortex).

Example 6. A patient is found to have neurologic deficits that include the following:

1. reduced joint position sense in the left foot,
2. reduced pinprick sensation on the palmar surface of the little finger of the right hand, and
3. reduced visual acuity in the left eye.

Where's the lesion?

The first two items are the same as in Examples 3 and 4 and imply a lesion localization somewhere between the low medulla and the C6/7 level of the spinal cord on the left (see Figure 1.20). This region is not even close to the line segment representing the patient's visual loss (see Figure 1.16). This means that no single lesion site could produce all of this patient's findings. By the rules of the game, the next objective is to explain all of the deficits on the basis of two lesion sites. This can obviously be achieved by assuming that one lesion is in the previously identified region of the medulla or spinal cord and the other lesion is in the left retina or optic nerve. The next step is to decide whether these two lesions are related or coincidental, using the approach to be presented in Chapter 3.

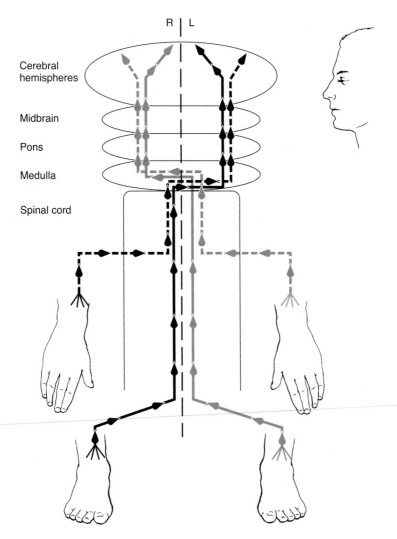

Fig. 1.21 Schematic drawing representing loss of joint position sense in all four limbs. Potential lesion sites lie in the midline and extend bilaterally, at the levels of the cortex, low medulla, or high cervical spinal cord.

Example 7. The findings on a patient's neurologic examination include the following:

1. reduced joint position and pinprick sensation in the left foot,
2. reduced joint position and pinprick sensation in the right foot,
3. reduced joint position and pinprick sensation in the left hand,
4. reduced joint position and pinprick sensation in the right hand, and
5. normal strength and sensation proximally in all four limbs.

Where's the lesion?

The deficits in joint position sense in all four limbs were discussed in Example 5. They imply a lesion site lying in the midline and extending bilaterally either in the cortex or in the region extending from the low medulla to the C7 level of the spinal cord. Within this latter region, the line segments representing pinprick sensation lie laterally (see Figure 1.3). Unlike the pathways for joint position sense, they are not contiguous across the midline, and only an extremely large lesion could affect them bilaterally. This is shown in Figure 1.22, which represents a cross section of the spinal cord (the reasoning would be the same for the medulla). Region A is the area corresponding to the loss of position sense in all four limbs and region B is the area corresponding to the loss of pinprick sensation. Because the lateral corticospinal tracts lie between these two regions, a single lesion large enough to encompass both regions A and B would necessarily result in weakness throughout the lower extremities. The preserved proximal strength (item 5) therefore eliminates this potential lesion site.

Similar reasoning eliminates the cortex as a potential localization. The representation of the body surface along the postcentral gyrus is organized in the following order from medial to lateral: distal lower extremity, proximal lower extremity, proximal upper extremity, distal upper extremity, face. The only way a single lesion could produce sensory deficits in both the distal upper extremity and the distal lower extremity would be to involve the proximal limbs also.

In short, no single lesion site can explain all of the findings in this patient. The findings cannot even be explained by positing two lesions. This patient has a multifocal or diffuse condition. By the rules of the game, the next goal is to identify some common characteristic unifying all of the lesion sites. In this case, all of the findings are sensory deficits restricted to the distal portions of the limbs. This suggests a process affecting peripheral nerves, specifically involving the longest sensory nerves. *Peripheral polyneuropathy* is the term for such a condition (see Chapter 6).

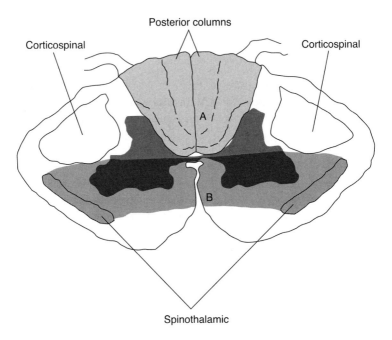

Fig. 1.22 Cross section of the high cervical spinal cord. Region A corresponds to the area that must be affected to produce loss of joint position sense in all four limbs. Region B corresponds to the area that would produce reduced pinprick sensation in all four limbs. Any lesion large enough to affect both region A and region B would also include the lateral corticospinal tracts, resulting in motor symptoms.

VI. Rules for Speed Play

Even in the limited number of examples presented in Part V, several themes emerge repeatedly. Many of these themes can be summarized as general principles that are often sufficient for localizing a lesion without actually drawing line segments for each symptom and looking for the points of intersection. Most neurologists have internalized these rules. When presented with a patient like the one described in Example 4, they immediately think of a spinal cord lesion; in fact, this is even a named syndrome (Brown-Séquard syndrome). The patient described in Example 7 is so typical of a patient with polyneuropathy that no neurologist would require diagrams to reach that conclusion.

The following principles summarize many of the "shortcuts" used by neurologists in localizing a lesion. They are useful in many clinical situations, but they are simplifications. If they are applied without thinking, they may result in errors or omissions. Even neurologists sometimes fall into this trap. When a case is confusing, it is always best to analyze it systematically as described in Part V. In fact, with more confusing cases, even the analysis of Part V may be inadequate, and the kind of detailed analysis presented in Part IV may be required.

With those caveats, the following principles may be presented. They are derived from the kind of reasoning already presented in analyzing Examples 1–7; a brief explanation follows each principle.

1. *If a patient has deficits of both strength and pain/temperature sensation in a single limb, and no other neurologic abnormalities, the lesion is either in the periphery (nerve/plexus/ root) or in the cortex.*

   Explanation: The pathway for pain and temperature sensation crosses the midline soon after entering the spinal cord. The motor pathways cross in the medulla: Below the site of this crossing they are on the opposite side of the nervous system from the sensory pathways; above the site of crossing, they are ipsilateral to the sensory pathways but not aligned with them until the cortex is reached (see Figures 1.4 and 1.9).

2. *If pain/temperature sensation is reduced in one limb and position/ vibration sensation is reduced in a contralateral limb, the lesion is somewhere in the spinal cord (on the same side as the position/vibration deficit).*

   Explanation: The pathway for pain and temperature sensation crosses the midline soon after entering the spinal cord; the pathway for position and vibration sense does not cross until it reaches the low medulla. Between the two sites of crossing (i.e., within the spinal cord), the pathway for pain and temperature in one limb lies on the same side of the nervous system as the pathway for position and vibration sense in the contralateral limbs (see Figure 1.20).

3. *Bilateral sensory and motor deficits throughout the body below a roughly horizontal level on the trunk, with normal function above that level, indicate a spinal cord lesion (at or above that level).*

   Explanation: A large spinal cord lesion will disrupt all ascending fiber tracts from all parts of the body below the lesion, and it will disrupt all descending fiber tracts traveling to those body parts. A smaller spinal cord lesion may spare portions of those fiber tracts. The tracts are arranged in

such a way that the spared portions typically contain the fibers corresponding to the uppermost part of the affected region of the body. Hence, a given
sensory/motor level can indicate a large spinal cord lesion at that level, or
a smaller lesion higher up in the spinal cord.

4. *Increased reflexes in a symptomatic limb suggest a central lesion; reduced
   reflexes in a symptomatic limb suggest a peripheral lesion.*

Explanation: The nerve root, plexus, peripheral nerve, and muscle are
all included in the reflex arc, which is tonically inhibited by descending
pathways from above (see Figure 1.15).

5. *Reduced pain/temperature sensation on one side of the face and the opposite side of the body implies a lesion between the pons and C2 (ipsilateral
   to the facial numbness). Reduced pain/temperature sensation on one side
   of the face and the same side of the body implies a lesion in the high brainstem or above.*

Explanation: The pathway for pain and temperature sensation from the
face enters the pons via the trigeminal nerve, descends on the same side to
about the C2 level of the spinal cord, crosses, and ascends on the opposite
side. The descending pathway (from the pons to C2) is close to the ascending pathway conveying pain and temperature sensation from the contralateral body. After crossing at the C2 level, the tract conveying facial
sensation is on the same side as the tract conveying ipsilateral trunk and
limb sensation, but the two tracts are not close to each other until reaching
the high brainstem (see Figures 1.6 and 1.11).

6. *Facial weakness ipsilateral to body weakness implies a lesion in the high
   pons or above.*

Explanation: The facial nerve (supplying the muscles of the face) exits
from the pons; no lesion below that level can affect facial strength.

7. *Both a third nerve palsy and Horner's syndrome can result in ptosis and
   pupillary asymmetry, but with a third nerve palsy, the ptosis is on the side
   of the large pupil; with Horner's syndrome, the ptosis is on the side of the
   small pupil.*

Explanation: A third nerve palsy often results in dysfunction of parasympathetic fibers traveling with the third nerve, causing a large pupil
because of impaired constriction. Horner's syndrome is due to damage to
the sympathetic system, causing inadequate pupillary dilation and therefore a small pupil. With either lesion, the ptosis is always on the same side
as the abnormal pupil.

8. *Diplopia is always due to a lesion in the brainstem or periphery (nerve/ neuromuscular junction/muscle), but not the cortex. A gaze palsy (impaired movement of both eyes in one direction, but both eyes move congruently and remain aligned in all positions of gaze) is due to a lesion in the cortex or brainstem but not in the periphery.*

Explanation: Cortical and brainstem gaze centers control movements of both eyes in parallel; individual eye movements are controlled by brainstem nuclei and mediated by individual cranial nerves. This is discussed further in Chapters 2, 11, and 13.

9. *Visual symptoms restricted to one eye imply a lesion anterior to the chiasm.*

Explanation: From the chiasm back to the occipital cortex, information from the two eyes is combined in the visual system, so that any lesion affecting the visual pathways at the chiasm or behind it will generally affect vision from both eyes. Only prior to the chiasm is visual information from each eye segregated (see Figure 1.16). This point is also discussed in Chapters 2 and 13.

10. *Aphasia or dysphasia (abnormal language processing resulting in difficulty understanding words, recalling words, or organizing words grammatically) implies a lesion in the dominant cerebral hemisphere. Dysarthria (abnormal motor control of speech resulting in disturbances of articulation, rate, rhythm, or voice quality) in the absence of dysphasia suggests a subcortical, brainstem, or cerebellar lesion.*

Explanation: The cognitive processing necessary for language comprehension and production takes place largely in the dominant cerebral hemisphere. The cerebral hemispheres are also involved in the specific motor sequences involved in speech, but there is enough redundancy of function that the unaffected hemisphere can often compensate for a unilateral hemispheric lesion as long as the areas involved in language processing are intact. There is less redundancy at lower levels, so a unilateral subcortical, brainstem, or cerebellar lesion can produce significant dysarthria.

11. *An altered level of consciousness indicates either dysfunction of both cerebral hemispheres or a lesion in the brainstem or the thalamus.*

Explanation: The physiologic basis of "consciousness" is not well understood. Even if it were, it would surely be too complicated to represent in terms of line segments. Suffice it to say that the thalamus and reticular activating system in the brainstem are critical elements, but there is no localized region in the cerebral cortex essential for maintenance of consciousness. A lesion that completely destroys the function of the cerebral cortex on one side will not affect consciousness as long as the brainstem, thalamus, and contralateral cortex are intact.

Chapter 2

The Neurologic Examination

I. More Localization Problems

Example 1. In the dark, a patient's right pupil is 3 mm larger than the left. In bright light, the right pupil is only 1 mm larger than the left.

Questions:

1. Which pupil is abnormal, the right or the left?
2. Which pathway is abnormal, the sympathetic or the parasympathetic?
3. Is this patient likely to have ptosis? If so, on which side?

Example 2. A patient has weakness of the right face, arm, and leg.

Question:

Which is likely to be weaker, the forehead or the lower face?

Example 3. A patient has weakness of hip flexion, knee flexion, and ankle dorsiflexion in the left lower extremity.

Questions:

1. Is this distribution of weakness consistent with a single nerve root lesion?
2. Is this pattern of weakness suggestive of any other lesion localization?

II. General Comments on the Neurologic Examination

A careful history can elicit most of the information necessary to localize a patient's lesion, especially if you follow up open-ended questions with questions that focus on specific nervous system pathways. For example, to investigate temperature sensation, you can ask patients if they have any problems detecting water temperature when washing their hands or stepping into a bathtub. Regarding fine touch discrimination, you can ask patients whether they have problems pulling the correct coin or other objects out of their pockets. Position sense can be explored by asking whether they have problems knowing where their feet are on the accelerator and brake pedals of their cars. Even a history of clonus may sometimes be deduced from patients who experience uncontrollable, rhythmic jerking of the foot when slamming on the brakes. Similarly, precise questions may differentiate between proximal and distal weakness, horizontal and vertical diplopia, monocular and binocular visual loss, aphasia and dysarthria, and so forth.

No matter how accurate and detailed the history, however, you will need to perform a neurologic examination. This is the most reliable way to identify certain abnormalities, such as subtle weakness, eye movement abnormalities, sensory deficits, and asymmetric reflexes. Moreover, the information obtained from a history depends on the reliability of the informant. If the informant is a poor observer, has trouble communicating, or for some reason provides misleading information, it is essential to have an independent source of information. The neurologic examination serves this purpose.

The nervous system has many functions, and there are many ways to test each function. The components of a standard neurologic examination are listed in Table 2.1. It would not be practical to perform all possible tests on each patient. Instead, the examination must be tailored to the situation. In patients with no neurologic symptoms, a screening examination is adequate (see Part VI of this chapter). In patients who do have neurologic symptoms, it is best to try to narrow the list of potential localization sites as much as possible based on the history. It will then be possible to focus the examination in order to verify the salient features of the history and to refine the localization even further.

One constraint on the neurologic examination is that it requires patient cooperation. Some patients are unable or unwilling to cooperate fully with the examination, so findings must be interpreted with caution and checked for internal consistency. A second constraint on the examination, even when cooperation is not an issue, is the fact that there is a range of normal findings. It is frequently difficult to determine whether a given finding is outside the range of normal. For example, one individual may be much stronger than another, but the weaker individual is not necessarily abnormal. Weakness that has developed recently is a much more significant indicator of neurologic disease than lifelong weakness. The same is true of hyperreflexia and many

Table 2.1 Organization of the Neurologic Examination

A. Mental status

    1. Level of alertness

    2. Language

        a. Fluency

        b. Comprehension

        c. Repetition

        d. Naming

        e. Reading

        f. Writing

    3. Memory

        a. Immediate

        b. Short-term

        c. Long-term

            i. Recent (including orientation to place and time)

            ii. Remote

    4. Calculation

    5. Construction

    6. Abstraction

B. Cranial nerves

    1. Olfaction (CN I)

    2. Vision (CN II)

        a. Visual fields

        b. Visual acuity

        c. Funduscopic examination

    3. Pupillary light reflex (CNs II, III)

    4. Eye movements (CNs III, IV, VI)

    5. Facial sensation (CN V)

    6. Facial strength

        a. Muscles of mastication (CN V)

        b. Muscles of facial expression (CN VII)

    7. Hearing (CN VIII)

(Continued)

Table 2.1 (continued)

---

    8. Vestibular function (CN VIII)

    9. Palatal movement (CNs IX, X)

    10. Dysarthria (CNs IX, X, XII)

    11. Head rotation (CN XI)

    12. Shoulder elevation (CN XI)

    13. Tongue movements (CN XII)

C. Motor

    1. Gait

    2. Coordination

    3. Involuntary movements

    4. Pronator drift

    5. Individual muscles

        a. Strength

        b. Bulk

        c. Tone (resistance to passive manipulation)

D. Reflexes

    1. Tendon reflexes

    2. Plantar responses

    3. Superficial reflexes

    4. "Primitive" reflexes

E. Sensory

    1. Light touch

    2. Pain/temperature

    3. Joint position sense

    4. Vibration

    5. Double simultaneous stimulation

    6. Graphesthesia

    7. Stereognosis

---

other neurologic findings. Unfortunately, it is not always clear whether an examination finding is new or old, because patients usually do not present for examination until they are already experiencing symptoms. When there is no baseline examination available for comparison, patients can sometimes be "used as their own controls." If a finding in one region of the body is different from corresponding findings elsewhere, it is likely to be significant. For this reason, the two sides of the body should be compared directly at each step of the examination. A finding on the right significantly different from the corresponding finding on the left is strong evidence of a neurologic lesion.

Even when the examination is asymmetric, it can be difficult to determine whether the abnormality is new or old. It may be completely irrelevant to the patient's current symptoms. Although the examination supplements the history, it cannot supplant it.

The neurologic examination can be performed in any order. Examiners may even change the sequence of the examination from one patient to the next, depending on the patient's symptoms, mobility, and ability to cooperate. Many subtle abnormalities are most evident by comparing one side of the body to the other, so it is generally best to follow each test with the same test on the other side, before moving on to a different test. Sensory testing and mental status testing are the parts of the examination most likely to make patients uncomfortable, so it is often wise to perform these tests last. These are only guidelines, however. Each examiner's style and preferences will differ.

The sequence in which the neurologic examination is presented is more standardized, primarily to make it easier for a listener or reader to focus and organize the information. If I am particularly interested in a patient's deep tendon reflexes, for example, it helps me to know when the presenter is likely to discuss them. Among other things, it helps me avoid interrupting the presentation to ask about details that the presenter was going to discuss in due course. It doesn't really matter what the sequence of presentation is, as long as it is consistent. A fairly standard sequence is shown in Table 2.1. It can be thought of as "zooming in" on the patient. The component presented first, mental status, could almost be tested by telephone. Little direct observation of the patient is necessary. Gait is tested by observing the patient, but no physical contact is required. The remainder of the motor examination requires some physical contact, but at a fairly crude level. The component presented last, the sensory exam, requires the closest and most refined physical interactions, such as the small limb movements required for testing joint position sense or the stimuli applied in testing pain sensation. The cranial nerves are inserted as a bridge between mental status and the rest of the examination, and the deep tendon reflexes are positioned between the motor and the sensory exams because the reflex arc includes both sensory and motor components.

The portion of the examination for which presentation in a consistent sequence is most important is the mental status examination. Certain findings on the mental status examination can only be interpreted by knowing a patient's ability to perform other, more fundamental tasks. For example, difficulty with simple calculations may have some localizing significance in a patient who is otherwise cognitively intact, but not in a patient who is unable to answer any questions because of impaired language function or a depressed level of consciousness. This ambiguity is avoided by presenting the level of alertness first, then language function, and then memory. The remainder of the mental status examination can be presented in any order.

III. How to Do the Neurologic Examination

Even though the neurologic examination outlined in Table 2.1 is seldom performed in its entirety, one must be able to perform each of the components of the neurologic examination when appropriate. This part of the chapter presents instructions for doing so.

A. Mental Status Examination

1. Level of alertness

No special testing is required. While taking the history and examining the patient, observe whether the patient is alert, attentive, sleepy, or unresponsive.

2. Language

a. Fluency

No special testing is required. Throughout the course of the patient interaction, assess whether the patient's phrases and sentences are of normal length, are spoken effortlessly and at a normal rate, and have normal grammatical structure. Note that fluency is independent of content; speech can be completely fluent and still be incomprehensible.

b. Comprehension

Comprehension is often adequately assessed through the routine history and physical but can also be tested explicitly. Give the patient progressively more complex commands, such as one step (e.g., "Touch your nose"), two steps (e.g., "Touch your nose, then stick out your tongue"), and three steps (e.g., "Touch your nose, then stick out your tongue, and then raise your right foot"). Commands that require a body part to cross the midline (e.g., "Touch your right ear with your left thumb") are more complex than those that don't. Increasingly complex grammatical structures can also be used (e.g., "Touch the coin with the pencil." "With the comb, touch the straw."). Ask the patient progressively more complex questions, either yes/no (e.g., "Does a stone sink in water?" "Do you put on your shoes before your stockings?") or otherwise. Again, more complex grammatical structures such as passive voice or possessive may be useful (e.g., "Is my aunt's uncle a man or a woman?" "If a lion was killed by a tiger, which one is still alive?").

c. Repetition

Ask the patient to repeat phrases or sentences of progressively greater length and complexity (e.g., "It is cold outside." "We all went over there together." "The lawyer's closing argument convinced the jury." "The final movement of the symphony was disappointing.").

d. Naming

In the course of routine conversation, observe whether the patient frequently pauses and struggles to think of words. In addition, test naming explicitly by asking the patient to name items as you point to them (e.g., shirt, shoe, phone, collar, lapel, shoelace, heel, receiver). Less common objects are generally harder to name, and parts of an object are harder to name than the entire object.

e. Reading

Ask the patient to follow a written command. This can be one of the same commands used to test comprehension of spoken language.

f. Writing

Ask the patient to write an original sentence, and to write a sentence from dictation. Look for omitted or added words, or for word substitutions.

3. Memory

a. Immediate memory

Tell the patient "repeat after me," and then recite a string of seven digits. Lengthen or shorten the string until you find the longest string the patient can repeat correctly. This is called the *digit span*. Note: Despite its categorization as "immediate memory," this is really more appropriately considered "attention."

b. Short-term memory

Ask the patient to memorize three unrelated words (e.g., horse, purple, anger), and then distract the patient for 5 minutes (usually by performing other parts of the exam). Then ask the patient to recall the list. If the patient misses an item, give clues (e.g., "One was an animal"), and if this isn't enough, offer a multiple choice (e.g., "It was a cat, a bear, or a horse").

c. Long-term memory

Long-term memory includes both *recent* and *remote* memory. Assess recent memory by testing the patient's orientation to time (e.g., day, date, month, season, year), and place (e.g., state, city, building), and by asking questions about events of the past few days or weeks (e.g., "Who are the current candidates for president?" or, assuming an independent source is available for verification, "What did you have for supper last night?"). Remote memory can be tested by asking for the names of the presidents in reverse order as far back as the patient can remember, or by asking about important historical events and dates. The patient can also be asked about details of personal life such as full name, birth date, names and ages of children and grandchildren, and work history, assuming independent verification is available.

4. Calculation

Ask some straightforward computation problems (e.g., $5 + 8 =?$; $6 \times 7 =?$; $31 - 18 =?$) and some "word problems" (e.g., "How many nickels are there in \$1.35?" "How many quarters in \$3.75?").

5. Construction

Ask the patient to draw a clock, including all the numbers, and to place the hands at 4:10. Ask the patient to draw a cube; for patients who have trouble doing so, draw a cube and ask them to copy it.

6. Abstraction

Ask the patient to explain similarities (e.g., "What do an apple and an orange have in common?...a basketball and a grapefruit?...a tent and a cabin?...a bicycle and an airplane?...a sculpture and a symphony?") and differences (e.g., "What's the difference between a radio and a television?... a river and a lake?...a baby and a midget?...character and reputation?").

B. Cranial Nerve Examination

1. Olfaction

Although I do not usually test olfaction, it can be assessed by having the patient occlude one nostril and identify a common scent (e.g., coffee, peppermint, cinnamon) placed under the other nostril.

2. Vision

a. Visual fields

Have the patient cover his or her left eye. Stand facing the patient from two arm's-lengths away, close your right eye, and stretch your arms forward and to the sides so that your hands are positioned at about 1:30 and 10:30 and just barely visible in your peripheral vision. They should be the same distance from you and the patient. Hold the index finger on each hand extended. Ask the patient to keep looking directly at your nose and indicate whether you move the finger on the left hand, the right hand, or both. Your finger movement should be a single, quick twitch. Use your own left eye's visual field as a control. Next, move your hands down to roughly 4:30 and 7:30 and test again. Then test analogous portions of the visual field of the patient's left eye (using your right eye as a control).

b. Acuity

Place a hand-held visual acuity card 14 inches in front of the patient's right eye, while the left eye is covered. The patient should wear his or her usual corrective lenses. Ask the patient to read the lowest line on the chart (20/20). If the patient cannot do so, move up a line, and continue doing so until you reach a line where the majority of items are read correctly. Note which line this is, and how many errors the patient makes on this line. Repeat the process for the left eye.

c. Funduscopic examination

Funduscopic examination is described in standard physical examination textbooks.

3. Pupillary light reflex

Reduce the room illumination as much as possible. Shine a penlight on the bridge of the patient's nose, so that you can see both pupils without directing light at either of them. Check that they are the same size. Now move the penlight so that it is directly shining on the right pupil, and check to see that both pupils have constricted to the same size. Next, move the penlight back to the bridge of the nose so that both pupils dilate, and then shine the light directly on the left pupil, again checking for equal constriction of the two eyes. Finally, move the penlight rapidly from the left pupil to the right; the pupil size should not change. Swing the light back to the left pupil; again, the pupil size should remain constant. Repeat this "swinging" maneuver several times to be sure there is no consistent tendency for the pupils to be larger when the light is directed at one eye than when it is directed at the other one.

4. Eye movements

Observe the patient's eyelids for *ptosis* (drooping). Have the patient fixate on your finger held about two feet away, in the vertical and horizontal midline. Observe for *nystagmus*—a quick movement of the eyes in one direction, alternating with a slower movement of the eyes in the opposite direction, repeated several times or more.

To evaluate smooth pursuit movements, ask the patient to avoid any movement of the head but to continue watching your finger as you slowly move it to the patient's right. Observe the smoothness and range of the patient's eye movements. Keep your finger at the far right of the patient's gaze for several seconds while observing again for nystagmus. Move your finger slowly to the patient's left and repeat the observations. Return your finger to the vertical and horizontal midline, and then move it slowly up, repeating the observations. Then move your finger slowly down and repeat the observations. Finally, return to the midline position, and move your finger diagonally down and to the left; then return to the midline and move your finger down and to the right.

To evaluate voluntary saccades, hold up your right index finger about 10° to the left of the patient's nose, and hold up your left thumb about 10° to the patient's right. Ask the patient to look at your nose. Then ask the patient to look at your finger. Then ask the patient to look back at your nose. Then ask the patient to look at your thumb. Continue to have the patient move from one target to another in random order several times, and observe whether there is a consistent tendency to overshoot or under-shoot the target.

5. Facial sensation

Lightly touch the patient's right forehead once, and then repeat on the opposite side. Ask the patient if the two stimuli feel the same. Repeat this procedure on the cheek and on the chin. This is usually adequate testing, unless the patient reports asymmetric facial sensation, in which case you should lightly touch each side of the forehead with a sharp pin and ask the patient if the stimuli feel equally sharp, then repeat the procedure on the cheek and on the chin. Testing of the corneal reflex is not routinely necessary, but it is useful in uncooperative patients or when the rest of the exam suggests that there may be a problem with facial sensation or strength. It is tested by having the patient look to the far left, then touching the patient's right cornea with a fine wisp of cotton (introduced from the patient's right, outside the field of vision) and observing the reflexive blink that occurs in each eye. The process is then repeated with the left eye.

6. Facial strength

a. Muscles of mastication

Have the patient open the jaw against resistance, and then close the jaw against resistance. Have the patient move the chin from side to side.

b. Muscles of facial expression

Have the patient close his or her eyes tightly. Observe whether the lashes are buried equally on the two sides and whether you can open either eye manually. Then have the patient look up and wrinkle the forehead; note whether the two sides are equally wrinkled. Have the patient smile, and observe whether one side of the face is activated more quickly or more completely than the other.

7. Hearing

For a bedside examination, it usually suffices to perform a quick hearing assessment by holding your fingers a few inches away from the patient's ear and rubbing them together softly. Alternatively, you can hold your hand up as a sound screen and ask the patient to repeat a few numbers that you whisper behind your hand while rhythmically tapping the opposite ear to keep it from contributing. Each ear should be tested separately.

8. Vestibular function

Ask the patient to fixate on your nose as you turn the patient's head to one side as quickly as possible, and observe the patient's eyes to see if they remain fixed on the target. This is called the *head impulse test* or the *head thrust maneuver*. It depends on the vestibulo-ocular reflex, which is the mechanism by which the nervous system keeps the eyes pointed in a stable direction even while the head is moving.

9. Palatal movement

Ask the patient to say "aaah" or to yawn, and observe whether the two sides of the palate move fully and symmetrically. The palate is most readily visualized if the patient is sitting or standing, rather than supine. There is generally no need to test the gag reflex in a screening neurologic examination. When you have reason to suspect reduced palatal sensation or strength, the reflex can be checked by observing the response when you touch the posterior pharynx on one side with a cotton swab; compare this to the response elicited by touching the other side.

10. Dysarthria

When the patient speaks, listen for articulation errors, abnormalities of voice quality, and irregularities of rate or rhythm.

11. Head rotation

Have the patient turn the head all the way to the left. Place your hand on the left side of the jaw and ask the patient to resist you as you try turning the head back to the right. Palpate the right sternocleidomastoid (SCM) muscle with your other hand at the same time. Repeat this maneuver in the other direction to test the left SCM.

12. Shoulder elevation

Ask the patient to shrug the shoulders while you resist the movement with your hands.

13. Tongue movement

Have the patient protrude the tongue and move it rapidly from side to side. Ask the patient to push the tongue against the left cheek from inside the mouth while you push against it from outside, and then do the same on the right side of the mouth.

C. Motor Examination

1. Gait

Observe the patient's casual gait, preferably with the patient unaware of being observed. Have the patient walk toward you while walking on the heels, then walk away from you walking on tiptoes. Finally, have the patient walk in tandem, placing one foot directly in front of the other as if walking on a tightrope (i.e., the "drunk-driving test"). Note if the patient is unsteady with any of these maneuvers, or if there is any asymmetry of movement. Also observe how the arms swing, and look for *festination,* an involuntary tendency for steps to accelerate and become smaller.

2. Coordination

a. Finger tapping

Ask the patient to make a fist with the right hand, then to extend the thumb and index finger and tap the tip of the index finger on the tip of the thumb as quickly as possible. Repeat with the left hand. Observe for speed, accuracy, and regularity of rhythm.

b. Rapid alternating movements

Have the patient alternately pronate and supinate the right hand against a stable surface (such as a table, or the patient's own thigh or left hand) as rapidly as possible; repeat for the left hand. Again, observe speed, accuracy, and rhythm.

c. Finger-to-nose testing

Ask the patient to use the tip of his or her right index finger to touch the tip of your index finger, then the tip of his or her nose, then your finger again, and so forth. Hold your finger so that it is near the extreme of the patient's reach, and move it to several different positions during the testing. Repeat the test using the patient's left arm. Observe for accuracy, smoothness, and tremor.

d. Heel-knee-shin testing

Have the patient lie supine, place the right heel on the left knee, and then move the heel smoothly down the shin to the ankle. Repeat using the left heel on the right shin. Again, observe for accuracy, smoothness, and tremor.

3. Involuntary movements

Observe the patient throughout the history and physical for *tremor, myoclonus* (rapid, shock-like muscle jerks), *chorea* (rapid, jerky twitches, similar to myoclonus but more random in location and more likely to blend into one another), *athetosis* (slow, writhing movements of the limbs), *ballismus* (large amplitude, flinging limb movements), *tics* (abrupt, stereotyped, coordinated movements or vocalizations), *dystonia* (maintenance of an abnormal posture or repetitive twisting movements), or other involuntary motor activity.

4. Pronator drift

Have the patient stretch out the arms so that they are level and fully extended, with the palms facing straight up, and then close the eyes. Watch for five to ten seconds to see if either arm tends to pronate (so that the palm turns inward) and drift downward.

5. Individual muscles

a. Strength

In the upper extremities, test shoulder abduction, elbow extension, elbow flexion, wrist extension, wrist flexion, finger extension, finger flexion, and finger abduction. In the lower extremities, test hip flexion, hip extension, knee flexion, knee extension, ankle dorsiflexion, and ankle plantar flexion.

For each movement, place the limb near the middle of its range, and then ask the patient to resist you as you try to move the limb from that position. For example, in testing shoulder abduction, the patient's arms should be horizontal, forming a letter "T" with the body, and the patient should try to maintain that position while you press down on both arms at a point between the shoulders and the elbows. When possible, place one hand above the joint being examined to stabilize the joint, and exert pressure with your other hand just below the joint, to isolate the specific movement you are trying to test.

b. Bulk

While testing strength, inspect the muscles active in each movement and palpate them for evidence of atrophy. You can usually do this with the hand you have placed above the joint to stabilize it. Fasciculations (random, involuntary muscle twitches) should also be noted.

c. Tone

Ask the patient to relax and let you manipulate the limbs passively. This is harder for most patients than you might imagine, and you may need to try to distract them by engaging them in unrelated conversation, or ask them to let their limbs go limp, "like a wet noodle."

D. Reflex Examination

1. Tendon reflexes

The biceps, triceps, brachioradialis, knee (patellar), and ankle (Achilles) reflexes are the ones commonly tested. The joint under consideration should be at about 90° and fully relaxed. It is often helpful to cradle the joint in your own arm to support it. With your other arm, hold the end of the hammer and let the head of the hammer drop like a pendulum so that it strikes the tendon (specifically, just anterior to the elbow for the biceps reflex, just posterior to the elbow for the triceps reflex, about 10 cm above the wrist on the radial aspect of the forearm for the brachioradialis reflex, just below the patella for the knee reflex, and just behind the ankle for the ankle reflex). You should strive to develop a technique that results in a reproducible level of force from one occasion to the next. When a patient has reflexes that are difficult to elicit, you can amplify them by using reinforcement procedures: Ask the patient to clench his or her teeth or (when testing lower extremity reflexes) to hook together the flexed fingers of both hands and pull. This is also known as the *Jendrassik maneuver.*

Clonus is a rhythmic series of muscle contractions induced by stretching the tendon. It most commonly occurs at the ankle, where it is typically elicited by suddenly dorsiflexing the patient's foot and maintaining light upward pressure on the sole.

2. Plantar response

Using a blunt, narrow surface (e.g., a tongue blade, key, or handle of a reflex hammer), stroke the sole of the patient's foot on the lateral edge, starting near the heel and proceeding along the lateral edge almost to the base of the little toe, then curve the path medially just proximal to the base of the other toes. This should take the form of a smooth "J" stroke. Always start by applying minimal pressure. This is usually adequate, but if no response occurs, repeat the maneuver with greater pressure.

The normal response is for all the toes to flex (a "flexor plantar response"). When there is damage to the central nervous system motor pathways, a normally suppressed reflex is disinhibited, so an abnormal response is observed: The great toe extends (dorsiflexes) and the other toes fan out. This is called an extensor plantar response; it is also known as a *Babinski sign.*

3. Superficial reflexes

The abdominal reflexes, cremasteric reflexes, and other superficial reflexes are described in standard physical examination textbooks. They are not usually relevant to standard screening examinations.

4. Primitive reflexes

The grasp, root, snout, and palmomental reflexes are known as primitive reflexes or frontal release signs. These tests do not fit easily into any examination category. They are reflex responses, but their pathways are far more complicated than the monosynaptic arcs of the deep tendon reflexes. I do not test these reflexes. They have very little localizing value, and, in particular, there is no convincing evidence that they reflect frontal lobe pathology. They are not even reliable indicators of abnormal function, because except for the grasp, all of these reflexes are present in a substantial proportion of normal individuals, especially older individuals.

E. Sensory Examination

1. Light touch sensation

To test for light touch sensation, have the patient close his or her eyes and tell you whether you are touching the left hand, right hand, or both simultaneously. Repeat this several times, using as a stimulus a single light touch applied sometimes to the medial aspect of the hand and sometimes to the lateral aspect. Note whether the patient consistently fails to detect stimulation in one location. Also note whether the patient consistently "extinguishes" the stimulus on one side of the body when both sides are *stimulated simultaneously*. Next, touch the patient once lightly on the medial aspect of each hand simultaneously, and ask if they feel the same. Ask the same question for the lateral aspect of each hand. If any abnormalities are detected, extend your region of testing proximally in the limb to map out the precise area of abnormality. Perform analogous testing on the feet.

2. Pain/temperature sensation

When preparing to test pain and temperature sensation explain to the patient that you will be touching each finger with either the sharp or the dull end of a safety pin, and demonstrate each. Be sure the safety pin is previously unused. Then, with the patient's eyes closed, lightly touch the palmar aspect of the thumb with the sharp point of the pin, and ask the patient to say "sharp" or "dull." Repeat this for each finger of each hand, usually using the sharp point but including at least one dull stimulus on each hand to be sure the patient is paying attention. Next, touch the patient with the pin once lightly on the medial aspect of each hand, and ask if they feel equally sharp. Ask the same question for the lateral aspect of each hand. If any abnormalities are detected, extend your region of testing proximally in the limb to map out the precise area of abnormality. Perform analogous testing on the feet. Discard the pin in a container for contaminated medical sharps.

It is not usually necessary to test both pain and temperature, as either will suffice. You can test temperature in a fashion analogous to pain; a reasonable stimulus is the flat portion of a tuning fork after it has been immersed in cold water and dried.

3. Joint position sense

With the finger and thumb of one hand, stabilize the distal interphalangeal joint of the patient's left thumb by holding it on the medial and lateral aspects. With the finger and thumb of your other hand, hold the medial and lateral aspects of the tip of the thumb and move it slightly up or down. Have the patient close his or her eyes and identify the direction of movement. Repeat several times. Most normal patients can identify movements of a few degrees or less. Perform analogous testing of the patient's right thumb and both great toes. If abnormalities are detected, proceed to more proximal joints in the same limb until a joint is found where position sense is intact.

The *Romberg* test also helps to assess position sense. Have the patient stand with both feet together, and then note whether the patient can maintain balance after closing his or her eyes.

4. Vibration sense

Vibration sense can be tested by tapping a 128-Hz tuning fork lightly against a solid surface to produce a slight (silent) vibration. With the patient's eyes closed, hold the base of the tuning fork firmly on the distal interphalangeal joint of the patient's left thumb and ask the patient if the vibration is detectable. Let the vibration fade until the patient no longer detects it, then apply the tuning fork to your own thumb to see if you can still feel any vibration. Repeat this testing on the patient's right thumb and both great toes. For one of the limbs, stop the vibration before applying the tuning fork to the limb to be sure that the patient is paying attention. If not, remind the patient to respond only when he or she feels a definite vibration, not just pressure. If any abnormalities are detected, apply the tuning fork to progressively more proximal joints until one is found where the vibration is detected normally.

5. Double simultaneous stimulation

The test for double simultaneous stimulation is performed while testing light touch sensation (see *1. Light touch sensation*, above).

6. Graphesthesia

To test for graphesthesia, ask the patient to close the eyes and identify a number from 0 to 9 that you draw on his or her index finger using a ballpoint pen (with the tip retracted). Repeat with several other numbers and compare to the other hand. There is rarely any need to test graphesthesia in the feet.

7. Stereognosis

To test for stereognosis, ask the patient to close the eyes and identify a small object (e.g., nickel, dime, quarter, penny, key, paper clip) you place in his or her right hand. Test the left hand in the same way.

IV. Additional Comments on Terminology and Examination Technique

When reporting examination findings, you must be familiar with some basic definitions and standard conventions. In this part of the chapter, I present some of the more commonly used terms, as well as some hints and comments regarding common sources of confusion. Many of these latter comments reflect my personal observations or opinions, and other neurologists might disagree.

A. Mental Status Examination

1. Terminology

A number of specialized terms often confuse students. Here is a partial glossary.

abulia, loss of initiative, willpower, or drive

acalculia, inability to calculate

agnosia, inability to recognize one or more classes of environmental stimuli, even though the necessary intellectual and perceptual functions are intact

agraphia, inability to write

alexia, inability to read for comprehension

amnesia, inability to retain new information

anomia, inability to name objects or think of words; in practice, often used as a synonym for *dysnomia*

anosognosia, inability to recognize one's own impairment

anterior aphasia, acquired language disorder in which verbal output is *nonfluent*. See *Broca's aphasia*, *expressive aphasia*, and *nonfluent aphasia*

aphasia, literally, a complete loss of language function, but in practice, used as a synonym for *dysphasia*

aphemia, complete loss of the ability to speak, but retained comprehension and writing ability

apraxia, inability to perform a previously learned set of coordinated movements even though the necessary component skills (including intellect, language function, strength, coordination, and sensation) remain intact

Broca's aphasia, acquired language disorder characterized by *nonfluent* verbal output with omission of relational words (prepositions, conjunctions, articles, and minor modifiers), abnormal *prosody,* impaired repetition, and relatively intact comprehension. See *anterior aphasia, expressive aphasia,* and *nonfluent aphasia;* see also Figure 1.19

conduction aphasia, acquired language disorder characterized by prominent impairment of repetition, relatively intact comprehension, and verbal output that is *fluent* but contains *literal paraphasias;* see Figure 1.19

delirium, an acute, transient, fluctuating confusional state characterized by impairment in maintaining and shifting attention, often associated with agitation, disorientation, fear, irritability, illusions, or hallucinations

dementia, an acquired, persistent decline of intellectual function that causes impaired performance of daily activities, without clouding of the sensorium or underlying psychiatric disease

dysnomia, difficulty naming objects or finding the desired words

dysphasia, acquired disorder of language not due to generalized intellectual impairment or psychiatric disturbance

expressive aphasia, acquired language disorder in which verbal output is *nonfluent.* See *anterior aphasia, Broca's aphasia,* and *nonfluent aphasia*

fluent, an adjective used to describe verbal output that is normal to excessive, easily produced, with normal phrase length (five or more words) and normal *prosody*

fluent aphasia, acquired language disorder in which verbal output is *fluent.* See *posterior aphasia, receptive aphasia, Wernicke's aphasia*

Gerstmann's syndrome, the constellation of (1) *agraphia,* (2) *acalculia,* (3) *right-left confusion,* and (4) *finger agnosia;* classically associated with lesions in the angular gyrus of the dominant hemisphere (but the subject of endless debate)

jargon, verbal output containing so many *literal paraphasias* that the words are unrecognizable

nonfluent, an adjective used to describe verbal output that is sparse, with only one to four words per phrase

nonfluent aphasia, acquired language disorder in which verbal output is *nonfluent*. See *anterior aphasia*, *Broca's aphasia*, and *expressive aphasia*

paraphasia, a substitution error in which the word produced is similar in sound or meaning to the intended word. A *literal* or *phonemic* paraphasia is a sound substitution error resulting in production of a word that is phonemically related to the intended word (e.g., "greed" or "greeb" instead of "green"). A *semantic* or *verbal* paraphasia is a word substitution error in which the word produced is semantically related to the intended word (e.g., "blue" instead of "green")

posterior aphasia, acquired language disorder in which comprehension is impaired. See *fluent aphasia*, *receptive aphasia*, and *Wernicke's aphasia*

prosody, the rhythm and tempo of speech

prosopagnosia, inability to recognize faces

receptive aphasia, acquired language disorder in which comprehension is impaired. See *fluent aphasia*, *posterior aphasia*, and *Wernicke's aphasia*

transcortical aphasia, acquired language disorder in which the ability to repeat is intact; see Figure 1.19

Wernicke's aphasia, acquired language disorder characterized by markedly impaired comprehension and repetition, with verbal output that is *fluent* but contaminated by numerous *paraphasias* or, in severe cases, *jargon*. See *fluent aphasia*, *posterior aphasia*, *receptive aphasia*; see also Figure 1.19

2. Patient cooperation

Many patients resist formal mental-status testing. Some find it threatening. Others are offended by it ("What do you mean, do I know my name?"), and some just don't see the point. In fact, formal mental-status testing is often unnecessary, and I generally reserve it for patients whose mental status is suspect, based on information I obtain in the history or the rest of the examination (see Part VI of this chapter). When I do see the need to do a formal mental status examination, I usually introduce it by saying, "Now I'm going to test your memory. I'm going to ask you to remember three things. Then I'm going to distract you with a bunch of questions, some of which will be easy and some will be hard. Then I'll test you on the three things." Most patients can understand the need for testing memory, and they are more willing to accept all the other components of the mental status examination if they are presented as "distractions."

Even so, some patients find the mental-status examination so annoying that they refuse to cooperate, and some even refuse to proceed with any other portion of the physical examination. For this reason, I usually defer formal mental-status testing until I have nearly completed the rest of the examination. By then, I will have observed the patient's ability to respond to some fairly complicated commands (for example, with visual field testing and finger-to-nose testing), and this will help me tailor my examination.

3. Tailoring the examination to the patient

Try to guess the approximate level of performance you expect from a patient and then ask a screening question that might be a little too tough. If the patient gets the correct answer, you can skip the easier questions. If the patient doesn't get the correct answer, you can gradually reduce the difficulty of your questions until you have reached the patient's level. This approach saves time. Try to stockpile questions of various levels of complexity, so you don't have to think them up on the spot. For example, it is useful to remember sentences of different word lengths for testing repetition. A reasonably tough math problem that I often use as my initial screening question is "How much change would you get from a dollar if you bought six apples at twelve cents each?"

4. Aphasia terminology

Note the confusing array of synonyms in the definitions listed in Section 1, above. For example, an *expressive* aphasia is one in which expression is impaired, yet a *fluent* aphasia is one in which fluency is preserved. These terms are often more trouble than they are worth. It is best to describe explicitly the pattern of language deficits, focusing especially on comprehension, fluency, and repetition.

Dysarthria is an impairment of the motor functions necessary for speech production. Dysarthria is not a language disorder, and it is not a component of the mental status examination.

5. Cultural and educational factors

A patient's background will obviously influence performance on mental status testing, and the examiner must try to take this into account. There is no reliable way to do this; it is ultimately a matter of gestalt. Some tests are affected more than others by background. For example, the ability to copy a sequence of repetitive hand movements is relatively independent of education. In contrast, the interpretation of proverbs is so dependent on an individual's cultural and educational background that I consider it practically useless and instead rely on the interpretation of similarities and differences as an assay of abstract thought.

6. Standardized screening tests

Don't confuse the mental-status examination with the Mini-Mental State Examination (MMSE), which is a specific battery of questions commonly used as a quick screening instrument. Its value lies in the fact that it is simple, does not take much time to administer, and yields a numerical value that can be followed over time, but it is no substitute for a thorough mental-status examination. Another commonly used battery is the Montreal Cognitive Assessment (MOCA), which is somewhat more comprehensive but still useful mainly as a screening instrument.

7. Reporting findings

It is most informative to report patients' actual responses, rather than interpretations such as "mildly abnormal" or "slightly concrete."

B. Cranial Nerve Examination

1. Olfaction

I almost never test the sense of smell. It is difficult to know whether patients who cannot identify a particular scent have a disturbance of olfaction or whether they are just not familiar with that scent. When patients give a history of olfactory problems, I take them at their word. Formal instruments for testing olfaction are available. They are particularly useful for research purposes.

2. Visual fields

There are many alternatives to the technique for testing visual fields described in Part III of this chapter. You can ask patients to tell you when they first see a test stimulus as you slowly move it in from the periphery at various orientations. You can ask patients to count the number of fingers you hold up at various spots in the field. You can ask patients to tell you when they can detect that a stimulus is red as you move it in from the periphery of the field (the "kinetic red target" method). Each of these techniques has advantages and disadvantages, and some neurologists have very strong opinions about which technique is best. According to one study, the kinetic red target technique was more sensitive than other methods, and the combination of the kinetic red target method with the method presented in Part III was superior to any individual testing technique. The reason I prefer the method described in Part III is that the visual stimulus can be presented very briefly, minimizing the opportunity for the patient to shift fixation and maximizing the likelihood that the stimulus is actually in the intended region of the visual field. Also, I find the other techniques harder to interpret when patients have mental status abnormalities. Regardless of the technique used, each eye must be tested separately. Otherwise, if there is a defect in a portion of the visual field of only one eye, the other eye will be able to compensate and the defect will not be detected. One example of this situation is the bitemporal hemianopia that can occur with a lesion in the optic chiasm (see Chapter 1, Part V)—the defective hemifield of each eye corresponds to the intact hemifield of the other eye, so the patient may be completely unaware of the deficit until each eye is tested separately.

3. Eye movements

Eye movement abnormalities may be masked by convergence if the target is too close to the patient, but if you stand too far away, it may be difficult for you to see subtle abnormalities. I often position my head close to the patient and off to the side while holding the target (my finger) as far away from the patient as possible.

4. Corneal and gag reflexes

Because testing of the corneal reflex and the gag reflex is uncomfortable for the patient, I only perform these tests when I am trying to answer a specific question. When I check the gag reflex, I always check it bilaterally. About 20% of normal individuals do not have a gag reflex, so the test is most informative when the responses are asymmetric.

5. Weber and Rinne tests

Most physical diagnosis textbooks advocate the Weber and Rinne tests for distinguishing conductive hearing loss from sensorineural deafness. I do not. I find that patients have difficulty understanding what is being asked, and they give inconsistent responses (especially on the Weber test). Even if these tests gave consistently reliable results, they would still not be as sensitive or as informative as an audiogram.

C. Motor Examination

1. Grading muscle strength

The most common convention for grading muscle strength is the 0 to 5 Medical Research Council (MRC) scale:

0 = no contraction

1 = visible muscle twitch but no movement of the joint

2 = weak contraction insufficient to overcome gravity

3 = weak contraction able to overcome gravity but no additional resistance

4 = weak contraction able to overcome some resistance but not full resistance

5 = normal; able to overcome full resistance

The most compelling feature of this scale is its reproducibility. For example, an examiner is unlikely to assign a score of 1 to a muscle that another examiner graded 3 or stronger. A major limitation of the scale is that it is insensitive to subtle differences in strength. In particular, grade 4 covers a wide range, so that in most clinical situations the MRC scale does not allow precise differentiation of the severity of weakness from one muscle to the next. Similarly, it is not a sensitive tool for documenting moderate changes in strength over time. Many clinicians try to compensate for this by using intermediate grades, such as 3+ or 5-, but at the expense of reproducibility, because there is no consensus on how these intermediate grades should be defined.

2. Terminology

a. Patterns of weakness

Weakness of a single limb is called *monoparesis*. *Hemiparesis* is weakness of one side of the body; *paraparesis* is weakness of both lower extremities; and *quadriparesis* is weakness of all four limbs. *Monoplegia, hemiplegia, paraplegia,* and *quadriplegia* are analogous terms that refer to complete or nearly complete paralysis of the involved limbs. *Diplegia* is a term that is best avoided because different authors use it differently.

b. Tone (resistance to passive manipulation)

Several forms of increased resistance to passive manipulation are distinguished. *Spasticity* depends on the limb position and on how quickly the limb is moved, classically resulting in a "clasp-knife phenomenon" when the limb is moved rapidly: The limb moves freely for a short distance, but then there is a "catch" such that the examiner must use progressively more force to move the limb until at a certain point there is a sudden release and the limb moves freely again. Spasticity is generally greatest in the flexors of the upper extremity and the extensors of the lower extremity. This pattern is easy to remember for anyone who has seen patients with long-standing hemiparesis (especially if the patients did not receive physical therapy): they hold the hemiparetic arm flexed at the elbow, wrist, and fingers and pressed tightly to the chest, and they walk with the hemiparetic leg stiffly extended and the ankle plantar flexed, forcing them to circumduct the leg. *Rigidity,* in contrast to spasticity, is characterized by increased resistance throughout the movement. *Lead-pipe* rigidity applies to resistance that is uniform throughout the movement. *Cogwheel* rigidity is characterized by rhythmic interruption of the resistance, producing a ratchet-like effect. Rigidity is usually accentuated by distracting the patient. *Paratonia,* or *"gegenhalten,"* is increased resistance that becomes less prominent when the patient is distracted; without such distraction, the patient seems unable to relax the muscle. This is particularly common in patients who are anxious or demented. When it is prominent, other abnormalities of tone are difficult to assess.

c. Coordination

Coordination testing is often referred to as cerebellar testing, but this is a misnomer. Although the cerebellum is very important in the production of coordinated movements and particular abnormal findings on coordination testing may suggest cerebellar disease, other systems also play critical roles. As an obvious example, severe arm weakness will prevent a patient from performing finger-to-nose testing, even though the cerebellum and its pathways may be intact.

3. Modifications of strength testing

a. Selection of muscles to test

The eight upper-extremity movements and six lower-extremity movements tested in the examination described in Part III of this chapter are sufficient for a screening examination. If some of these muscles are weak, or if the patient complains of focal weakness, additional testing may be necessary to determine if the weakness is in the distribution of a specific nerve or nerve root.

b. Limb position

The position of the joint during strength testing is important, because it determines the mechanical advantage of the patient relative to the examiner. For example, it is much easier to overcome patients when they are trying to extend the elbow from a fully flexed position than it is when they are starting from a position of nearly maximal extension. In most cases it is reasonable to test the muscle with the joint at about mid-position, although positions that increase the patient's mechanical advantage may be preferable for particularly strong examiners or frail patients.

Some examiners test corresponding muscles on both sides (e.g., the left and right biceps muscles) simultaneously. I usually do not do this because it prevents me from using one hand to stabilize the joint and palpate the muscle.

An alternative to the strength examination technique presented in Part III in this chapter is to position the patient's limb and then ask the patient to move the limb steadily in a specified direction while the examiner resists the movement. The main reason I generally prefer to follow the format presented in Part III is that I can give essentially the same instruction ("Don't let me move your limb") for all movements. This is especially helpful when patients are confused, aphasic, or demented, or when we are communicating through an interpreter. It may take them a while to understand the instruction initially, but once they understand the task for one or two muscles they usually comprehend it much more readily for subsequent muscles.

D. Reflex Examination

1. Grading reflexes

The most common convention for grading deep tendon reflexes is simple but imprecise:

0 = absent

1 = reduced (hypoactive)

2 = normal

3 = increased (hyperactive)

4 = clonus

Some examiners use a grade of 5 to designate sustained clonus, reserving 4 for unsustained clonus that eventually fades after 2 to 10 beats. Also, some examiners include a reflex grade of 1/2 to indicate a reflex that can only be obtained using reinforcement.

The obvious limitation of this terminology is that it provides no guidelines for determining when reflexes are reduced, normal, or increased. This is left up to individual judgment, based on the examiner's sense of the range of reflexes present in the normal population.

2. Detection of subtle asymmetry

Comparison between reflexes in one part of the body and another is much more important than the absolute reflex grade. The most important comparison is between corresponding reflexes on the right and left, where even subtle asymmetry may be significant. For example, patients with an S1 radiculopathy may have an ankle jerk that would be considered normal, yet it is clearly less brisk than the ankle jerk on the other side. This is another limitation of the reflex grading scale: It does not express subtle distinctions that may be clinically important. For this reason, many examiners augment the scale by using '+' or '−' to designate intermediate grades. These grades have very little reproducibility from one examiner to another (or even from one examination to the next by a single examiner). They are only useful for indicating that asymmetry exists, not for quantifying it in any meaningful way.

When reflexes are brisk, it is difficult to detect slight asymmetry. For the most sensitive comparison, it is best to reduce the stimulus until it is just barely above threshold for eliciting the reflex. In patients with brisk reflexes, I can often set the reflex hammer aside and elicit the reflex by tapping lightly with my fingers. Once I have found the threshold stimulus for a given reflex, I look for two manifestations of asymmetry. First, is the threshold stimulus the same on each side, or do I consistently need to hit harder on one side than the other? Second, if the threshold stimulus is the same on each side, does it elicit the same magnitude of response on each side? Such subtle distinctions are most readily made by testing the reflex on one side immediately after testing the corresponding reflex on the other side, rather than testing all reflexes in one limb before testing the contralateral limb.

Another technique I use to heighten sensitivity to subtle reflex asymmetry is to place my finger on the patient's tendon and strike my finger rather than striking the tendon directly. This helps me aim more accurately and allows me to feel the tendon contraction. Moreover, it demonstrates to patients that I am willing to "share the pain," thereby gaining their sympathy and cooperation.

3. Relaxing the patient

Relaxation is critical in the reflex examination. Tendon reflexes are difficult to elicit when patients tense the muscles being tested. It is helpful to distract patients by engaging them in conversation while testing their reflexes. I take this opportunity to ask questions that I forgot to ask earlier, or if I have decided that formal mental status testing is necessary, I often do it while testing reflexes.

4. Significance of a Babinski sign

The Babinski sign is not graded. It is an abnormal finding that is either present or not. It is one of the few neurologic examination findings that can be interpreted without comparison to the contralateral response or consideration of patient compliance.

E. Sensory Examination

The sensory examination can be the most frustrating part of the neurologic examination. The instructions often must be repeated several times or more before patients understand what they are being asked to do. Even then, some patients over-interpret insignificant distinctions while others have difficulty attending to the task and fail to report important abnormalities. This part of the examination is also tiresome and somewhat uncomfortable for patients. For these reasons, the sensory examination is usually one of the last things I test. That way, I have a fairly good sense of whether the patient is likely to over-interpret small differences, and I can adjust accordingly. Furthermore, if a patient gets exasperated and insists on terminating the exam altogether (which sometimes happens), I already have most of the other information I need.

V. Interpretation of the Neurologic Examination

The general principles governing lesion localization were discussed in Chapter 1. The following discussion presents some additional principles that are often helpful in deducing lesion localization based on specific examination findings.

A. Mental Status Examination

Cognition is poorly understood. All of the categories used to describe mental status (e.g., calculation, abstraction) are convenient simplifications, but they do not necessarily reflect the way in which the brain actually functions. For example, it is very unlikely that any region or circuit in the brain is devoted specifically or exclusively to calculation.

This complicates the interpretation of the mental status examination. For example, students often ask whether the subtraction of serial sevens ("Count backwards from 100 by 7") is a test of calculation or of attention. The answer is both, and neither. For patients to subtract serial sevens successfully they must (1) be alert, (2) comprehend language well enough to understand a fairly abstract command, (3) retain the command in memory long enough to process it, (4) possess the necessary calculation skills, (5) be able to verbalize the response, and (6) maintain attention on the task so that the current result can be taken as the basis for generating the next one. It is not possible to assign a one-to-one correlation between a task on the mental status examination and a single cognitive function in the same way that abduction of an eye correlates to the function of a single lateral rectus muscle. When a patient is unable to perform a specific cognitive task, there are always several possible explanations. The examiner must observe the response to a variety of tasks, determine which ones are difficult for the patient, and try to determine the kinds of cognitive processing common to those tasks. Inferences about lesion localization are then possible.

Decreased level of alertness occurs only with dysfunction of both cerebral hemispheres, the thalamus, or the ascending reticular activating system in the brainstem (see Speed Rule 11 in Chapter 1). The usual cause is a generalized metabolic abnormality, such as hypoxia or hyperglycemia. Less commonly, appropriately placed structural lesions (especially expanding ones) may produce the same result. The implications and management options are very different for structural causes and metabolic causes, and a major goal of the examination is to distinguish between these two possibilities (see Chapter 11).

Mental status changes in alert patients can result from either focal or generalized processes. Generalized processes usually affect all cognitive functions about equally, although the initial manifestations may just be inattention or word-finding difficulty. Focal lesions typically affect some cognitive functions more than others, and the pattern of cognitive deficits can have some localizing significance.

The most common examples of selective mental status abnormality involve language function. As discussed in Chapter 1, language fluency, comprehension, and repetition each have rough anatomic correlates within the dominant cerebral hemisphere. Language disorders can be separated into broad categories depending on the degree to which each of these three functions is involved. For example, a classic Wernicke's aphasia (lesion site #1 in Figure 1.19 C) is characterized by fluent verbal output but impaired comprehension and repetition. Any aphasia in which repetition is spared is called *transcortical:* transcortical *sensory* when comprehension is impaired, transcortical *motor* when verbal output is nonfluent, and *mixed* transcortical when both comprehension and fluency are abnormal (lesion sites #4, #5, and #6 in Figure 1.19C).

Other cognitive abnormalities that may be seen in relative isolation include *acalculia, agraphia, alexia,* and *apraxia.* Each of these deficits is associated with focal lesions in the dominant hemisphere. The left hemisphere is dominant for language in almost all right-handed individuals. The left hemisphere is also language-dominant in most left-handed subjects, but the relationship is less predictable.

Neglect of one side of the environment can be seen with a focal lesion in either hemisphere, but it is much more common and tends to be more severe when the lesion is in the non-dominant hemisphere, especially the non-dominant parietal lobe. Non-dominant parietal lesions may also produce anosognosia, which is the inability to recognize the existence or severity of one's own impairment.

Unilateral disease of the prefrontal cortex often has surprisingly few clinical consequences, but bilateral prefrontal disease is typically associated with difficulty maintaining and shifting attention. Such patients will demonstrate both *impersistence* (an inability to stick with a task or topic of conversation) and *perseveration* (a tendency to continue returning to tasks and topics of conversation even when they are no longer appropriate).

None of these focal findings has any localizing significance unless it occurs out of proportion to other cognitive deficits. Each of them can occur as part of a general dementing illness such as Alzheimer's disease. In fact, it is often impossible to assess language function or other "focal" functions when significant dementia is present, or when there is reduction in the level of alertness. Patients with generalized cognitive impairment perform poorly on all aspects of the mental status examination, and it is usually futile to try to determine if one function is more severely affected than another.

B. Cranial Nerve Examination

1. Visual field defects

Because of the precise spatial organization of the visual pathways throughout their course, visual field defects can be exquisitely localizing at times.

Date: 5/30/2014 11:23
Member: Elizabeth M Friedrichsen

Title   Author
                               Due

ILL - Introduction to c|
6/27

Wow! In 2014, you have saved $78.

Storm Lake Public Library
Call 712-732-8026 with any issues.
60 days overdue is considered theft.

The most basic principles of visual field defects and their localizing value are discussed in Chapter 1 (see Figure 1.16) and Chapter 13.

2. Pupillary abnormalities

a. Asymmetric pupils (anisocoria)

The sympathetic and the parasympathetic pathways that determine pupillary size were discussed in Chapter 1 (see Figures 1.17 and 1.18). In most circumstances, the sympathetic and parasympathetic systems are both active simultaneously, and pupillary size is determined by the relative activity in the two systems. This results in potential ambiguity when one pupil is larger than the other (*anisocoria*): there could be a lesion in the sympathetic pathway (and therefore reduced dilating activity) on the side of the smaller pupil or a lesion in the parasympathetic pathway (and therefore less constriction) on the side of the larger pupil. To decide, the pupils should be examined both in bright light and in the dark. If the pupillary asymmetry is greatest in the dark, then the lesion is in the sympathetic system, because this is the system responsible for dilating the pupils, and darkness induces maximal dilation (Figure 2.1A). Conversely, pupillary asymmetry that is greatest in the light indicates a lesion in the parasympathetic pathway (Figure 2.1B). When the pupillary asymmetry is of equal magnitude in dark and in light, it is generally physiologic (i.e., a normal variant).

Another clue to the lesion site in a patient with anisocoria may be provided by ptosis. Because the parasympathetic fibers travel with the third cranial nerve for much of their course, a parasympathetic lesion often produces other signs of third nerve dysfunction, including eye movement abnormalities or pronounced ptosis (because the levator palpebrae muscle is innervated by the third nerve). Sympathetic lesions also produce ptosis, because they innervate Müller's muscle in the eyelid, but this is a much smaller muscle than the levator palpebrae, so the ptosis is much less dramatic. Thus, ptosis on the side of the larger pupil indicates a parasympathetic lesion on that side. Mild ptosis on the side of the smaller pupil indicates a sympathetic lesion on that side (Horner's syndrome). This is a restatement of Speed Rule 7 in Chapter 1.

b. Afferent pupillary defect

The pupillary reflex has both an afferent and an efferent limb. Anisocoria indicates an efferent defect (i.e., a lesion in the efferent fibers supplying the pupillary sphincter and dilator muscles). In contrast, an afferent defect

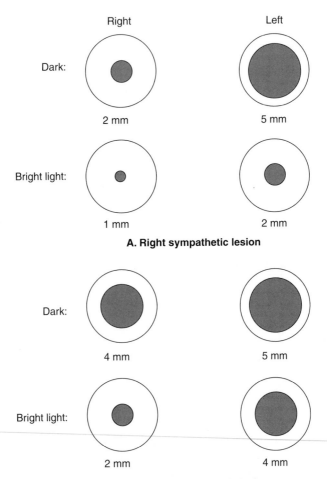

Fig. 2.1 Diagram illustrating the distinction between sympathetic and parasympathetic lesions producing anisocoria. When the left pupil is larger than the right, it could mean a right sympathetic lesion (A) or a left parasympathetic lesion (B). With sympathetic lesions, the pupillary asymmetry is greatest in the dark, whereas with parasympathetic lesions, the asymmetry is greatest in bright light.

(i.e., a lesion in the retina or optic nerve) does not produce anisocoria. Instead, an afferent defect produces abnormal findings on the "swinging flashlight test." To understand this test, you must recognize two facts. First, pupillary size is determined by an average of the illumination detected by each eye. For a simple demonstration of this, observe a normal subject's right pupil while covering the left eye: The pupil enlarges, because the average illumination has been effectively halved. Second, the efferent limb of the pupillary reflex is bilateral, so in normal subjects both pupils receive the same command and they are always the same size. Even if there is an afferent problem, so that one of the eyes registers less light than it should, this input projects bilaterally in the brainstem and affects both pupils equally, so the pupils are still equal in size. The pupils will only be unequal in size when the efferent pathways are not working properly.

Now consider what happens when a patient has an optic nerve lesion. For purposes of illustration, assume the lesion is in the left optic nerve and that it halves the amount of illumination that eye registers. If you shine a bright light directly in the left eye, it will register less illumination than it should, but it will still register more illumination than it did in the ambient room light, so the average of the illumination registered by the two eyes will increase. As a result, both pupils will constrict. Assume that this produces a change in pupil size from 5 mm to 3 mm (Figure 2.2A and B). A bright light directed at the right eye will produce a similar response: In this case, the brain will register an even greater increase in average illumination compared to ambient room light, because it will register the "full" effect of the bright light, not just half of it. The resulting pupillary constriction will be even stronger—producing a change in pupil size from 5 mm to 2.5 mm, for example (Figure 2.2C). It is difficult for an examiner to appreciate this subtle a distinction in the magnitude of the pupillary response. But now consider what happens when you swing the bright light back and forth between the two eyes. When you shine it in the left eye, both pupils are 3 mm. When you swing the light to the right eye, both pupils constrict to 2.5 mm. When you swing it back to the left eye, both pupils dilate back to 3 mm, and so forth. Because the examiner usually can observe the pupil under the bright light more readily than the other pupil, you will note the left pupil dilating each time you shine the light in it. This result might seem paradoxical, as if the pupil were dilating in response to bright light, but not when you recognize that the dilation only occurs when the light is swung from the right eye to the left one. In effect, by swinging the bright light back and forth, you are simply varying the intensity of the light perceived by the brain, and the pupils are constricting and dilating appropriately in response. This finding is termed a left afferent pupillary defect, or a left Marcus Gunn pupil.

3. Eye movement abnormalities

a. Gaze palsy

An eye movement abnormality in which the two eyes move conjugately but they have limited movement in one direction is called a *gaze palsy*. It is due to malfunction of one of the "gaze centers" (cortical and brainstem regions responsible for conjugate gaze) or to interruption of the pathways leading from them. When the lesion is in a brainstem gaze center, the neurons there cannot be activated either voluntarily or via the vestibulo-ocular reflex (discussed in Part VI of this chapter). This is called a *nuclear* gaze palsy. When the lesion is in a cortical gaze center, only voluntary gaze is impaired; the vestibular connections with the brainstem neurons responsible for gaze remain intact, so the vestibulo-ocular reflex is preserved. This is called a *supranuclear* gaze palsy.

b. Internuclear ophthalmoplegia

Lesions distal to the brainstem gaze centers (for example, in the nucleus of cranial nerve VI, or in the inferior oblique muscle on one side) produce disconjugate eye movement abnormalities. Specific patterns of eye movement abnormalities and their localizing significance are discussed in Chapter 13. One particular eye movement abnormality merits special recognition. Isolated impairment of adduction in one eye could conceivably result from damage to a single medial rectus muscle, a lesion in one tiny branch of one third nerve, or a focal neuromuscular junction problem, but it is much more commonly due to a lesion in the ipsilateral *median longitudinal fasciculus (MLF)*. This pathway runs from the sixth nerve nucleus on one side up to the third nerve nucleus on the other. This allows one eye's lateral rectus muscle and the other eye's medial rectus muscle to be activated synchronously, producing conjugate horizontal gaze (whether activated voluntarily or by reflex). A lesion in the MLF unlinks these two nuclei, so that the brainstem gaze center is able to get its message to the sixth nerve nucleus but not to the contralateral third nerve nucleus. The third nerve and medial rectus muscle continue to function normally in situations that do not require conjugate eye movements (e.g., convergence on a near object), but they cannot be activated by the horizontal gaze center. A lesion of the MLF is termed an *internuclear ophthalmoplegia, or INO*. The adduction difficulty is accompanied by nystagmus in the other eye as it abducts; in fact, in subtle cases, this may be the most prominent finding.

4. Facial weakness

In the same way that hyperactive deep tendon reflexes or a supranuclear gaze palsy indicate a central lesion whereas hypoactive reflexes or disconjugate eye movement abnormalities imply a peripheral lesion, the pattern of facial weakness can help differentiate between central and peripheral lesions. When one entire side of the face is weak, the lesion is usually peripheral. With a central lesion (such as a stroke in one cerebral hemisphere), the forehead muscles are often spared. This is because the portion of the facial nerve nucleus containing the cell bodies of neurons that innervate the forehead muscles typically gets input from the motor strips of both cerebral hemispheres, so it can still be activated by the cortex contralateral to the lesion. The portion of the facial nerve nucleus innervating the lower face does not have the same bilateral input; its input is predominantly from the contralateral cortex.

5. Hearing loss and vertigo

As explained in Chapter 1, a central lesion affects hearing in both ears almost equally. The only way to produce hearing loss restricted to one ear is with a peripheral lesion. The interpretation of the head impulse test described in Part III, and other examination findings that help to distinguish between central and peripheral vertigo, are discussed in Chapter 14.

6. Dysarthria and dysphagia

Unilateral weakness of muscles of the palate, pharynx, or larynx indicates a peripheral lesion (i.e., at the level of lower motor neuron, neuromuscular junction, or muscle). These muscles are innervated by fibers that originate in the nucleus ambiguus in the medulla and that travel in the glossopharyngeal and vagus nerves (cranial nerves IX and X, respectively). The nucleus ambiguus receives descending input from both cerebral hemispheres. A unilateral central lesion does not usually produce focal palatal, pharyngeal, or laryngeal weakness, because input to the nucleus ambiguus from the other hemisphere remains intact.

Dysarthria and dysphagia are prominent symptoms of lower motor neuron lesions of cranial nerves IX and X. These symptoms tend to be less prominent after unilateral cortical lesions because of the bilateral cortical input to the nucleus ambiguus. Bilateral cortical lesions often produce dramatic speech and swallowing problems, however. This is known as *pseudobulbar palsy* because the interruption of bilateral descending input to the brainstem simulates a lesion in the brainstem itself (a "bulbar" lesion). On close examination, the character of the dysarthria is different in patients with upper motor neuron lesions and patients with lower motor neuron lesions. There is classically a strained, strangled character to the speech of the former, whereas the latter typically sound breathy, hoarse, and hypernasal. In fact, dysarthria can result from any conditions that damage motor control of the structures necessary for speech production, including cerebellar or basal ganglia disorders, and the specific characteristics of the dysarthria may be useful in localization and differential diagnosis.

7. Neck weakness

The accessory nerve (cranial nerve XI) is a prime candidate for the most confusing of all the cranial nerves. The motor nerves innervating the SCM and trapezius muscles originate in the cervical spinal cord (at the C1-2 level for the SCM and the C3-4 level for the trapezius). They then ascend alongside the spinal cord and enter the skull through the foramen magnum, only to exit the skull again (through the jugular foramen) as the accessory nerve. The nerve cells in the spinal cord at C3-4 that control the trapezius muscle receive descending cortical input that originates almost exclusively in the contralateral cerebral hemisphere. The cortical input to the neurons that control the SCM muscle comes from both hemispheres, but predominantly the ipsilateral one. An additional confounding feature is that the left SCM rotates the head to the right (and vice versa).

As a result, peripheral lesions produce weakness of the ipsilateral SCM and trapezius muscles, resulting in weakness of shoulder elevation on that side and impaired head rotation to the opposite side. Central lesions produce weakness of the ipsilateral SCM and the contralateral trapezius, resulting in weakness of shoulder elevation on the side opposite the cortical lesion, and impaired head rotation away from the cortical lesion. Consequently, patients with hemiparesis have weakness of shoulder elevation on the side of the hemiparesis and weakness of head rotation toward the side of the hemiparesis.

8. Tongue weakness

The hypoglossal nerve (cranial nerve XII) receives descending cortical input from both hemispheres about equally, except that the fibers destined for the genioglossus muscle receive their cortical input only from the contralateral hemisphere. There appears to be variability in this pattern, so unilateral central lesions sometimes produce ipsilateral tongue weakness, more often produce contralateral tongue weakness, and most often produce no significant tongue weakness at all. Unilateral peripheral lesions produce weakness of the ipsilateral tongue muscles, resulting in difficulty protruding the tongue to the opposite side. Thus, when the patient is asked to protrude the tongue in the midline, it deviates toward the side of the lesion. Atrophy and fasciculations are often prominent with peripheral lesions, as with lower motor neuron lesions throughout the body (see the discussion of the motor examination in Section C).

C. Motor Examination

1. Upper motor neuron vs. lower motor neuron lesions

Several examination findings help to distinguish central from peripheral lesions in the motor system. Deep tendon reflexes provide one clue, as discussed in Chapter 1 (Speed Rule 4): Reflexes are typically hyperactive with a central lesion and hypoactive with a peripheral one. The Babinski sign is a reliable indicator of a central lesion. Spasticity (described in Part IV) is also characteristic of a central lesion, whereas tone is normal or reduced with a peripheral lesion. Atrophy and fasciculations are common with *lower motor neuron (LMN)* dysfunction and unusual with *upper motor neuron (UMN)* dysfunction. The pattern of muscle involvement is also helpful. A central lesion usually results in weakness that is more pronounced in the flexors of the lower extremities than in the extensors, but in the upper extremities the extensors are weaker than the flexors. Note that the muscles in which strength is relatively preserved (the flexors of the upper extremities and the extensors of the lower extremities) are the same ones in which spasticity is usually most pronounced. This is often called pyramidal weakness, but it does not occur with pure lesions of the pyramidal tracts. Instead, it is the net result of disrupting all the descending motor tracts and is probably most appropriately called the UMN pattern of weakness. The UMN pattern of weakness also causes supination of the upper extremity to be weaker than pronation; this accounts for the finding of a pronator drift, in which the arm pronates and drifts downward when the patient is asked to hold it extended with palms up (supinated). This is a fairly sensitive indicator of subtle UMN weakness. It is also useful as a test for internal consistency, because patients with nonorganic weakness will often allow their arm to drift downward but fail to pronate it.

To summarize, UMN lesions are characterized by the pattern of weakness (most prominent in the extensors of the upper extremity and the flexors of the lower extremity), spasticity (most pronounced in the opposite muscles), hyperreflexia, and the Babinski sign. LMN lesions are characterized by weakness, hypotonia, hyporeflexia, atrophy, and fasciculations.

2. Patterns of lower motor neuron weakness

For patients with weakness due to *diffuse* disease of the peripheral nervous system, the specific pattern of muscle involvement often provides useful localizing information (see Chapter 6). For example, predominantly distal weakness usually suggests a disease of peripheral nerves, but predominantly proximal weakness typically occurs in muscle disorders and neuromuscular junction diseases.

For patients with weakness due to *focal* lesions in the peripheral nervous system, the most reliable approach to localization is to consult a reference book, but in most cases adequate localization can be achieved by remembering a few simple patterns. In each extremity, consider three principal joints: the hip, knee, and ankle in the lower extremities, and the elbow, wrist, and knuckle in the upper extremities (it really doesn't matter which knuckle; the pattern applies equally well to interphalangeal joints and metacarpophalangeal joints). At each joint, consider flexion and extension separately. This gives six principal movements in each limb. Most localization problems can be solved by remembering the innervation patterns for these six principal movements (plus shoulder abduction and finger abduction in the upper extremities).

Figure 2.3 shows which nerve roots provide innervation for each of these principal movements. In the upper extremities, the pattern can be remembered by ordering the movements in a kind of spiral that proceeds down the arm: shoulder abduction (A), elbow flexion (B), elbow extension (C), wrist extension (D), wrist flexion (E), finger flexion (F), finger extension (G), and finger abduction (H). The corresponding roots then proceed in order: C5 (A), C5-6 (B), C6-7 (C), C6-7 (D), C7-8 (E), C8 (F), C8 (G), and T1 (H).

In the lower extremities, the pattern is even simpler (Figure 2.4). The movements can be considered in sequence down the front first and then the back: hip flexion (A), knee extension (B), ankle dorsiflexion (C),

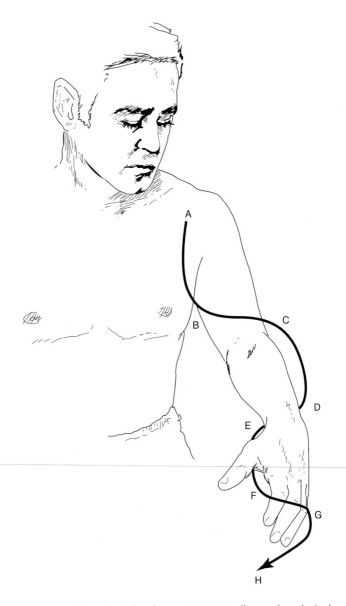

Fig. 2.3 Nerve roots and peripheral nerves corresponding to the principal movements of the upper extremity. The letters labeling the movements form a spiral down the extremity. The nerve roots and peripheral nerves corresponding to each movement are listed in the accompanying table.

Table for Figure 2.3

Movement	Roots	Peripheral Nerve
A. Shoulder abduction	5	Axillary
B. Elbow flexion	5/6	Musculocutaneous
C. Elbow extension	6/7	Radial
D. Wrist extension	6/7	Radial
E. Wrist flexion	7/8	Median
F. Finger flexion	8	Median
G. Finger extension	8	Radial
H. Finger abduction	T1	Ulnar

hip extension (D), knee flexion (E), and ankle plantar flexion (F). The corresponding roots are: L2-3 (A), L3-4 (B), L4-5 (C), L4-5 (D), L5-S1 (E), and S1-2 (F).

The peripheral nerves providing innervation for these same principal movements are listed in Figures 2.3 and 2.4. There is no simple pattern, but fortunately, there aren't many nerves to remember. In the upper extremities, all the extension movements in Figure 2.3 (C, D, and G) are innervated by the radial nerve. The two distal flexion movements (E and F) are supplied by the median nerve, and the proximal one (elbow flexion, B) by the musculocutaneous nerve. The axillary nerve supplies the deltoid muscle, which is the main shoulder abductor (A), and the interosseous muscles (H) are innervated by the ulnar nerve.

In the lower extremities, the sciatic nerve innervates the muscles responsible for knee flexion (E); its peroneal branch supplies ankle dorsiflexion (C), while its tibial branch supplies ankle plantar flexion (F). The femoral nerve innervates knee extensor muscles (B). The innervation of the iliopsoas muscle, which flexes the hip (A), arises very proximally from the L2 and L3 nerve roots; some consider this to be part of the femoral nerve, and others simply call it the "nerve to iliopsoas." The gluteus muscles, responsible for hip extension (D), are innervated by the gluteal nerves.

The nerve root corresponding to each commonly tested deep tendon reflex can also be derived from Figures 2.3 and 2.4. In particular, the biceps and brachioradialis reflexes are mediated by the C5-6 roots, the

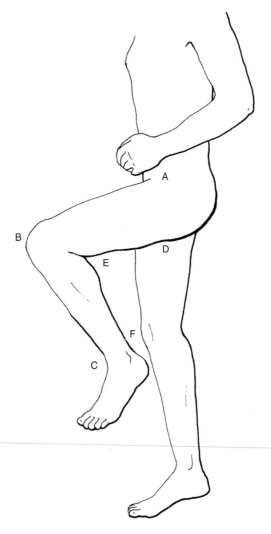

Fig. 2.4 Nerve roots and peripheral nerves corresponding to the principal movements of the lower extremity. The letters labeling the movements proceed in order from proximal to distal down the front of the limb, and then repeat from proximal to distal down the back of the limb. The nerve roots and peripheral nerves corresponding to each movement are listed in the accompanying table.

Table for Figure 2.4

Movement	Roots	Peripheral Nerve
A. Hip flexion	2/3	Femoral ("nerve to iliopsoas")
B. Knee extension	3/4	Femoral
C. Ankle dorsiflexion	4/5	Peroneal
D. Hip extension	4/5	Gluteal
E. Knee flexion	5/1	Sciatic
F. Ankle plantar flexion	1/2	Tibial

triceps reflex by the C6-7 roots (mainly C7), the knee jerk by the L3-4 roots (mainly L4), and the ankle jerk by the S1 root. The internal hamstring reflex is less often tested, but the L5 nerve root mediates it.

D. Reflex Examination

The localizing significance of the tendon reflexes has been discussed in Section C and in Chapter 1.

E. Sensory Examination

As explained in Chapter 1, the pathways for different sensory modalities cross at different levels in the nervous system, making them very useful for localizing lesions. Unlike the features that help to distinguish UMN lesions from LMN lesions in the motor pathways, there are not really any examination findings that differentiate the central portion of a sensory pathway from the peripheral portion.

For most localization problems, precise knowledge of the sensory fields of specific peripheral nerves and nerve roots is unnecessary. It is usually sufficient to remember the following facts (refer to Figures 2.5 and 2.6):

1. Sensation from the thumb and index finger travels via the C6 nerve root, the C7 root carries sensory information from the middle finger, and the C8 root conveys sensory information from the fourth and fifth fingers.

2. For the remainder of the upper extremity, the root innervation "fans out" from the hand (see Figure 2.5).

3. These innervation patterns cover both the anterior and posterior aspects of the upper extremity.

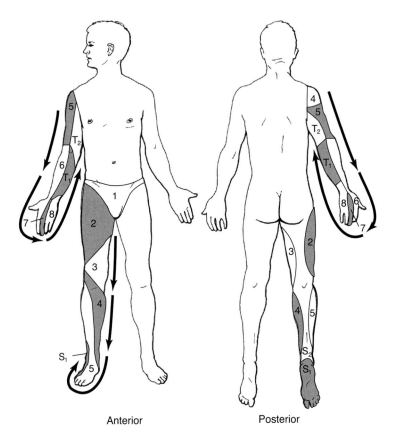

Anterior   Posterior

Fig. 2.5 Diagram illustrating the nerve roots corresponding to the principal dermatomes in the upper and lower extremities.

4. The **L**5 dermatome includes the **l**arge toe and the **l**ateral **l**ower **l**eg; the **S**1 dermatome includes the **s**mall toe and **s**ole. Roots L4, L3, and L2 cover the region fanning out medially and proximally from the L5 dermatome. The S2 dermatome extends from the S1 dermatome up the back of the leg (see Figure 2.5).

5. The median nerve carries sensation from all fingers except the fifth finger and half of the fourth, which are served by the ulnar nerve. These nerve territories extend proximally up to the wrist on the palmar aspect of the hand. On the dorsal aspect, the ulnar nerve territory still

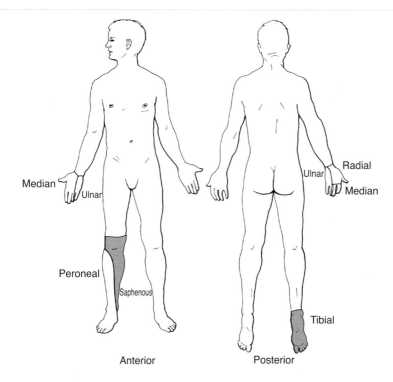

Fig. 2.6 Diagram illustrating the territories of sensory innervation for the principal peripheral nerves of the distal upper and lower extremities.

extends to the wrist, but the median nerve territory fades into radial nerve territory at the metacarpal-phalangeal joints (see Figure 2.6).

6. The common peroneal nerve innervates the lateral leg and the dorsum of the foot; the tibial nerve innervates the sole.

For the peripheral nerve innervations of more proximal limb regions, it is best to consult diagrams in reference books.

VI. Modifications of the Neurologic Examination

A. Screening Neurologic Examination

Medical students should always try to perform complete physical examinations (including complete neurologic examinations) on all patients they evaluate, so they can gain a sense of the range of normal variation and ask questions about the findings they observe. House officers and practicing physicians usually do not have the time to perform complete examinations on all patients, however. They must be able to perform a rapid examination that screens for most common abnormalities. They can then use the results of this screening examination—together with the history—to decide whether certain components of the examination must be conducted in more detail. For such screening purposes, the following neurologic examination is generally adequate and can be completed in five minutes or less. It may be performed in any order. This examination is offered as a suggestion for students to use in future practice; it is not adequate for students examining patients during a neurology clerkship.

Mental status

Make sure patients can follow at least one complicated command, taking care not to give them any nonverbal cues. Test them for orientation to person, place, and time. If their responses are appropriate and they are able to relate a detailed and coherent medical history, no further mental status testing is necessary (unless they are reporting cognitive problems).

Cranial nerves

Test visual fields in one eye, both pupillary responses to light, eye movements in all directions, facial strength, and hearing to finger rub.

Motor system

Test strength in the following muscles bilaterally: deltoids, triceps, wrist extensors, hand interossei, iliopsoas, hamstrings, ankle dorsiflexors. Test for a pronator drift. Test finger tapping, finger-to-nose, and heel-knee-shin performance. Test tandem gait and walking on the heels.

Reflexes

Test plantar responses and biceps, triceps, patellar, and ankle reflexes bilaterally.

Sensation

Test light touch sensation in all four distal limbs, including double simultaneous stimulation. Test vibration sense at the great toes.

Remember, this examination must be expanded when an asymmetry or other abnormality is found. For example, if the triceps muscle is weak in one arm, other muscles innervated by the radial nerve must be tested, as well as other muscles in the distribution of the C7 nerve root. Patients' specific complaints may also compel modifications in the examination. For example, patients complaining of memory loss need thorough mental status testing even if their performance on the screening examination is perfectly normal.

B. Examination of Stuporous or Comatose Patients

Many parts of the neurologic examination must be modified or elimi-nated in comatose patients, because they cannot answer questions or follow commands. Fortunately, there is no great mystery regarding the location of nervous system dysfunction in these patients; it is in the brainstem or above. The neurologic examination is directed mainly at determining whether this pathology is due to a structural lesion or due to metabolic dysfunction (including drug effects). The basis for this determination is discussed in Chapter 11; the most pertinent examination findings are a consistent asymmetry between right- and left-sided responses or abnormal reflexes that indicate dysfunction in specific regions of the brainstem.

Mental status

The mental status examination in a comatose patient is simply an assess-ment of the patient's responses to visual, auditory, and noxious stimuli. In addition to reflex responses that involve circuitry confined to the spinal cord, a comatose patient may demonstrate motor responses that reflect reflex pathways mediated by the brainstem. Two specific patterns of motor activity are classically described (Figure 2.7). *Decorticate posturing* consists of upper extremity adduction and flexion at the elbows, wrists, and fingers, together with lower extremity extension. *Decerebrate posturing* consists of upper extremity extension, adduction, and pronation together with lower extremity extension. This terminology reflects the analogy that has been drawn between these postures and the postures maintained by experimen-tal animals after specific lesions, but in fact, these postures do not have reliable localizing value in human patients. In general, patients with deco-rticate posturing in response to pain have a better prognosis than those with decerebrate posturing.

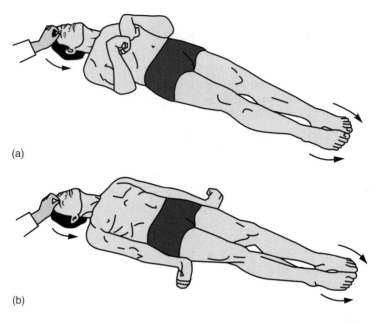

(a)

(b)

Fig. 2.7 a) Decorticate posturing (flexion and adduction of upper extremities, extension of lower extremities). b) Decerebrate posturing (pronation, adduction, and proximal extension of upper extremities, with wrist flexion; extension of lower extremities).

Cranial nerves

In comatose patients, visual acuity cannot be tested and formal testing of visual fields is impossible. A rough assessment of visual field defects may be obtained by assessing response to visual threat, such as a finger or small object introduced suddenly into the visual field. Pupillary reflexes can be tested in the same manner as in a conscious person.

Eye movements can be assessed by activating them using the *vestibulo-ocular reflex*. One way to test this reflex is with the *oculocephalic* maneuver, or *doll's eyes* maneuver. This is similar to the head thrust maneuver described in Part III, except that it does not require patient cooperation. Holding the patient's eyes open with one hand, turn the patient's head quickly to one side, and observe how the eyes move relative to the head. If there is any chance that there has been a traumatic injury to the cervical spine, plain films of the cervical spine must be obtained before performing

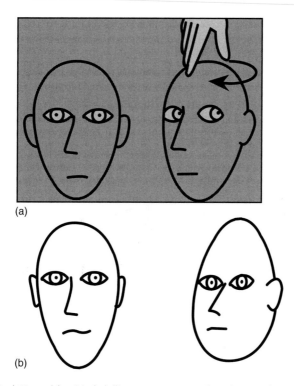

(a)

(b)

Fig. 2.8 a) Normal (positive) doll's eyes response: when the examiner rotates the patient's head in one direction, the patient's eyes stay fixed in space (as if the patient were trying to keep the eyes focused on a distant object)—thus, relative to the head, the eyes move in the opposite direction. b) Absent doll's eyes response: when the examiner rotates the patient's head in one direction, the patient's eyes rotate with the head—thus, relative to the head, the eyes remain fixed.

this maneuver. Doll's eyes are considered to be positive (Figure 2.8) when the vestibulo-ocular reflex is intact: the eyes remain fixed on the same point in space during head rotation (i.e., they do not turn with the head; instead, they appear to be moving relative to the head in the direction opposite to the head movement). Absence of this response in a comatose patient indicates dysfunction somewhere in the vestibulo-ocular reflex pathway: in the afferent limb (from the labyrinth and vestibular nerve), the efferent limb (cranial nerves III and VI and the muscles they innervate), or the pathways connecting them in the pons and medulla. Technically, the oculocephalic maneuver also stimulates neck proprioceptors, so it is not a pure test of the vestibulo-ocular reflex, but in practice, this is not a major consideration.

Another maneuver that stimulates the vestibulo-ocular reflex more strongly is the *cold caloric* procedure. Place the patient in the supine position, with the head or upper body tilted forward so that the neck forms an angle of 30° with the horizontal. Fill a syringe with 50–100 ml of ice-cold water and attach a small catheter. Inject the water against the tympanic membrane (checking with an otoscope first to be sure the membrane is intact). In this position, cold water has the same effect on the horizontal semicircular canal as sustained turning of the head in the opposite direction; the result is sustained deviation of both eyes toward the ear being cooled. If the eyes remain stationary, there is a problem in the vestibulo-ocular reflex pathway—usually in the pons or medulla, but occasionally in the afferent or efferent limbs (cranial nerves III, VI, or VIII). In conscious subjects, the cold caloric procedure produces not only deviation of the eyes toward the cooled ear but also nystagmus, with the fast component away from the cooled ear. Caloric testing is usually not performed in conscious patients, however, because it can cause severe vertigo and nausea, and the same elements of the nervous system can be tested in much less noxious ways. Even in comatose patients, you do not need to perform the cold caloric procedure if the doll's eyes response is normal.

Cranial nerves V and VII can be assessed in comatose patients by testing corneal reflexes and by observing facial grimacing in response to noxious stimulation (supraorbital pressure or nasal tickle, for example). Cranial nerves IX and X can be assessed by testing the gag reflex, but remember that the gag reflex may be absent in 20% of normal subjects.

Motor and sensory systems

Formal strength testing is impossible in comatose patients, but deep tendon reflexes and resistance to passive manipulation can still be tested in the usual manner. The strength with which the patient moves each limb in response to pain should be assessed, and also the degree to which the movement is purposeful. Noxious stimulation of the lower extremity (produced by squeezing a nailbed or pinching the skin) may produce *triple flexion* (dorsiflexion of the ankle, with flexion of the knee and hip) purely as a local withdrawal reflex. To look for purposeful withdrawal, the stimulus should be applied in a location where triple flexion would be an inappropriate response, such as the anterior thigh: Hip flexion would indicate purely reflex withdrawal, whereas hip extension would indicate a purposeful movement. In contrast, hip flexion in response to a noxious stimulus applied to the posterior thigh could be either a reflex or a purposeful response. In both upper and lower extremities, reflex withdrawal produces limb adduction, so to differentiate reflex withdrawal from purposeful movement, the noxious stimulus should be applied to the medial aspect of the limb.

Pain sensation in comatose patients can be assessed by observing the response to noxious stimulation (and noting whether the response varies depending on which limb is stimulated). Other sensory modalities cannot be tested.

VII. Discussion of Localization Problems

Example 1. The magnitude of this patient's pupillary asymmetry is greatest in the dark, so the sympathetic system is not functioning normally. The smaller pupil is therefore the abnormal one (see Figure 2.1A). Thus, this patient has a sympathetic lesion on the left, and mild left-sided ptosis would be expected.

Example 2. For a patient to have face, arm, and leg weakness all on the same side of the body, there must be an upper motor neuron lesion (see Chapter 1, Speed Rule 6). An upper motor neuron lesion typically spares forehead muscles, because there is bilateral cortical input to the portion of the facial nerve nucleus controlling those muscles.

Example 3. The L2-3 roots correspond to hip flexion, the L5-S1 roots to knee flexion, and the L4-5 roots to ankle dorsiflexion (see Figure 2.4). Thus, no single nerve root lesion could produce this pattern of weakness. No single peripheral nerve lesion could do so, either. This pattern is typical of an upper motor neuron lesion, which usually produces more weakness in the flexors of the lower extremity than in the extensors.

Chapter 3

What's the Lesion?

James W. Albers and Douglas J. Gelb

I. Case Histories

For each of the following cases, answer the following questions:

1. Where's the lesion?
2. Is the lesion focal, multifocal, or diffuse?
3. Is this a mass lesion or a non-mass lesion?
4. What is the temporal profile?
5. What diagnostic category is most likely?

Case 1. A 55-year-old woman has been brought to the emergency room by her husband because she seems confused and is having progressively more difficulty expressing her thoughts. For at least the last 10 weeks, she has had increasing clumsiness and weakness in her right arm and leg, and she is bumping into objects in her home. On examination, she has a right visual field defect (homonymous hemianopia), aphasia, a mild right hemiparesis (face, arm, leg), and increased reflexes on the right side with an extensor plantar response (Babinski sign) on the right.

Case 2. A 72-year-old right-handed man noted the abrupt feeling of heaviness in his left arm while watching television. His left leg gave out when he tried to stand, and he fell to the floor. He called for help, and when his wife came into the room, she noted that the left corner of his face was sagging. He could still speak. He had no symptoms other than the weakness of his entire left side. Over the next several hours he improved slightly.

Case 3. A 22-year-old man was well until 2 days ago, when he developed fever, severe headache, nausea, and vomiting. He became progressively

more obtunded over the next day. He had two generalized seizures in the morning and was brought to the emergency room, where he was found to have a fever and stiff neck. He was stuporous, and he had generalized hyperreflexia and bilateral Babinski signs.

Case 4. A 47-year-old man developed ringing in his right ear several years ago, and it has grown worse over time. Over the same time period, his hearing in that ear has gradually deteriorated, and he has developed weakness and loss of feeling on the right side of his face. Over the past few months, he has developed stiffness, weakness, and numbness of his left arm and leg.

Case 5. A 28-year-old accountant and part-time boxer has been brought to the urgent care clinic by his wife because he has become irritable and abusive. She reports that he has had intermittent headaches for 3 months, and the headaches have become more severe and constant in the past month. He has been unable to work for about a week because of excessive drowsiness, and he sleeps for up to 24 hours if not awakened. The patient is poorly cooperative and says only that he has a headache.

On neurologic examination, he is drowsy and irritable but able to follow commands. He has mild to moderate weakness in his left arm and leg, and a left pronator drift. Tendon reflexes are hyperactive on the left. There is a left Babinski response. The lower part of his face droops slightly on the left side.

Case 6. A 21-year-old right-handed woman experienced a sensation of numbness and tingling over her abdomen and in her legs. The next day, her legs began to feel stiff and tight, and she experienced difficulty in initiating her urinary stream and incomplete voiding. As the day progressed, the numbness and tingling became more pronounced in her mid-abdomen and below, and she began to have trouble walking. She went to bed early that evening, and when she awoke the next morning, she was unable to stand.

Case 7. A 69-year-old right-handed retired executive is seeing her internist for a routine checkup. Her husband mentions that she has undergone a marked personality change over the past several months. He also notes that she has been forgetful for about a year and keeps asking the same things over and over. She no longer seems interested in her personal appearance. The mental status examination confirms these observations. Her language output is fluent, but she frequently pauses because she can't think of a word. She has difficulty following complicated commands. She can remember only one of three items after a 5-minute delay,

and she recalls no current events. She is unable to subtract two-digit numbers in her head. The remainder of her examination is normal.

Case 8. A 44-year-old left-handed woman suddenly developed a severe bilateral temporal and occipital headache. She also complained of a stiff neck. When she tried to lie down, she experienced severe nausea and vomited twice. She was taken immediately to the hospital, where she was noted to be somnolent, but when she was stimulated she responded appropriately and moved all four limbs equally. Her level of consciousness deteriorated over the next 4 hours, to the point where she could not be aroused even with vigorous stimulation.

Case 9. A 57-year-old woman has come to the emergency room because in the middle of a business meeting earlier today she suddenly became dizzy and experienced nausea and vomiting. On examination, she is dysarthric and has weakness of the left palate. She starts to cough when she tries to swallow water. There is loss of pinprick sensation over the left side of her face and the right side of her body, and ataxia of her left arm and leg. Seven hours have passed, and there has been no progression or improvement.

Case 10. Over the course of a few days, a 30-year-old man with Hodgkin's disease began to experience severe pain beginning in his back and encircling the left side of his chest in a band 3 cm wide just below his breast. The pain was very intense at first but subsided somewhat, coincident with a rash that appeared in precisely the same distribution. He is still having pain in that area two weeks later, and notes diminished touch sensation in the region of pain.

Case 11. A patient reports a pain that is similar to the one described in Case 10. The pain involves the left side of her chest. No rash is present, and for many months the pain has been getting worse. It remains localized to a narrow and circumscribed area of her chest, making her think that it might be "heart trouble." In addition, she complains of difficulty walking and says that her left leg seems to be weak and stiff.

II. Beyond Localization

Chapters 1 and 2 presented strategies for localizing the site of nervous system dysfunction. Although lesion localization is fundamental to the process of generating a differential diagnosis, it is only the first step. It might seem as if the next step, once the lesion site has been identified, would simply be to obtain an imaging study of that region. This is not

always the most appropriate diagnostic strategy, however. Even when it is, a prior determination of the diagnoses that are plausible on clinical grounds will be important for guiding decisions regarding which imaging modality to order, how urgently to do it, and how to interpret ambiguous results. Anyone who has ever read a radiologist's report knows that "clinical correlation is required."

In this chapter, we present a systematic way to analyze the history and examination in order to generate a reasonable hypothesis about the pathophysiologic process underlying the patient's problem. Many of the concepts and clinical vignettes were adapted by Dr. Albers from material developed by neurologists at the Mayo Clinic. The approach is based on addressing the following three features in order:

A. *Localization*: Where's the lesion?

B. *Temporal profile*: How did the symptoms begin, and how have they changed over time?

C. *Epidemiology*: Does the patient have risk factors for specific conditions?

Before explaining how this information is used to draw conclusions about etiology, a few terms must be defined.

A. Localization

The principles of localization were presented in Chapters 1 and 2. For the purposes of clinical decision making, it is often sufficient to determine whether the lesion is supratentorial, in the posterior fossa, in the spinal cord, or in the peripheral nervous system. When considering potential etiologies, the most important question is whether the problem is a focal lesion, multifocal, or diffuse.

A *focal* lesion is confined to a single circumscribed area. Focal lesions are usually unilateral, but not always—a lesion that extends from one side to the other across the midline is also focal.

A *multifocal* process is made up of two or more focal lesions distributed randomly. These lesions may all be at the same level of the nervous system (for example, many different cortical lesions, or many lesions of individual peripheral nerves), or they may be at different levels (for example, one in the spinal cord and one in the cerebral cortex).

A *diffuse* process involves symmetric parts of the nervous system without extending across the midline as a single circumscribed lesion. Diseases causing generalized dysfunction of neurons, or just of neurons in the basal

ganglia, or just of peripheral nerves, or just of sensory nerves, or just of long nerves, would all be examples of diffuse processes.

B. Temporal Profile

The first consideration in describing the temporal profile is whether symptoms are *transient* or *persistent*. *Transient* symptoms resolve completely; *persistent* symptoms do not. There are three types of persistent time course:

Static (stationary) symptoms reach a maximum level of severity and then do not change.

Improving symptoms reach a maximum level of severity and then begin to resolve.

Progressive symptoms continue to worsen.

These categories are mutually exclusive at any instant, but they are not immutable. For example, consider a patient who develops symptoms that continue to get worse for a week, remain unchanged for a month, and then start to improve so that by 6 months the patient is completely back to normal. If evaluated at 3 days, the symptoms would be progressive, but at 3 weeks they would be static, and at 3 months they would be improving. For diagnostic purposes, the most important information about the temporal profile is the rapidity with which changes occur:

Acute symptoms evolve over minutes to days.

Subacute symptoms evolve over days to weeks.

Chronic symptoms evolve over months to years.

These categories overlap, and they are intended as rough guidelines. Diseases that typically have a chronic time course may at times present acutely, conditions that ordinarily would be considered subacute sometimes evolve over years, and so forth. Nonetheless, these broad definitions turn out to be useful in most cases.

C. Epidemiology

Lesion localization and temporal profile are the most important factors in generating a list of potential etiologies. Epidemiologic considerations are used mainly to arrange the list in order of likelihood. For example, thyroid disease and brucellosis can both cause subacute diffuse processes, but a physician treating an affluent adult patient in an urban area would be

much more concerned about thyroid disease because it is much more common in that setting. As another example, an elderly patient with a stroke is more likely to have atherosclerotic disease than an arterial dissection, but dissection becomes a serious consideration if the same patient has recently sustained trauma to the neck. The relevant epidemiologic factors vary from one disease to the next, so they will not be discussed in detail in this chapter.

III. Etiology

There are seven general categories of persistent neurologic disease that can be distinguished, each with a characteristic spatial-temporal profile.

A. Degenerative Diseases

In degenerative disorders, one or more components of the nervous system begin to malfunction after functioning normally for many years. Once the deterioration begins, it doesn't stop. Two common examples are Alzheimer's disease and Parkinson's disease. Degenerative diseases are *diffuse, chronic,* and *progressive.*

B. Neoplastic Diseases

In practice, the term *neoplasm* is applied mainly to collections of cells that are multiplying uncontrollably because of some genetic transformation (i.e., cancer). The rules presented here apply to the more general, literal meaning of neoplasm, "new growth." This means that any new structural lesion that is growing (including a slowly enlarging hematoma or a herniating intervertebral disc) will be classified as a neoplasm. This makes sense clinically, because when these processes are in the differential diagnosis, cancer is usually a possibility also, and it is appropriate to direct the diagnostic evaluation at the most serious potential diagnosis. Neoplastic diseases are characterized as *focal, chronic* (or, less often, *subacute*), and *progressive.*

C. Vascular Diseases

Disruption of the cerebrovascular system can produce either ischemia (resulting from obstructed blood vessels) or hemorrhage (resulting from ruptured blood vessels). Either way, the symptoms are almost always *acute.* Ischemic lesions are always *focal.* Hemorrhagic lesions may be either *focal* or *diffuse,* depending on whether the blood escapes into a freely interconnecting space (e.g., subarachnoid hemorrhage) or a confined space (e.g., subdural hematoma, parenchymal hemorrhage). Ischemic events are typically *static* or *improving*, whereas hemorrhagic events are typically *progressive*.

D. Inflammatory Diseases

Inflammation in the nervous system is most often a response to an infection or some other insult. As with hemorrhage, an infection in a confined space (such as an abscess) results in a *focal* lesion, whereas in an unrestricted space the result is a *diffuse* lesion (e.g., meningitis or encephalitis). Either way, the time course is usually *subacute* and *progressive*. In some cases, the immune system appears to become activated even without external provocation (autoimmune diseases); *multifocal* deficits typically result, with a *chronic* or *subacute* time course, usually *progressive*. Multiple sclerosis and vasculitis are examples.

E. Toxic and Metabolic Diseases

In one sense, all diseases are metabolic, because the only way to damage any organ is to interfere with cellular metabolism. For example, occlusive vascular disease deprives cells of oxygen and energy sources, ultimately resulting in complete termination of all cellular processes. This would not generally be considered a metabolic disease, however, because there is an underlying structural lesion: an obstructed blood vessel. The term metabolic disease is reserved for processes that disrupt cellular metabolism at a molecular level without any underlying structural lesion evident macroscopically. Diseases caused by toxic substances, both endogenous (e.g., uremia) and exogenous (e.g., drug overdose), are included in this category. Diabetes mellitus, thyroid disease, vitamin B12 deficiency, abnormal liver function, electrolyte abnormalities, and hypoxemia are some other metabolic disorders that commonly produce neurologic symptoms. Since structural lesions are excluded by definition, metabolic diseases are *diffuse*. Their time course can be *acute, subacute,* or *chronic*. They can be *static* or *progressive*.

F. Traumatic Diseases

The main feature distinguishing traumatic disease from vascular disease is an epidemiologic consideration: the onset in the setting of trauma. Traumatic disorders are always *acute* in onset. Nonhemorrhagic traumatic lesions are generally *static* or *improving*; they may be *diffuse* (concussion) or *focal* (contusion, encephalomalacia). Traumatic hemorrhage has the same spatial-temporal profile as nontraumatic hemorrhage: It is *progressive* and may be *diffuse* or *focal*.

G. Congenital and Developmental Diseases

Congenital and developmental disorders are conceptually very similar to degenerative diseases, except that the deterioration begins early in life. In some cases, the affected element of the nervous system never develops at all. Like degenerative disease, developmental disorders are characteristically *chronic* and *diffuse*. They may be *progressive* or (unlike degenerative disease) they may be *static*.

Table 3.1 summarizes the way in which these diagnostic categories can be distinguished on the basis of focality and time course.

It is often helpful to distinguish between mass lesions and non-mass lesions. *Mass lesions* alter cellular function not only at the site of the lesion but also in the surrounding area, by compression or destruction of neighboring tissue. *Non-mass lesions* alter cellular function at the site of the lesion but spare adjacent tissue. Mass lesions cause *focal, progressive* symptoms. Diffuse processes, regardless of time course, are non-mass lesions; so are lesions that are focal but not progressive. It is clear from Table 3.1 that circumscribed hemorrhages, abscesses, and neoplasms are all mass lesions; all the other processes listed in the chart are non-mass lesions.

The categories listed in Table 3.1 easily generalize to multifocal conditions. Thus, an acute multifocal process that is static or improving is still most likely vascular (and probably embolic, in particular). Trauma can also produce multifocal lesions with this temporal profile, just as it can produce focal lesions. Acute, progressive multifocal lesions are rare, but the analogy with focal lesions still applies: This combination of focality and temporal course suggests multifocal hemorrhage, which in turn suggests a bleeding diathesis. Just as subacute focal processes are generally inflammatory, so are subacute multifocal processes. Multiple sclerosis is the most common specific diagnosis when the lesions are all in the central nervous system. Other diagnoses in this category include vasculitis and endocarditis. Finally, when symptoms are chronic, and multifocal rather than focal, neoplastic disease remains the prime diagnostic consideration. Specifically, a metastatic tumor is the most likely diagnosis in this setting.

Table 3.1 Characteristic Spatial-Temporal Profiles of Major Disease Process Categories

	Acute: Static or Improving	Acute: Progressive	Subacute	Chronic
Focal	1. Vascular (ischemic) 2. Traumatic (contusion, encephalomalacia)	1. Vascular (intraparenchymal hemorrhage) 2. Traumatic (intraparenchymal, subdural, or epidural hemorrhage)	Inflammatory (abscess)	Neoplastic
Diffuse	1. Toxic-metabolic (including anoxic) 2. Traumatic (concussion)	1. Vascular (subarachnoid hemorrhage) 2. Toxic-metabolic 3. Traumatic (subarachnoid hemorrhage)	1. Inflammatory (meningitis, encephalitis) 2. Toxic-metabolic	1. Degenerative 2. Congenital-developmental 3. Toxic-metabolic

This approach is less useful for transient symptoms, where the distinction between acute, subacute, and chronic symptoms becomes less meaningful. Moreover, the symptoms often resolve so quickly that it is impossible to distinguish between multifocal and diffuse lesions. Even so, it is often possible to distinguish focal transient symptoms from diffuse transient symptoms, especially in patients with paroxysmal disorders, who have episodic recurrence of transient symptoms and over time may learn to identify and describe their symptoms in detail. The three most common causes of focal transient symptoms are seizures, transient ischemic attacks, and migraines. Diffuse transient symptoms are typically caused by transient hypoperfusion (e.g., a cardiac arrhythmia), seizures, or metabolic processes (e.g., hepatic encephalopathy, hypoglycemia, and intoxication).

IV. Discussion of Case Histories

Case 1. The aphasia, right hemianopia, and right hemiparesis localize the lesion to the left cerebral cortex (if this is not clear, review Chapter 1). The lesion is therefore **focal**. It is also **progressive**, so it is a mass lesion. The time course is **chronic**, making a *neoplasm* most likely.

Comment: An appropriate summary note might read: "55-year-old woman with a 10-week history of progressive symptoms and neurologic findings suggestive of a left cortical mass lesion, likely neoplasm." In this case, magnetic resonance imaging (MRI) and biopsy confirmed the diagnosis of glioma. The patient was treated with radiation therapy and chemotherapy.

Case 2. Facial weakness ipsilateral to body weakness suggests a **focal** lesion in the high pons or above (see Speed Rule 6 in Chapter 1). There has been **no progression**, so this is not a mass lesion. The symptoms developed **acutely**. A focal lesion that developed acutely and is improving is usually an *ischemic vascular* lesion (unless there is a history of trauma).

Comment: A computed tomography (CT) scan demonstrated a small infarct in the right internal capsule. The patient had his antihypertensive medications adjusted and was started on aspirin.

Case 3. The altered level of consciousness indicates dysfunction in the brainstem, thalamus, or both cerebral hemispheres (see Speed Rule 11 in Chapter 1). The generalized seizures are indicative of bihemispheric disease. All of the abnormal neurologic findings (e.g., hyperreflexia and Babinski signs) are symmetric. Thus, the condition is **diffuse**. It follows that it is not a mass lesion. The symptoms developed over 2 days, making them **subacute**. A diffuse, subacute process could either be *toxic–metabolic* or *inflammatory* (meningitis or encephalitis). In this case, the fever and stiff neck make meningitis or encephalitis most likely.

Comment: The patient was started empirically on ceftriaxone and a lumbar puncture was performed immediately. Cerebrospinal fluid examination demonstrated greater than 200 white blood cells, predominantly lymphocytic. Acyclovir was added, and when cerebrospinal fluid cultures remained negative at 48 hours, the ceftriaxone was stopped. The patient gradually recovered, and polymerase chain reaction testing of the spinal fluid confirmed the diagnosis of herpes simplex encephalitis.

Case 4. The right facial numbness and left body numbness indicate a lesion on the right between the pons and the C2 level of the spinal cord (see Speed Rule 5 in Chapter 1). The left arm and leg weakness and stiffness further restrict the possible localization to the region between the pons and the low medulla (if this is not evident, draw the pathways). Finally, the right facial weakness and the tinnitus and hearing loss in the right ear localize the lesion further, to the right pons or pontomedullary junction. Such a precise unilateral localization implies a **focal** lesion. It is **progressive**, so it is a mass lesion. The progression has taken place over several years, making it **chronic**. A focal, chronic lesion is a *neoplasm*.

Comment: In this case, the neoplasm was a schwannoma—a benign tumor. It was resected, and the patient continues to do well 15 years later.

Case 5. As with Case 2, the weakness of left face, arm, and leg imply a right-sided **focal** lesion at the level of the high pons or above. It is a mass lesion, because it is **progressive**. The time course is **chronic** (3 months). Again, a focal, chronic lesion signifies a *neoplasm*.

Comment: In this case, a CT scan demonstrated a right subdural hematoma (SDH). This shows how the rules are only approximations. Still, SDH represents a "new growth" that slowly expands, so for practical purposes it behaves like a benign tumor. The patient had the SDH evacuated, and he recovered fully.

Case 6. Even though no information about the physical examination is available, the likely lesion localization can be inferred from this patient's history alone. The abnormal sensory and motor function below a level in the mid-abdomen implies a **focal** lesion in the spinal cord, at the thoracic level or above (see Speed Rule 3 in Chapter 1). Since the symptoms are **progressive**, this is a mass lesion. The time course is **subacute**. A focal, subacute lesion is typically *inflammatory*—specifically, an abscess.

Comment: An MRI scan of the cervical and thoracic spine failed to demonstrate an abscess, but a lumbar puncture revealed a pleocytosis in the spinal fluid. All cultures were negative. This patient was thought to have transverse myelitis, an inflammatory (possibly autoimmune) disorder that behaves like a mass lesion within the spinal cord. Her symptoms gradually resolved without treatment. This is another example of how the rules can fail. In this case, they pointed to the correct diagnostic category but the wrong specific diagnosis. As it happens, it is often impossible to distinguish between transverse myelitis and a spinal cord abscess on clinical grounds, so it is appropriate to direct the evaluation at the possibility of an abscess, which would require urgent treatment.

Case 7. This patient has personality changes and deficits in several different cognitive functions, including language comprehension, short-term and long-term memory, and calculations. This implies a **diffuse** cortical localization. Since it is diffuse, this is not a mass lesion. The deficits have **progressed** over several months, making this a **chronic** problem. A diffuse, chronic disorder can be a *degenerative* disease, a *congenital/developmental* problem, or a *toxic–metabolic* disorder. The patient is too old to be presenting with a congenital or developmental disease, and there is nothing to suggest any specific metabolic abnormality, so a degenerative disease is most likely.

Comment: Even though a degenerative disease is the most likely diagnosis, potential toxic-metabolic causes should be investigated. In fact, neoplasms can sometimes break the rules and produce a diffuse picture rather than focal. This patient had a head CT scan and a number of blood and urine tests to investigate these possibilities. All of the tests were normal, and her subsequent course was consistent with Alzheimer's disease.

Case 8. This case is similar to Case 3, except that the time course is **acute** rather than subacute. The lesion is **diffuse** (and therefore not a mass lesion), and it is **progressive***:* This means it is either *vascular* (specifically, subarachnoid hemorrhage), *toxic-metabolic*, or *traumatic*. There is no history of trauma and no reason to suspect a toxic–metabolic disorder, so subarachnoid hemorrhage is the most likely diagnosis.

Comment: A head CT scan was normal, but a lumbar puncture revealed subarachnoid hemorrhage. A cerebral angiogram demonstrated an aneurysm of the anterior communicating artery. The aneurysm was successfully coiled, and the patient has returned to her baseline level of function.

Case 9. The reduced pinprick sensation over the left face and right body imply a *focal* lesion on the left, between the pons and the C2 level of the spinal cord (see Speed Rule 5 in Chapter 1). The weakness of the left palate confines the lesion to the medulla, because only lower motor neuron lesions produce unilateral palatal weakness (see Chapter 2). Ataxia of the left arm and leg is also consistent with a focal lesion in this location, because a lesion in the medulla can disrupt cerebellar connections. The symptoms began *acutely*, and they have *not progressed*, so this is not a mass lesion. A focal, acute lesion with a *static* time course implies either a *vascular (ischemic)* or a *traumatic* etiology, and there is no history of trauma in this case.

Comment: This patient had a normal head CT scan, but MRI revealed a small infarction in the left lateral medulla. In the emergency room, she was found to have atrial fibrillation, which had never been noted before. The stroke was presumed to be embolic, so anticoagulant therapy was begun. Further evaluation revealed hyperthyroidism. She was converted to normal sinus rhythm, her hyperthyroidism was treated, and after 6 months the anticoagulation was stopped. By that time, her symptoms had completely resolved except for minimal ataxia of the left arm.

Case 10. This patient has symptoms confined to the distribution of a single nerve root. This makes a lesion in the nerve root itself most likely, but, theoretically, the lesion could be anywhere from the level of the nerve root on up the sensory pathway to the cortex. Additional symptoms would be expected with any of these higher localizations, however. In any case, the lesion is *focal*. It is *not progressive*, so it is not a mass lesion. The time course is *subacute*, so the process is probably *inflammatory*, and specifically, an abscess.

Comment: This is another situation in which the rules indicate the correct diagnostic category (inflammatory) but the wrong specific diagnosis. In this case, epidemiologic factors are important. A rash in a dermatomal distribution is very suggestive of herpes zoster reactivation, which can produce sensory symptoms (especially pain) in the same distribution. This occurs particularly often in immunocompromised individuals, including those receiving chemotherapy for cancer. The patient received famciclovir and pain treatment, and the symptoms gradually resolved.

Case 11. In addition to chest wall symptoms like those described by the patient in Case 10, this patient has left leg weakness, which could not be explained by a lesion in a thoracic nerve root. Instead, the most plausible localization is within the thoracic spinal cord on the left, in the one or two segments where the spinothalamic pathway has not yet crossed to the right side of the cord. This is a **focal** lesion, and since it is **progressive**, it is a mass lesion. The time course is **chronic**. A chronic focal lesion is a *neoplasm*.

Comment: An MRI scan revealed a meningioma compressing the left T4 nerve root and the spinal cord at that level. This benign tumor was resected, and the patient's only residual symptom was mild stiffness of the left leg.

II

Common Diseases

Chapter 4

Stroke

I. Case Histories

Case 1. A 65-year-old man drove himself to the emergency room at 9 a.m. after experiencing a 4-minute episode of word-finding difficulty and right hand weakness. He had experienced four similar episodes in the last 3 weeks. He had undergone coronary bypass surgery for unstable angina a year ago, and he had a long history of hypertension and diabetes. He was taking aspirin, propranolol, and glyburide daily. He was afebrile, his blood pressure was 140/80, his pulse was 85 per minute and regular, and a left carotid bruit could be heard in systole and diastole. There were no murmurs and his neurologic examination was normal.

Case 2 A 59-year-old woman came to the emergency room at her family's insistence at 9 p.m. after she mentioned that she had been having trouble seeing out of her left eye since awakening that morning. She had been in good health except for long-standing hypertension and occasional "rapid heartbeats." She denied previous visual symptoms or other episodic neurologic symptoms. She was taking captopril. The patient was alert, her blood pressure was 170/95, her pulse was 130 per minute and irregular, and there were no murmurs or bruits. The only abnormality on neurologic exam was a left homonymous hemianopia.

Case 3. A 73-year-old man was brought to the emergency room by paramedics after he fell down on the way back from the bathroom and discovered that he could not move his left side. His symptoms had not progressed in the 90 minutes that had elapsed since the initial event. He had been hypertensive for 20 years and was taking hydrochlorothiazide, and he had been taking lovastatin for a year because of hyperlipidemia. He denied previous episodes of focal neurologic symptoms. He was alert, with a blood pressure of 180/100 and a pulse that was 80 per minute and regular. There were no bruits or murmurs. Neurologic exam showed normal mental status (with no neglect); dysarthria; left hemiparesis involving face, arm, and leg; left-sided hyperreflexia; a left extensor plantar response (Babinski sign); and normal sensation.

Questions:

1. What are the causes of these patients' symptoms?
2. How would you manage these patients in the emergency room?
3. Would you admit these patients to the hospital?
4. What tests would you order?
5. What treatment would you initiate?

II. Approach to Stroke

In managing a patient who has had a stroke or TIA (transient ischemic attack), four questions are fundamental:

1. Is the diagnosis correct?
2. What can be done to restore blood flow (if the stroke was ischemic)?
3. What can be done to limit the damage?
4. What can be done to reduce the patient's risk of future strokes?

Question 4 has two components:

4a. What can be done to reduce the risk of cerebrovascular disease? In fact, this question applies to everyone with risk factors for vascular disease, even those who have never had a stroke or TIA. The term *"primary prevention"* refers to measures that can reduce the risk of stroke in patients who have never had a stroke or TIA (although these same measures are also beneficial for patients who have already experienced at least one stroke or TIA).

4b. What can be done to reduce the risk of stroke in patients who have already had at least one stroke or TIA? These measures are referred to as *secondary prevention*.

Question 1 is addressed in Part IV, Questions 2 and 3 in Part V, Question 4a in Part VI, and Question 4b in Parts VII and VIII. Part III presents some definitions and necessary background information.

III. Background Information

A. Definitions

stroke sudden onset of a focal neurologic deficit caused by cell death in a localized region of the nervous system resulting from a disturbance of the cerebral circulation

ischemic stroke a stroke caused by inadequate blood flow. (synonym: cerebral infarction)

hemorrhagic stroke a stroke caused by bleeding through a ruptured blood vessel wall; the location can be parenchymal, subarachnoid, subdural, or epidural

transient ischemic attack (TIA) a transient episode of neurologic dysfunction caused by focal brain, spinal cord, or retinal ischemia, without acute infarction

B. Classification of Strokes by Etiology

About 80% of strokes are ischemic, and 20% are hemorrhagic. Cerebral ischemia may be global, as in the case of cardiac arrest, or focal, as a result of obstruction of an individual artery. Local obstruction, in turn, can occur when an embolus flows downstream from the heart or some other proximal site in the vascular tree and lodges in an artery, or it can result from local disease in the artery itself. The most common cause of local obstruction is atherosclerosis, but other potential causes include fibromuscular dysplasia, arteritis, dissection of the arterial wall, migraine, coagulopathies, and lipohyalinosis. Lipohyalinosis is a vasculopathy affecting small arteries that penetrate the brain substance. It occurs in patients with hypertension. Occlusion of a single penetrating artery to the brain results in a small (less than 1.5 cm) subcortical infarct, often called a *lacunar infarct*, or *lacune.*

In addition to global or focal arterial obstruction, ischemic strokes can occur when there is obstruction to the venous drainage from a brain region, caused by thrombosis in a cerebral sinus or vein. This most commonly occurs in patients who have a coagulopathy or who are severely dehydrated.

Ischemia damages not only the neurons and glial cells in the affected region, but also the blood vessels in that region, rendering them more prone to rupture. This can result in "hemorrhagic transformation" of an ischemic stroke, which sometimes causes a recognizable deterioration in the patient's clinical condition, or smaller petechial hemorrhages that can be detected with sensitive imaging techniques but may have no clinical consequences. In contrast to hemorrhage into an ischemic stroke, primary hemorrhage into the brain parenchyma is usually due to rupture of small dilatations of penetrating arteries in the brain. These dilatations are most common in patients with chronic hypertension.

Hemorrhage into the subarachnoid space usually occurs after rupture of a congenital aneurysm known as a *berry aneurysm*. These are typically located on major arteries in the circle of Willis. Rupture of a vascular malformation can result in either parenchymal or subarachnoid hemorrhage (or both). Vascular malformations are classified into four categories. *Arteriovenous malformations* (AVMs), consisting of direct communication between arteries and veins with no intervening capillary bed, are the ones most likely to produce hemorrhage. *Cavernous angiomas* (also known as *cavernous hemangiomas* or *cavernomas*) are small collections of closely packed, distended blood vessels of varying wall thickness without any intervening brain parenchyma; they are low pressure systems that are often clinically silent, but they may result in hemorrhage. *Venous angiomas* (also known as *deep venous anomalies*) consist of one or more dilated veins, with no arterial component. They are very low pressure systems that generally have no clinical significance. *Capillary telangiectases* are made up of multiple small caliber, very thin-walled vessels within normal brain; they are almost never hemorrhagic.

C. Pathophysiology

Ischemic stroke occurs when a localized area in the nervous system is deprived of glucose and oxygen because of inadequate cerebral blood flow. The severity of injury is a function of how much the blood flow has been reduced and for how long. In the center of a region of focal ischemia, blood flow is typically less than 20–30% of normal. If this degree of ischemia persists for more than an hour, all tissue elements in the region undergo complete necrosis. Surrounding this maximally affected zone is an area known as the *ischemic penumbra,* in which the blood flow reduction is less profound. Cells in this area revert to anaerobic glycolysis, triggering an *ischemic cascade.* Tissue lactate, hydrogen ions, and inorganic phosphate concentrations rise. Neurons lose their electrical excitability and their ability to regulate intracellular calcium. This precipitates release of the excitatory amino acids glutamate and aspartate into the extracellular space, and suppresses their reuptake. At high concentrations, these amino acids have a variety of harmful effects, including a further increase in intracellular calcium, which affects protein phosphorylation, leading to alterations in gene expression and protein synthesis. At the same time, the transmembrane ionic gradients begin to deteriorate and water flows passively into the neurons, resulting in cellular edema. Increased lipolysis leads to release of arachidonic acid and the production of free radicals, which are highly reactive species that damage proteins, DNA, and the fatty acids in cell membranes. These processes trigger specific derangements of genomic expression that result in apoptosis (programmed cell death).

If blood flow is restored early enough, the ischemic cascade can be terminated, but beyond a certain time window the destructive cycle becomes self-sustaining and cell death becomes inevitable. The duration of that time window depends on the extent to which blood flow is reduced. The availability of collateral blood supply generally increases with increasing distance from the center of the stroke, so the time window for salvaging cells lasts longer in the periphery of the ischemic penumbra than in the more central regions, but the specifics vary widely.

Ischemic stroke is most often due to an obstruction of the arterial system. Less commonly, it can occur as a result of obstruction to the cerebral sinuses or veins. The pathophysiology is less well understood, but most likely the obstruction in venous outflow produces a sudden mass effect in a localized region of brain, compressing the tiniest vessels in the arterial tree and compromising their ability to deliver oxygen to the brain tissue. This precipitates the same ischemic cascade that occurs when the disruption of blood supply is at the level of a larger, more proximal artery. The mechanism of cellular injury in hemorrhagic stroke is probably similar—a sudden increase in local pressure compresses all the end-arteries in the region, triggering the ischemic cascade—but this is less well established.

IV. Diagnosis

A. Clinical Features

In most cases, strokes can be diagnosed purely on the basis of the history and examination. As discussed in Chapter 3, vascular disease presents with acute, focal symptoms. Focality is the key feature. Many patients with syncope, delirium, and even heart attacks have been erroneously diagnosed with a stroke because their symptoms developed acutely. The diagnosis of stroke should only be considered when the symptoms and signs can be explained on the basis of a single lesion in the CNS. For ischemic strokes, not only is the lesion focal, but it also lies within the territory of a single

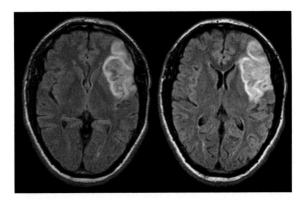

Fig. 4.1 MRI (FLAIR sequence, axial plane) images showing an ischemic stroke in the distribution of the superior division of the left middle cerebral artery (MCA). (*Source:* Preston DC, Shapiro BE. Neuroimaging in neurology: an interactive CD. Elsevier, 2007).

artery (see Figures 4.1, 4.2, and 4.3). Thus, recognition of ischemic stroke requires some knowledge of the typical syndromes produced by occlusion of the various arteries (Table 4.1).

Occlusion of the ophthalmic artery, the first branch of the internal carotid artery (ICA), results in loss of vision in the ipsilateral eye. The vision may go totally black, or it may just be dim, dark, or obscured. The episodes are usually transient, and patients sometimes describe the onset and resolution as "like a shade," first closing and later opening.

Occlusion of the middle cerebral artery (MCA) typically produces contralateral numbness and weakness affecting face and arm more than leg, a contralateral visual field deficit, and difficulty turning both eyes contralaterally. MCA occlusion on the dominant side results in aphasia. MCA occlusion on the nondominant side can produce visuospatial deficits. Contralateral neglect can result from MCA occlusion on either side, but it is usually more prominent with lesions on the nondominant side.

Anterior cerebral artery (ACA) occlusion typically produces numbness and weakness of the contralateral leg, with less involvement of the arm. ICA occlusion results in a combination of the MCA and ACA syndromes. Conversely, occlusion of a branch of the MCA or ACA produces only a portion of the full syndrome.

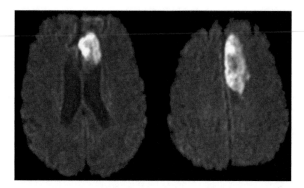

Fig. 4.2 MRI (diffusion-weighted sequence, axial plane) images showing an ischemic stroke in the distribution of the left anterior cerebral artery (ACA). Note that the diffusion-weighted sequences offer less spatial resolution than T1, T2, or FLAIR images, but they are more sensitive for identifying ischemia early in the course. (*Source:* Preston DC, Shapiro BE. Neuroimaging in neurology: an interactive CD. Elsevier, 2007).

Posterior cerebral artery (PCA) occlusion produces a contralateral visual field defect. PCA occlusion in the dominant hemisphere can lead to alexia without agraphia—these patients can write, but can't read (even things they just wrote themselves). Occlusions of the basilar or vertebral arteries or their branches produce infarcts in portions of the brainstem or cerebellum

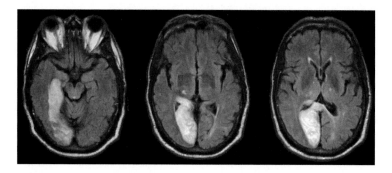

Fig. 4.3 MRI (FLAIR sequence, axial plane) images showing an ischemic stroke in the distribution of the right posterior cerebral artery (PCA). (*Source:* Preston DC, Shapiro BE. Neuroimaging in neurology: an interactive CD. Elsevier, 2007).

Table 4.1. Clinical features associated with ischemic strokes in the distribution of major cerebral arteries.

Artery	Weakness	Sensory Loss	Visual Field Deficit	Other
MCA	Contralateral face, arm > leg	Contralateral face, arm > leg	Contralateral hemifield	1. Impaired gaze in contralateral direction 2a. Dominant hemisphere MCA: Aphasia 2b. Non-dominant hemisphere MCA: Visuospatial impairment 3. Neglect (especially with non-dominant hemisphere MCA strokes)
ACA	Contralateral leg > arm	Contralateral leg > arm		Deficits of attention and/or motivation
PCA			Contralateral hemifield	Dominant hemisphere PCA: alexia without agraphia

Vertebrobasilar A. Lateral Medulla	Usually minimal	1. Ipsilateral face 2. Contralateral arm, leg, trunk	1. Ipsilateral Horner's syndrome 2. Ipsilateral ataxia 3. Dysarthria, dysphagia 4. Nystagmus 5. Vertigo
Vertebrobasilar B. Medial Medulla	Contralateral arm, leg	Contralateral arm, leg (especially proprioception)	Ipsilateral tongue weakness
Vertebrobasilar C. Pons	1. Ipsilateral face 2. Contralateral arm, leg	1. Contralateral arm, leg, trunk 2. Ipsilateral face (sometimes contralateral also)	1. Impaired gaze in ipsilateral direction 2. Nystagmus 3. Ipsilateral Horner's syndrome 4. Ataxia (ipsilateral or contralateral)
Vertebrobasilar D. Midbrain	Contralateral face, arm, leg		1. Ipsilateral third nerve palsy 2. Contralateral ataxia (in some cases)

and corresponding clinical syndromes that reflect the cranial nerves in the affected territory, as well as the ascending and descending tracts passing through the infarcted region. One classic syndrome is the lateral medullary syndrome ("Wallenberg's syndrome"), consisting of reduced pain and temperature sensation in the ipsilateral face and the contralateral limbs and trunk, an ipsilateral Horner's syndrome, dysarthria, dysphagia, ataxia, vertigo, and nystagmus. Another classic syndrome is produced by infarction of the midbrain affecting the cerebral peduncle and the oculomotor nerve, resulting in an ipsilateral third nerve lesion and contralateral hemiparesis.

Lacunar infarcts most frequently occur in the basal ganglia, thalamus, pons, or internal capsule, and they are associated with several classic clinical syndromes: pure motor (hemiparesis with no sensory deficit), pure sensory (numbness on one entire side of the body, but normal strength throughout), ataxic hemiparesis (ataxia and mild weakness on one side of the body), and "clumsy hand–dysarthria" (as the name implies). These "*lacunar syndromes*" are not specific, however. The same clinical syndromes can result from many other mechanisms, including large vessel occlusion, cardioembolism, vasculitis, and even compression from tumors or hematomas.

Subarachnoid hemorrhage does not routinely invade the brain parenchyma, so unlike other stroke symptoms it does not typically present with focal symptoms and signs. The usual presenting symptoms are headache and meningeal signs, so it is discussed in Chapter 12. Venous infarcts are difficult to distinguish clinically from arterial ischemia, except that they need not conform to the distribution of an individual artery, and they typically occur in patients who are predisposed to coagulation disorders. Patients with venous infarcts often report headache. Recent head trauma is the main clue suggesting epidural or subdural hemorrhage. Parenchymal, subdural, and epidural hemorrhages usually produce greater mass effect than ischemic strokes do in the acute setting, so they are more likely to cause headache or a reduced level of consciousness. They can also produce signs and symptoms that overlap more than one arterial territory. At times, however, they can be indistinguishable from ischemic strokes—the only reliable way to differentiate ischemic stroke from parenchymal, subdural, or epidural hemorrhage is with imaging studies.

B. Imaging

Most ischemic strokes are evident on the diffusion-weighted sequences of an MRI scan within minutes, but in most medical centers MRI scans are difficult to obtain acutely, during the time window in which immediate intervention is possible. CT scans are much more readily available in the acute setting, but ischemic strokes are often undetectable on CT scans for hours or days. Parenchymal, subdural, and epidural hemorrhages are visible on CT scans immediately, however. That is why it is standard practice to obtain a CT scan immediately in the setting of an acute stroke—not to diagnose an ischemic stroke, but to be sure the patient has not had an acute hemorrhage (or, rarely, some other condition).

After a stroke occurs, it will continue to manifest as a region of impeded diffusion (also referred to as "restricted diffusion") on MRI for about two weeks, but MRI scans are unnecessary when the history and examination provide compelling evidence of a stroke and the mechanism of stroke is apparent. In some cases, however, visualization of the stroke can help guide clinical decisions. For example, the history and examination are sometimes insufficient to conclude whether the stroke is in the anterior or the posterior circulation, which could be critical in deciding whether or not to recommend carotid endarterectomy.

MRI scans sometimes show findings consistent with an acute ischemic stroke even in patients whose symptoms resolved completely within minutes or hours of onset. For this reason, some stroke experts advocate obtaining MRI scans in all patients whose clinical presentation is consistent with TIA, because this is the only way to be sure that these patients have not experienced an acute infarction. I disagree with this approach for two reasons. First, although the sensitivity of an MRI scan for stroke is very high, it is not 100%, especially for small strokes—in other words, ischemia on an MRI scan can prove that an event was a stroke rather than a TIA, but a normal MRI scan does *not* prove that an event was a TIA rather than a stroke. Second, and more importantly, the distinction between TIA and stroke has minimal impact on patient management. For patients whose clinical manifestations have resolved, no acute intervention is required. The goal is to reduce the risk of future stroke, and in this regard the implications of a TIA and a stroke are identical.

In some cases, visualization of cerebral blood vessels may be important in management decisions. Magnetic resonance angiography (MRA) and computed tomographic angiography (CTA) are noninvasive techniques for evaluating cerebral arteries. Traditional intra-arterial (catheter) angiography can provide better resolution in some cases. In situations where venous infarcts are a consideration, magnetic resonance venography (MRV) or computed tomographic venography (CTV) can be performed.

V. Management of Acute Stroke

A. Restoration of Blood Flow in Ischemic Stroke

After ensuring that a patient with an acute ischemic stroke is adequately oxygenated and hemodynamically stable, the most urgent goal is to restore blood flow to salvageable areas of the brain. If blood flow can be restored before the ischemic cascade reaches an irreversible stage, portions of the ischemic penumbra can recover. If the ischemia persists beyond that point, the ischemic cascade will proceed even if blood flow is successfully restored. In fact, restoration of blood flow after that point can actually be harmful, because the sudden increase in perfusion pressure can overwhelm the already-impaired blood vessels in the ischemic zone, resulting in hemorrhage. Hemorrhage is an even greater concern when the restoration of blood flow involves administration of a thrombolytic agent. The result is that restoration of blood flow is beneficial only during a narrow window of opportunity.

Patients who receive recombinant tissue plasminogen activator (tPA) intravenously within 4.5 hours of the onset of ischemic stroke symptoms are significantly more likely than untreated patients to have minimal or no neurologic deficit 3 months later. Although tPA treatment also increases the likelihood of intracerebral hemorrhage in the first 36 hours, the beneficial effect of the treatment outweighs the risk. Every effort should be made to start infusing the tPA within a 3-hour window, and the earlier in that window the better, because the likelihood of benefit is time-dependent.

Unfortunately, it is often difficult to evaluate and treat patients within 3 hours (or even 4.5 hours) of symptom onset. Unlike patients with myocardial ischemia, whose pain often convinces them of the urgency of their condition, patients with cerebral ischemia may misinterpret or minimize their symptoms. In some cases, the time of symptom onset is unknown. For example, patients whose symptoms are first noticed on awakening could have suffered their stroke at any time during their sleep. They are only eligible to receive tPA if they were awake and asymptomatic at some point in the preceding 4.5 hours. Even when patients receive medical attention quickly, their evaluation (including a CT scan to be sure there is no intracerebral hemorrhage) must be rapid and efficient if they are to receive treatment within the required time frame. It may someday be possible to identify patients in whom portions of the ischemic penumbra are still viable beyond 4.5 hours (for example, by using specialized imaging modalities such as perfusion scans), but these techniques are still investigational.

Two other methods to restore blood flow to an ischemic region are available, but only when the thrombus is lodged in a blood vessel large enough to be accessible with an endovascular catheter. The first is to inject a thrombolytic agent intra-arterially, directly into the thrombus. This allows titration to the lowest dose required to dissolve the clot, and it also reduces the risk of systemic hemorrhage because much less of the drug is delivered to the rest of the body. By reducing the risk and increasing the benefit, intra-arterial administration may extend the time window for thrombolytic therapy. For example, intra-arterial administration of prourokinase directly into an intracranial thrombus is beneficial if treatment is begun within 6 hours of symptom onset. Prourokinase is not commercially available, but many stroke experts believe that intra-arterial tPA can also be given within a 6-hour time window. This prolongation of the therapeutic window is counterbalanced to some degree by the fact that it takes longer to mobilize the staff necessary for intra-arterial treatment than it does to administer IV tPA. The second alternative to intravenous tPA is to remove the clot with an intra-arterial device. The FDA has approved two types of endovascular clot retrieval device for use up to 8 hours after symptom onset. It is not yet known whether these devices improve clinical outcomes, so intravenous tPA remains the treatment of choice for eligible patients presenting within the 4.5-hour time window. For patients seen outside this time window (or patients who are not eligible to receive tPA for some other reason), endovascular clot retrieval may be a reasonable option, as long as the patients understand that it has not yet been proven to be effective.

Other approaches under investigation (with the goal of increasing the likelihood of reperfusion or reducing the risk of hemorrhage) include the use of newer fibrinolytics, the combination of fibrinolytics with anti-thrombotic medications, the use of ultrasound with fibrinolytics to enhance recanalization, and the combination of intravenous and intra-arterial fibrinolytics. All of these approaches remain experimental. Aspirin provides a small but statistically significant benefit in the treatment of acute stroke. It is not clear whether this benefit relates to improved blood flow or some other effect of aspirin.

For patients with cerebral venous infarction, one small prospective study and several retrospective studies support the use of intravenous heparin. If this is ineffective, direct installation of a thrombolytic agent into the thrombus is sometimes attempted, although no controlled trials have been conducted.

No matter how much the risk of hemorrhage is reduced, and no matter how reliably blood flow can be restored, there are limits to how long the therapeutic window for reperfusion therapy can be extended, because the ischemic cascade eventually becomes irreversible. Thus, while reperfusion therapy is important, simultaneous therapy directed at halting or reversing the ischemic cascade may be critical for the preservation of brain function. Attempts to limit free radical formation, excitatory amino acid release, trans-membrane ion shifts, or programmed cell death are currently the subject of intense study, but every agent tried so far has been disappointing.

B. Limitation of Deficits

Even though the neuronal injury that results from a stroke cannot yet be treated successfully, factors that exacerbate the damage can be addressed. Both neurologic and systemic complications must be considered.

1. Neurologic complications

The most important neurologic complication of acute stroke is increased intracranial pressure. Strokes produce significant edema, which may result in mass effect on the brainstem, affecting level of consciousness and autonomic functions. There is debate about whether the typical measures used to treat increased intracranial pressure (see Chapter 11) are effective in the setting of ischemic stroke, but they may be lifesaving in the setting of impending transtentorial herniation due to mass effect from a hemorrhagic stroke. Intuition might suggest that clot removal would improve outcome, but in a large clinical trial in which patients with supratentorial hemorrhage were randomized either to have surgical evacuation of the hematoma within 96 hours or to receive medical management, the outcomes were the same in the two groups. Most clinicians advocate clot evacuation for patients who have a large parenchymal hemorrhage *in the cerebellum*, because swelling in this location can rapidly compress the brainstem and impair life-sustaining autonomic functions. Large ischemic strokes in the cerebellum can also swell and compress the brainstem, and most clinicians agree that the appropriate treatment is a decompressive suboccipital craniotomy with removal of the necrotic tissue. Hemicraniectomy—removal of the lateral-coronal portion of the skull—can decompress a rapidly swelling cerebral hemisphere in patients with severely increased intracranial pressure due to large ischemic strokes. Although this procedure may be lifesaving, it may also leave the patient with severe residual deficits. Patients and families must be thoroughly informed of the risks and benefits before proceeding with this intervention. The best clinical outcomes have been reported with younger patients. Moderate hypothermia has also been proposed as a treatment for patients with increased intracranial pressure after a stroke, but controlled trials are necessary.

Ischemic or hemorrhagic brain regions may serve as seizure foci. Seizures may even be the presenting symptom of infarction or hemorrhage on rare occasions. Patients who have seizures in the setting of a stroke should be loaded promptly with an anti-epileptic drug (AED), because seizures produce a transient rise in intracranial pressure, and this can be particularly dangerous in stroke patients who already have increased intracranial pressure due to edema. Status epilepticus is even more ominous in that regard and requires urgent treatment (see Chapter 5). The consequences of a seizure may be particularly dire in patients who have had an intraparenchymal hemorrhage (who almost always have elevated intracranial pressure to some degree) or in patients who have had a subarachnoid hemorrhage (who are at high risk of rebleeding), so some clinicians begin prophylactic AED treatment in these patients even if they have not had a seizure, but controlled trials have not been conducted. There is no evidence that prophylactic AED treatment is beneficial after an ischemic stroke.

Any patient with an intracranial lesion is at risk for hyponatremia, due to either SIADH (syndrome of inappropriate secretion of antidiuretic hormone) or cerebral salt wasting. Hyponatremia may in turn produce further neuronal injury, either directly or by provoking seizure activity. Serum sodium should be measured regularly, and appropriate testing and treatment undertaken if hyponatremia develops.

Patients who have suffered strokes (especially left hemisphere strokes) develop depression at a rate higher than would be predicted simply on the basis of a situational response to their deficits. It appears that depression may be a direct manifestation of injury to particular regions of the brain. When severe, the depression may significantly impede clinical recovery from a stroke. Some studies indicate that these patients respond to antidepressant medications, whereas others fail to observe a reliable response to any of the usual treatments for depression. There is no indication for the routine use of antidepressant medication to prevent depression after stroke.

2. Systemic factors

Hypoxia, hypotension, hyperthermia, and hyperglycemia may all exacerbate the neuronal injury that results from stroke. Patients should be monitored closely for the development of any of these conditions and treated promptly if they occur. One common mistake is to lower blood pressure too aggressively immediately after an acute stroke. In normal brain regions, autoregulatory mechanisms preserve a constant level of cerebral blood flow across a wide range of blood pressure, but these mechanisms are impaired in the ischemic penumbra, so that a relatively small drop in blood pressure can reduce perfusion to the point where the tissue suffers permanent damage. This can occur even at blood pressures that might seem normal or high, because patients who have had longstanding hypertension have often accommodated over time to their high baseline blood pressure, adjusting their autoregulatory mechanisms to a higher set point. Thus, although blood pressure control is an important long-term goal, high pressures do not necessarily require treatment in the acute setting.

Stroke patients often have impairment of their airway protection mechanisms and may need elective intubation to limit aspiration. A bedside evaluation of swallowing should be routine after stroke, and if the patient has problems, more extensive testing may be necessary. Some patients need feeding tubes until they can safely take in adequate nutrition by mouth.

Patients should be mobilized as soon as possible after a stroke, but fall precautions are essential. Patients who are rendered nonambulatory by a stroke should be treated prophylactically to prevent deep venous thrombosis. They should also receive vigorous skin care to prevent skin breakdown and decubitus ulcers, and monitored closely for the development of pneumonia or urinary tract infections.

C. Rehabilitation

Some studies have shown that early rehabilitation allows stroke patients to recover more quickly and perhaps to a higher level of function. Patients should be trained to maximize their function based on their current abilities. Speech pathologists can teach patients strategies to improve communication skills. They can also evaluate the ability of patients to swallow and suggest interventions to reduce the risk of aspiration. Physical therapists can teach patients exercises designed to increase range of motion and prevent contractures in weak muscles, as well as exercises to strengthen both the affected muscles and the unaffected muscles that may be required to compensate for the weak muscles. Constraint-induced movement therapy, in which patients are prevented from using their intact limbs and thereby forced to use their affected limbs, is a promising approach. Occupational therapists can also help to determine whether patients might benefit from facilitative or prosthetic devices.

VI. Primary Prevention

Despite many advances in the management of acute stroke, many patients present too late for treatment, and even those who receive timely, optimal treatment sometimes have poor outcomes. Unless medical science advances far beyond its current state, stroke prevention will continue to be the cornerstone of stroke management. Primary prevention is directed toward the early recognition and treatment of risk factors that predispose to the development of cerebrovascular disease.

A. Hypertension

Hypertension is a major risk factor for both ischemic and hemorrhagic stroke, and the higher the blood pressure, the greater the stroke risk. There is convincing evidence that control of hypertension substantially reduces the risk of stroke, even for mild hypertension (systolic blood pressure 140–159 mm Hg). Some studies suggest that certain medications or classes of medication—in particular, ramipril, an angiotensin converting enzyme (ACE) inhibitor, and losartan, an angiotensin receptor blocker—offer special protection beyond what can be explained on the basis of blood pressure reduction alone, but this has not been established.

B. Smoking

Smoking also increases the risk of both ischemic and hemorrhagic stroke. The risk increases with the number of cigarettes smoked, and varies with stroke subtype, but the overall stroke risk is about twice that of nonsmokers. Smoking cessation is associated with a rapid reduction in stroke risk.

C. Diabetes

Patients with diabetes have an increased risk of stroke, independent of their other cardiovascular risk factors. It is not clear whether tight glycemic control modifies stroke risk (although it has other beneficial effects). Tight blood pressure control in diabetic patients reduces the risk of stroke, and it appears that ACE inhibitors and angiotensin receptor blockers may be particularly beneficial. There is also evidence that HMG-CoA reductase inhibitors (statins) reduce the risk of stroke in patients with diabetes, especially those with at least one other vascular risk factor (hypertension, current tobacco use, retinopathy, or albuminuria), even if they do not have dyslipidemia.

D. Dyslipidemia

The relationship between stroke risk and serum lipids is complicated, but dyslipidemia appears to be associated with a reduced risk of hemorrhagic stroke and an increased risk of ischemic stroke. It remains unclear whether lipid modification affects stroke risk in patients with isolated dyslipidemia, but in patients with symptomatic cardiovascular disease, statins have been shown to reduce the risk of stroke. This is true even in patients with normal lipid profiles, suggesting that these medications may have beneficial cardiovascular effects independent of their lipid-lowering properties. As already discussed, a similar benefit has been reported in patients with diabetes.

E. Mechanical Heart Valves

Patients with mechanical heart valves have a very high risk of stroke. Treatment with warfarin reduces this risk by a factor of 4 or 5. For patients who can not take warfarin, antiplatelet agents cut the risk of stroke roughly in half.

F. Atrial Fibrillation

Atrial fibrillation is associated with an overall four-fold increase in the risk of stroke, but the risk varies greatly, with the highest risk in older patients and those with associated vascular diseases. Treatment with warfarin reduces the risk of stroke by a factor of 3. Aspirin is also effective, but less so. In patients younger than 75 with no associated risk factors (stroke, TIA, congestive heart failure, hypertension, or diabetes), the risk of stroke is low enough to recommend treatment with aspirin, but warfarin is the treatment of choice for all other patients with atrial fibrillation. In one randomized controlled trial, patients taking dabigatran (a direct thrombin inhibitor that is not FDA-approved) had a lower risk of major hemorrhage than patients taking warfarin, with both groups having a similar risk of stroke.

G. Carotid Stenosis

Atherosclerotic plaques in the carotid artery can lead to strokes or TIAs in at least two ways. First, plaques can serve as a site of thrombus formation, and pieces of thrombus or plaque can subsequently break off and flow downstream until they reach a blood vessel too small to accommodate them, get stuck in it, and block blood flow beyond that point. Second, plaques (and associated thrombus) can grow in place within the carotid to the point where they reduce blood flow through the carotid below some critical level. It is usually difficult to determine which of these two mechanisms is more important in an individual patient, but either way, it might seem obvious that endarterectomy (surgical excision of the plaque and associated thrombus) would be beneficial.

Intuition can be misleading with respect to stroke, however. I find it instructive to recall that some patients with complete occlusion of both carotid arteries live a completely normal life and never experience a single TIA or stroke. This fact highlights the ability of collateral blood vessels to compensate for the obstructed carotids. Of course, collateral blood vessels would not prevent pieces of plaque or thrombus from breaking off and lodging in smaller vessels downstream, but they could protect the region of brain supplied by those vessels by providing an alternate blood supply. Moreover, the likelihood of such plaque fragmentation undoubtedly varies from one patient to another, influenced by such factors as the precise composition of the plaque, the degree of local turbulence, the systemic blood pressure, and so forth. Thus, while carotid atherosclerosis can clearly lead to TIA and stroke, the risk may actually be quite low as a result of mitigating factors. Carotid endarterectomy itself can cause stroke and other complications. If the risk of endarterectomy exceeds the risk of stroke from the underlying carotid disease, the procedure will cause more harm than good. It is impossible to deduce these relative risks and benefits of surgery from first principles; they must be measured in clinical trials.

Several clinical trials have explored these issues, and the results have been roughly the same. Among individuals with at least a 60% reduction in the diameter of the internal carotid artery who have not had a TIA or stroke in the distribution of that carotid (*asymptomatic* carotid stenosis), about 11% of medically treated patients will experience an ipsilateral stroke or die within 5 years, compared to 5% of surgically treated patients. This result is statistically significant, but not robust. It represents an absolute risk reduction of 6% over 5 years, or 1.2% per year, a benefit that could easily be negated in circumstances in which the surgical morbidity is less than ideal. Furthermore, subgroup analysis suggests that women benefit less than men from the surgery, that patients over 75 years of age may not benefit, and that the degree to which the surgery is beneficial does not correlate with the severity of stenosis, a result that is counterintuitive. In brief, for individuals who have at least 60% carotid stenosis with no evidence that it has ever produced symptoms, endarterectomy is sometimes beneficial, but not always – the younger and healthier the patients are, the more likely they are to benefit from the procedure, especially if they are male.

Endovascular treatment of carotid stenosis is a potential alternative to endarterectomy. In principle, carotid angioplasty (while using a distal protection device) followed by stenting could result in a lower procedural risk than endarterectomy, because it can be performed under light anesthesia and avoids neck incision. Although study results have been mixed, the largest study to date of patients with asymptomatic carotid stenosis found no significant difference between endarterectomy and angioplasty/stenting with respect to the accumulated risk of stroke over the 2.5 years following the procedure. The incidence of stroke at the time of the procedure was greater with angioplasty/stenting, and the incidence of peri-procedural myocardial infarction was greater for endarterectomy. Patients who were younger than 70 years tended to do better with angioplasty/stenting, and older patients did better with endarterectomy.

Thus, for patients with asymptomatic carotid stenosis of at least 60%, endarterectomy, angioplasty/stenting, and medical management (without performing any procedure to correct the blockage) are all reasonable options. The relative indications for the three alternative approaches remain uncertain. For patients treated with a procedure, endarterectomy is currently standard, especially for patients who are at low surgical risk, but angioplasty is a viable alternative, particularly in younger patients or patients with established cardiac disease or other major surgical risk factors. In principle, angioplasty could also be an option in patients with stenosis of some arteries in which endarterectomy is not feasible, such as the vertebral or basilar arteries, or potentially even the proximal MCA, ACA, or PCA, but no evidence is available.

H. Sickle Cell Disease

Stroke is very common in patients with homozygous sickle cell disease, and the highest rate of stroke is in early childhood. Patients with this disease should be screened starting at age 2 using transcranial Doppler (TCD) ultrasound, which can identify the patients at highest risk of stroke. Those patients should be treated with periodic blood transfusions, which can dramatically reduce the risk of stroke in this disease.

I. Other Factors

Dietary factors associated with a reduced risk of stroke include fruits and vegetables, omega-3 fatty acids, whole grains, and nonhydrogenated unsaturated fats. Compared to abstinence, heavy alcohol intake is associated with an increased risk of all types of stroke, but intake of small to moderate amounts of alcohol is associated with a reduced risk of ischemic stroke. Elevated levels of homocysteine are associated with an increased risk of stroke. The same may be true of lipoprotein(a) and lipoprotein-associated phospholipase A_2, but the evidence is less convincing. A sedentary lifestyle is associated with an increased risk of stroke, and regular exercise with a lower risk. Obesity appears to be associated with an increased risk of stroke, independent of other cardiovascular risk factors, but the results are not conclusive. Obstructive sleep apnea is an independent risk factor for stroke. Interventions to modify any or all of these risk factors could be beneficial, but at this point, such benefit is unproven.

VII. Secondary Prevention of Ischemic Stroke

Any patient who has had a TIA or stroke is at risk for future strokes, with potentially devastating consequences. Strokes and TIAs are equivalent in this regard. If anything, a TIA merits even more urgent attention than a stroke, because if the cause of the TIA can be determined and effective secondary prevention instituted, the patient may be protected from experiencing any permanent neurologic deficit. About 10% of patients with TIAs have strokes within 90 days, and half of those are within the first 48 hours.

As discussed in Part VI, it can be difficult to predict the likelihood of future stroke in patients with known risk factors, because mitigating factors (such as the development of collateral blood vessels or the presence of features that reduce the risk of plaque fragmentation and embolism) may be present. In some patients, those mitigating factors may be so strong that the risk of stroke is practically nonexistent. Patients who have experienced a TIA or stroke, however, have already demonstrated that this is not the case for them. This shift in probabilities is the main feature distinguishing secondary prevention from primary prevention. All of the measures known to be effective for primary prevention are also effective for secondary prevention, but in addition, some interventions that have little or no value as primary prevention have proven benefit as secondary prevention.

Many of the fundamental features of the secondary prevention of ischemic stroke can be summarized in five general principles:

A. Patients with a cardioembolic source of stroke should be anticoagulated with warfarin.

B. Patients who have had a TIA or ischemic stroke in the distribution of an internal carotid artery with high-grade stenosis should have an endarterectomy.

C. All patients who have had a TIA or ischemic stroke, and who are not taking warfarin, should take an anti-platelet agent.

D. All patients who have had a TIA or ischemic stroke, and who have LDL levels of 100 mg/dL or higher, should take a statin.

E. All of the principles of primary prevention also apply to patients with established cerebrovascular disease.

With stroke, nothing is ever simple. All of these principles require clarification and qualifications.

A. Cardioembolic Disease

As discussed in Part VI, chronic anticoagulation with warfarin is the treatment of choice for all patients with atrial fibrillation, except those who are young and have no associated risk factors. Patients who have had a TIA or stroke have thereby demonstrated that they have associated risk factors, so they should be treated with warfarin (although dabigatran may prove to be a reasonable alternative, based on subgroup analysis of the study mentioned in Part VI). Warfarin is indicated for primary stroke prevention in patients with artificial heart valves, so it is certainly indicated for secondary prevention. Patients who have a stroke or TIA due to an acute myocardial infarction, and who have a mural thrombus in their left ventricle, should also receive warfarin. Less information is available about anticoagulation in patients with stroke due to embolism from other cardiac conditions, such as rheumatic valvular disease or cardiomyopathy, but it is still commonly used, primarily on the basis of analogy and anecdotal evidence. Because of a high risk of cerebral hemorrhage (see Chapter 10), bacterial endocarditis (in a patient without an artificial heart valve) is the one cardioembolic condition for which anticoagulation is generally considered to be contraindicated.

Patients who have had a stroke or TIA should be admitted to the hospital and placed on a cardiac rhythm monitor, in part because strokes can cause serious arrhythmias and partly to evaluate for intermittent atrial fibrillation. In some cases, atrial fibrillation is extremely sporadic so if the cause of stroke remains obscure after the standard evaluation (described below), it is often useful to arrange for a short-term cardiac event monitor for the patient to wear after discharge. In addition, patients who have had a stroke or TIA should have an echocardiogram to evaluate for cardiac lesions that predispose to embolism (unless they are already known to have atrial fibrillation or some other condition requiring chronic anticoagulation). Transesophageal echocardiography (TEE) is a more sensitive and specific test for many of these lesions than conventional transthoracic echocardiography (TTE), but it is more invasive and has associated morbidity. One analysis indicated that TEE was more cost effective than TTE, but this was based primarily on the likelihood of finding a thrombus in an intra-atrial appendage, and the results depended on some assumptions that have subsequently been challenged.

Anticoagulation should be maintained as long as the cardioembolic source remains; for many patients this means life-long anticoagulation. These patients need to be monitored regularly to maintain the correct degree of anticoagulation. An INR in the range of 2.0–3.0 is the usual goal, although a target range of 2.5–4.0 is standard for patients with mechanical heart valves. Anticoagulation with direct thrombin inhibitors such as dabigatran may eliminate the need to monitor coagulation parameters, but these medications remain investigational.

Two opposing risks govern the timing of anticoagulation in patients who have just had a cardioembolic stroke. On the one hand, these patients are clearly at risk for recurrent stroke, since the cardioembolic source is still present. On the other hand, the propensity for hemorrhagic transformation is particularly high after cardioembolic strokes. This is especially true when the anticoagulation goal is exceeded, which most often occurs when patients receive a bolus of heparin to initiate therapy. The risk of recurrent stroke in the acute setting is not high enough to justify administration of a heparin bolus. In fact, there is no proof that heparin in this setting is beneficial at all. Many experts recommend that patients simply be anticoagulated with warfarin after a delay of hours, days, or even weeks. The evidence on this question remains unclear, but if heparin is used at all in the days immediately following a stroke, it should only be in patients with a clear embolic source who are deemed to be at particularly high risk of recurrent events, and the dose should be titrated upward gradually, with no bolus, erring on the side of undershooting the anticoagulation target. Patients with cardioembolic disease who cannot take warfarin (e.g., patients who fall frequently because of disequilibrium) are usually treated with aspirin, but the evidence is weak.

It is difficult to interpret the finding of a *patent foramen ovale* (PFO) in a patient who has had a TIA or stroke. On the one hand, a PFO can be demonstrated on surface echocardiography in about 20% of normal individuals, suggesting that most patients with PFO are asymptomatic. On the other hand, the incidence of PFO is higher in patients with stroke (40%) than in the general population, especially in patients with stroke and no other identifiable cause (54%). It remains to be determined whether such patients should be treated with chronic anticoagulation, antiplatelet agents, cardiac surgery, or percutaneous transcatheter closure of the PFO. Based on the studies that have been done to date, patients with a PFO who take aspirin have a very low risk of recurrent stroke, so this appears to be a reasonable approach for most patients.

B. Carotid Stenosis

Carotid stenosis is a prime example of the distinction between primary and secondary prevention of stroke. Patients who have had a TIA or stroke in the distribution of a carotid artery with a high-grade (70–99%) stenosis (*symptomatic* carotid stenosis) have a very high risk of recurrence: 26% of such patients will have another stroke on the same side within 2 years, even if they receive appropriate medical therapy. Carotid endarterectomy reduces this risk to 9% over the same time period. This is an absolute risk reduction of 17% in 2 years, or 8.5% per year. Recall from Part VI that about 11% of medically treated patients with *asymptomatic* carotid stenosis will experience an ipsilateral stroke or die within 5 years; this translates roughly into a 4% risk within 2 years. In other words, among patients with high-grade carotid stenosis, the risk of future stroke is six times higher for those patients who have had at least one TIA or stroke attributable to the stenosis than it is for asymptomatic patients. In both groups, carotid endarterectomy reduces the risk of future stroke, but because the baseline risk of stroke is so much higher in symptomatic patients, the absolute benefit is dramatically greater for them (8.5% per year) than for asymptomatic patients (1.2% per year). Whereas in asymptomatic patients with high-grade carotid stenosis a variety of factors can result in the risks of endarterectomy outweighing the benefits, in symptomatic patients the benefit almost always outweighs the risk.

In symptomatic patients with only *moderate* carotid stenosis (50–69%), the situation is similar to that for asymptomatic patients: 22% of patients treated medically will have another stroke on the same side within 5 years, compared to 16% of patients treated with endarterectomy. This is an absolute risk reduction of 6% over 5 years, or 1.2% per year, which is low enough that individual circumstances must be considered carefully in deciding whether to recommend the surgery. For example, these statistics come from a study that was done at centers selected for their high level of expertise, where the risk of disabling stroke or death from the endarterectomy was 2%. In centers with less experience, a higher complication rate could easily negate the small benefit of surgery. Similarly, patients with multiple medical problems may have a greater than average risk of surgical complications that would outweigh the benefit of the procedure. For symptomatic patients with less than 50% stenosis, endarterectomy does not provide a significant benefit.

There is some debate about the appropriate time for performing endarterectomy after a stroke. As already discussed with respect to thrombolytic therapy, the blood vessels in an area of ischemic brain are fragile and have an increased propensity to hemorrhage. A sudden surge of blood at high pressure resulting from the opening of a previously narrow carotid artery might exacerbate this risk. For this reason, some physicians delay endarterectomy until at least 6 weeks after a stroke. Unfortunately, this is a period when the risk of recurrence is high. A pooled analysis of results from two large, controlled trials suggests that the benefits of endarterectomy are greatest if the surgery is performed within 2 weeks of the onset of symptoms.

As discussed in Part VI, endovascular treatment (carotid angioplasty and stenting) is a less invasive alternative to endarterectomy. As with asymptomatic stenosis, mixed results have emerged from studies comparing angioplasty/stenting to endarterectomy in patients with symptomatic carotid stenosis. The same study discussed in Part VI included a symptomatic carotid stenosis arm, and the results were similar to those for asymptomatic carotid stenosis. In another large, randomized trial, the risk of stroke, death, or peri-procedural myocardial infarction was significantly higher in the stenting group than in the endarterectomy group. The endovascular credentialing requirements were less stringent for this trial than for the trial discussed in Part VI, which may be one reason that the stenting outcomes were worse. At this point, endarterectomy remains the standard treatment for patients with symptomatic high-grade carotid stenosis, but angioplasty is a viable option in some cases, especially in younger patients or patients with established cardiac disease or other major surgical risk factors. The role of angioplasty/stenting for symptomatic stenosis of other cerebral blood vessels is unknown.

C. Anti-Platelet Medications

All patients who have had a TIA or stroke, and who are not taking warfarin, should receive anti-platelet therapy (regardless of whether or not they have had an endarterectomy). The three anti-platelet medications currently available are aspirin, clopidogrel (Plavix), and a combination of low-dose aspirin with extended-release dipyridamole (Aggrenox). A fourth anti-platelet agent, ticlopidine, is similar to clopidogrel but produces more adverse effects, so it is almost never used. Cilostazol (Pletal), a phosphodiesterase inhibitor, was reportedly more effective than aspirin for secondary stroke prevention in a randomized trial, but the results of that study have not yet been published in a peer-reviewed journal.

Aspirin is the antiplatelet agent that has been used most extensively. Studies have shown that it reduces the risk of subsequent stroke in patients presenting with a TIA or stroke, and that it is as effective as warfarin in patients who have no cardioembolic source. The ideal dose is unknown. Laboratory research has suggested that doses on the order of 30 mg per day should be adequate to block the thromboxane pathway, as desired, whereas higher doses also block the prostacyclin pathway, which may partially negate the beneficial effect. The dose of aspirin used in many of the large clinical stroke trials, however, was 1300 mg per day. Randomized trials comparing high-dose to low-dose aspirin have shown similar efficacy. Because higher doses are associated with a greater risk of gastrointestinal hemorrhage, the recommended dose for secondary stroke prevention is 50–325 mg per day.

Clopidogrel inhibits platelet aggregation by blocking the binding of adenosine diphosphate to its receptor on platelets. In one study comparing clopidogrel to aspirin, patients who were treated with clopidogrel had a lower combined risk of ischemic stroke, heart attack, or vascular death than did patients treated with aspirin. The difference was statistically significant, but small, and the largest benefit occurred in patients whose primary problem was peripheral vascular disease. For cerebrovascular disease per se, it is still not known whether clopidogrel is more or less effective than aspirin. In one study, combination therapy with aspirin and clopidogrel resulted in a slight reduction in the risk of stroke compared to treatment with clopidogrel alone, but the effect was not statistically significant, and it was outweighed by a statistically significant increase in the rate of major bleeding complications.

Possible mechanisms by which dipyridamole inhibits platelet function include inhibition of phosphodiesterase in platelets or inhibition of red blood cell uptake of adenosine (which suppresses platelet reactivity). Early studies of dipyridamole in cerebrovascular disease revealed no benefit relative to placebo, and the combination of dipyridamole with aspirin was no more effective than aspirin alone. In a study that included many more patients than previous studies and that used a higher daily dipyridamole dose in a slow-release preparation, the opposite results were found: The use of either aspirin or dipyridamole alone produced a statistically significant reduction in the risk of stroke or death, and the combination of aspirin and dipyridamole was more effective than either drug alone.

In short, each of the currently available anti-platelet agents—aspirin, clopidogrel, and aspirin/extended-release dipyridamole—reduces the risk of subsequent stroke in patients who have already had a TIA or stroke. The relative risk reduction is 28% for nonfatal stroke and 16% for fatal stroke. Although there is general agreement that anyone who has had a TIA or stroke (and who does not need to take warfarin) should take one of these three agents, experts disagree on whether one is preferable to the others. Clopidogrel and aspirin/extended-release dipyridamole have both been demonstrated to be more effective than aspirin, but the benefit from clopidogrel is more convincing for peripheral vascular disease than for cerebral vascular disease, and methodologic concerns have been raised regarding the aspirin/dipyridamole trial. A study comparing clopidogrel to aspirin/extended-release dipyridamole (with or without an angiotensin-receptor blocker) failed to show a statistically significant difference in efficacy. It is conceivable that certain subgroups of patients respond differentially to these medications, so if patients continue to have TIAs or strokes despite treatment with an anti-platelet agent it is probably reasonable to try changing to a different one (even though no evidence is available to support this practice).

D. Statin Therapy

As explained in Part VI, statins reduce the risk of stroke in patients with symptomatic cardiovascular disease, possibly because of effects independent of their lipid-lowering properties. Only one study to date has evaluated statin treatment after a TIA or stroke (in patients with no known coronary disease). To be enrolled in this study, patients had to have serum LDL levels of 100—190 mg/dL, and they were randomized to receive either placebo or atorvastatin at a dose of 80 mg per day. Patients in the treatment group had a 16% relative reduction in the risk of stroke over the following 5 years (although their risk of hemorrhagic stroke was slightly increased). They also had a significantly reduced rate of cardiovascular events. Without additional studies, there is no way to know whether patients with LDL levels below 100 mg/dL also benefit from atorvastatin, or whether other doses or other statins are also effective (though evidence from one study suggests that simvastatin at a dose of 40 mg per day may be effective for secondary stroke prevention in patients with total cholesterol levels of 135 mg/dL or higher).

E. Risk Factor Modification

In general, any risk factor modification that is effective for primary stroke prevention is also indicated for a patient who has already had a stroke or TIA. Patients who have experienced an episode of hemiparesis, aphasia, or some other dramatic deficit may be particularly amenable to major life-style changes (such as smoking cessation) that they had previously resisted. Clinicians should do everything possible to exploit the window of opportunity provided by this "wake-up call."

As noted in Part VI, some studies indicate that certain anti-hypertensive medications, notably ACE inhibitors and angiotensin receptor blockers, may be particularly effective for primary stroke prevention, and some evidence suggests that the same may be true for secondary stroke prevention. Despite the importance of controlling blood pressure in patients with cerebrovascular disease, this goal should be achieved gradually. As discussed in Part V, over-aggressive treatment of blood pressure too soon after a stroke may expand the region of irreversible damage.

F. Stroke Mechanisms Other Than Cardioembolism and Carotid Stenosis

Even though the optimum treatment has yet to be established for most of the specific mechanisms of stroke, it is likely that different treatments will eventually be established for different mechanisms. Several broad categories merit consideration.

1. Occlusive disease of large intracranial arteries

The large intracranial arteries (such as the carotid siphon, middle cerebral artery, and basilar artery) are not accessible for endarterectomy. Endovascular procedures, especially angioplasty with or without stenting, are a promising alternative, but they remain investigational, as discussed earlier. At one time, extracranial-intracranial bypass surgery was popular for intracranial disease in the anterior circulation, but a large, prospective, randomized study showed no difference between patients treated with bypass surgery plus aspirin and patients treated with aspirin alone. It is still possible that this approach could be beneficial for carefully selected patients, especially if it is possible to identify patients whose symptoms are related to hemodynamic compromise distal to the arterial obstruction, rather than emboli, but further studies are necessary. Bypass surgery has also been performed on the extracranial vertebral arteries, but the efficacy of this procedure has never been studied in a controlled way. A study comparing warfarin to aspirin in patients with significant stenosis of a large intracranial artery was terminated because of excessive hemorrhagic complications in the warfarin group. Thus, anti-platelet agents are the mainstay of secondary prevention for patients with stenosis of large intracranial arteries.

2. Penetrating artery disease

As with disease of the large intracranial vessels, there is no surgical option in patients with occlusive disease of the penetrating arteries. Endovascular techniques are not feasible either. Anti-platelet agents are typically prescribed.

3. Arterial dissection

With modern imaging techniques, arterial dissection is recognized much more often than in the past. It is most common in the setting of neck trauma or chiropractic manipulation, but the trauma may be surprisingly mild (such as an abrupt neck movement), and there is often no history of trauma at all. Clinicians should be especially alert to the possibility of arterial dissection in younger patients without traditional risk factors for stroke. The optimal management approach has not been established, but these patients are often anticoagulated for 3–6 months to allow time for thrombotic material to organize and recanalize.

4. Aortic arch disease

Atherosclerotic disease of the aortic arch is also increasingly recognized as a cause of stroke. Optimal treatment is unknown. Some clinicians use anticoagulation rather than anti-platelet agents for patients with large plaques in the aorta, particularly if the plaques are mobile or if there have been multiple recurrent events. A clinical trial is in progress.

5. Hematologic disorders, including coagulopathies

For patients with a predisposition to thrombosis, treatment is aimed at the underlying disorder. For example, patients with polycythemia vera are typically treated with phlebotomy and hemodilution; patients with antithrombin deficiency are treated with warfarin. Patients with significantly elevated titers of antiphospholipid antibodies are sometimes treated with warfarin, but the only evidence to support this practice is retrospective.

G. Determining the Underlying Mechanism of Stroke

It can be difficult, and sometimes impossible, to identify the mechanism underlying a patient's stroke. Patients with risk factors for atherosclerosis often have vascular pathology at several different sites, and all may be equally plausible causes of stroke. For example, a patient may have both atrial fibrillation and carotid stenosis – which one was responsible for the stroke? In some cases, clinical features help to narrow the list of possible stroke mechanisms. For example, penetrating artery disease cannot cause a dominant hemisphere MCA syndrome, with weakness, numbness, visual field defect, and aphasia. Similarly, if a patient with a stroke in the posterior circulation (such as a lateral medullary stroke) has carotid stenosis, the carotid disease was not the cause of the stroke. Imaging studies may supplement clinical inferences regarding the mechanism of stroke. For example, if the stroke is visualized by CT or MRI in an area supplied by the posterior circulation, carotid occlusive disease is clearly not the cause. Penetrating artery disease does not produce a lesion larger than 2 cm in diameter. Multiple cortical infarcts in different vascular territories are most suggestive of cardioembolism. Rarer causes of multiple infarcts are diffuse atherosclerosis, coagulopathy, or vasculitis. Wedge-shaped cortical infarcts, particularly in the distribution of the middle cerebral artery, are usually caused by an embolic mechanism, whereas irregular, patchy infarcts in the border zones between the territories of the middle cerebral artery and the anterior cerebral artery or posterior cerebral artery are typically caused by low flow from carotid occlusive disease or global hypoperfusion.

Even when the clinical and imaging features are most consistent with a particular stroke mechanism, they usually are insufficient to exclude other potential mechanisms. In most patients, the carotid arteries and heart must still be imaged directly. As already discussed, patients who have had a TIA or stroke should have a TTE or TEE, unless they already have a known indication for anticoagulation and cardiac imaging would not change their management. Several techniques are available for imaging the extracranial and intracranial arteries. Intra-arterial angiography is considered the gold standard, although magnetic resonance angiography (MRA) and computed tomographic angiography (CTA) are noninvasive and offer comparable resolution for many purposes. Duplex carotid ultrasound is a useful screening test for detecting carotid occlusive disease. Normal carotid ultrasound results are usually reliable, but patients with abnormal carotid ultrasound results usually need further studies, because ultrasound estimates of the magnitude of stenosis are sometimes inaccurate, and a more detailed definition of the cerebral vascular anatomy may be needed if endarterectomy is a consideration. Transcranial Doppler is another technique for examining the intracranial circulation. The choice of vascular imaging modality depends on such factors as whether or not the patient has renal disease (because the dye load associated with a CTA or intra-arterial angiogram could precipitate renal failure, and the dye load associated with an MRA of the neck vessels could precipitate nephrogenic systemic fibrosis), whether the patient needs an MRI anyway (in which case it is usually relatively easy to include MRA at the same time), and—most importantly—which information is likely to change patient management. For example, whereas identification of carotid stenosis frequently affects management decisions, stenosis of intracranial arteries often has little or no impact on treatment.

In some cases, even after appropriate investigations, two or more mechanisms of stroke remain plausible. In those cases, it may be appropriate to treat for both. For example, if a patient with a stroke in the territory of the internal carotid artery has high-grade carotid stenosis on that side and also has atrial fibrillation, both endarterectomy and warfarin may be indicated. Conversely, when no stroke mechanism is identified—especially in young individuals with none of the common risk factors for stroke—it may be reasonable to test for relatively rare mechanisms, such as coagulopathy, other hematologic disorders, arterial dissection, connective tissue diseases, and certain infections (such as syphilis or Herpes varicella-zoster).

In general, it is even more difficult to determine the underlying mechanism in patients who have had a TIA than it is in patients who have had a stroke. By definition, TIAs resolve completely, and in many cases, the patients have already returned to their baseline by the time of medical evaluation. As with strokes, the clinical features may narrow the list of possible mechanisms. For example, a detailed description of the event can make it very likely that it was in the distribution of the vertebrobasilar system, not the carotid. Identification of a single mechanism is often impossible, however, and it may be necessary to evaluate or even treat a patient for more than one plausible mechanism.

VIII. Secondary Prevention of Cerebral Hemorrhage

The principal methods for avoiding recurrent subarachnoid hemorrhage from an aneurysm are to occlude the neck of the aneurysm at open surgery with a clip, or to introduce a coil into the aneurysm via endovascular catheter, with the intent of inducing thrombosis of the aneurysm. A randomized trial demonstrated a better outcome for coiling than for clipping at 1 year. Patients in the coiling group were more likely to require subsequent re-treatment and had an increased risk of rebleeding, but even so, the risk of death within 5 years was lower in the coiling group than in the clipping group. Not all aneurysms are amenable to coiling, so clipping is still indicated in certain cases. Either way, the ideal is to perform the intervention within 3 days of the initial hemorrhage, so that there will be less risk of rebleeding if pressors and fluids are required to treat vasospasm.

Techniques aimed at reducing the risk of recurrent hemorrhage from an arteriovenous malformation include resection, embolization, and radiation. In patients with hypertension-related intraparenchymal hemorrhage, blood pressure control is the key to reducing the risk of recurrent hemorrhagic events.

IX. Discussion of Case Histories

Case 1. A 65-year-old man drove himself to the emergency room at 9 a.m. after experiencing a 4-minute episode of word-finding difficulty and right hand weakness. He had experienced four similar episodes in the last 3 weeks. He had undergone coronary bypass surgery for unstable angina a year ago, and he had a long history of hypertension and diabetes. He was taking aspirin, propranolol, and glyburide daily.

Comment: Episodic focal neurologic symptoms can be vascular, epileptic, psychogenic, metabolic, or migrainous in origin. In a 65-year-old "vasculopath," however, these spells most likely represent TIAs. Furthermore, the spells are consistent with the clinical syndrome produced by ischemia in the dominant MCA territory.

He was afebrile, his blood pressure was 140/80, his pulse was 85 per minute and regular, and a left carotid bruit could be heard in systole and diastole. There were no murmurs and his neurologic examination was normal.

Comment: The normal neurologic exam signifies that the patient has had a TIA, not a stroke. The bruit suggests carotid stenosis. This in itself does not mean that the TIA was due to carotid disease—after all, this patient has multiple risk factors for atherosclerotic disease, and it would not be surprising for it to involve his carotid arteries, but he could have simultaneous disease of his intracranial arteries or his heart. Nonetheless, given that the syndrome is typical of left MCA ischemia and the bruit is on the same side, all the evidence points to carotid disease as the cause of the patient's TIAs.

An intravenous (IV) line was inserted and normal saline was infused at 75 ml/hour. A CT scan of the head and carotid ultrasound were performed that day. The CT scan was normal and the carotid ultrasound suggested greater than 80% stenosis of the left internal carotid artery. The patient was admitted to the neurology service and a cerebral angiogram was scheduled for the next day.

Comment: Patients with cerebral ischemia should be well hydrated to avoid hypotension. The IV fluid should not contain dextrose (even in non-diabetics) because hyperglycemia is associated with increased infarct size in patients who suffer stroke. This patient has a high risk of stroke in the near future, and admission to the hospital will facilitate rapid evaluation and definitive treatment to prevent stroke. Hospital admission will also make it easier to evaluate the patient for treatment with tPA within the appropriate time window if his symptoms recur and persist while his evaluation is in progress (there is no indication for tPA at this point, because his symptoms have resolved). Some neurologists use heparin in patients with TIAs and high-grade arterial stenosis, hoping to prevent thrombosis at the stenotic site, but this has not been adequately studied. Furthermore, if he were to develop a stroke while on heparin, an elevated partial thromboplastin time would make him ineligible to receive tPA, for which there is more compelling evidence of benefit.

Angiography showed 90% stenosis of the left internal carotid artery, mild plaque without stenosis of the right internal carotid artery, and normal intracranial vessels bilaterally. Surgery was planned for the following day. The surgery was successful and the patient was discharged 5 days later. In addition to the medications he was taking on admission, he was discharged on atorvastatin, 80 mg/day, because of his history of diabetes and symptomatic vascular disease (both cardiac and cerebrovascular). He reported no new symptoms at a follow-up visit 6 weeks later.

Case 2. A 59-year-old woman came to the emergency room at her family's insistence at 9 p.m. after she mentioned that she had been having trouble seeing out of her left eye since awakening that morning. She had been in good health except for long-standing hypertension and occasional "rapid heartbeats." She denied previous visual symptoms or other episodic neurologic symptoms. She was taking captopril. The patient was alert, her blood pressure was 170/95, her pulse was 130 per minute and irregular, and there were no murmurs or bruits. The only abnormality on neurologic exam was a left homonymous hemianopia.

Comment: Patients with homonymous hemianopia frequently think their visual loss is monocular. Covering one eye at a time will often reveal the binocular visual loss to the patient. This patient had an acute, focal lesion with no history of trauma. This suggests a vascular etiology, and the specific syndrome is consistent with ischemia in the right PCA territory. The irregular heartbeat suggests the possibility of atrial fibrillation, and therefore, a cardioembolic mechanism.

An IV line was inserted and normal saline was infused at 75 ml/hour. An electrocardiogram confirmed atrial fibrillation, and a CT scan of the head was normal. Her blood pressure remained slightly elevated at 170–180/90–100.

Comment: Even if this patient had come to the emergency room as soon as she noticed her problem, tPA would not have been an option because her stroke could have occurred at any time after she fell asleep. Her mildly elevated blood pressure was left untreated to avoid relative hypotension and diminished cerebral perfusion. Warfarin (5 mg orally) was started the day after her admission to the hospital. Evaluation for the cause of atrial fibrillation revealed evidence of a prior myocardial infarction, but no acute ischemia. She had normal thyroid function. Diltiazem was started for rate control.

Comment: Although warfarin is clearly indicated for long-term stroke prophylaxis in patients with chronic atrial fibrillation who have had a stroke, experts differ on the timing. Some clinicians would defer anticoagulation for several days or even weeks, because of the risk that the infarct could undergo hemorrhagic transformation in the acute setting. This risk was considered acceptable in this patient because her clinical syndrome suggested a relatively small stroke; the CT scan showed no edema or hemorrhage, and her blood pressure was only mildly elevated.

The patient's hemianopia persisted, but she developed no new deficits. Her blood pressure had normalized by the time of discharge without any specific intervention. She was discharged on captopril, diltiazem, and warfarin. She was given specific instructions to obtain a repeat INR in one week, and scheduled for follow-up in an anticoagulation clinic; outpatient evaluation was also scheduled for her coronary artery disease.

Comment: Warfarin is a potentially dangerous drug. All patients discharged on warfarin should know who is going to monitor their warfarin therapy as an outpatient. They should be given clear instructions on what dose to take daily, and they should be told when to get blood drawn for the next INR measurement.

Case 3. A 73-year-old man was brought to the emergency room by paramedics after he fell down on the way back from the bathroom and discovered that he could not move his left side. His symptoms had not progressed in the 90 minutes that had elapsed since the initial event. He had been hypertensive for 20 years and was taking hydrochlorothiazide, and he had been taking lovastatin for a year because of hyperlipidemia. He denied previous episodes of focal neurologic symptoms. He was alert, with a blood pressure of 180/100 and a pulse that was 80 per minute and regular. There were no bruits or murmurs. Neurologic exam showed normal mental status (with no neglect); dysarthria; left hemiparesis involving face, arm, and leg; left-sided hyperreflexia; a left extensor plantar response (Babinski sign); and normal sensation.

Comment: The neurologic exam suggests a right-sided lesion at the level of the pons or above. An acute, focal, nonprogressive lesion is generally ischemic. The pure motor syndrome and the absence of features of cortical involvement (such as neglect or a visual field defect) suggest penetrating artery disease.

The patient was a candidate to receive tPA, so blood was sent for electrolytes, glucose, platelet count, and coagulation studies. He was taken immediately for a CT scan, which showed an old, small (1 cm) basal ganglia infarct on the left. The blood test results were normal, and IV tPA was administered. He was admitted to the neurology service, and his blood pressure was monitored in an intensive care unit for the next 24 hours, following an institutional protocol. By the time the patient was transferred out of the intensive care unit, he had recovered "approximately 75%" of the function on his left side but he still had significant weakness.

Carotid ultrasound and TEE performed the next day were both normal. An MRI scan of the brain 2 days after admission showed a small (1 cm) infarct in the right internal capsule and the previously noted left basal ganglia infarct. The patient was transferred to the rehabilitation service, and an ACE inhibitor was prescribed in addition to the diuretic for better long-term blood pressure control, and because of the potential for additional protective activity against stroke.

Comment: This patient might very well have improved even without tPA, but his chances of improvement were better with treatment. The use of tPA is recommended in acute ischemic stroke regardless of the underlying cause. In this case, the clinical syndrome suggested a lacunar infarct, and the MRI scan confirmed it, so the likely stroke mechanism was intrinsic disease of a penetrating artery, but thromboembolism was another possible mechanism. The MRI scan reassured the clinicians managing this patient that their diagnosis was correct, but did not really change management, so it was not really necessary. With no evidence of carotid disease or a cardioembolic source, long-term stroke prophylaxis in this patient consisted of more aggressive blood pressure control together with an anti-platelet medication. When the available anti-platelet drugs were reviewed with the patient, he requested aspirin because he had to pay for his medications himself.

Chapter 5

Seizures

I. Case Histories

Case 1. A 7-year-old boy was noted by his teacher to be intermittently inattentive in the classroom. He would stare with a blank expression on his face for several seconds at a time. He would not respond to his name being called and sometimes had rapid fluttering movements of his eyelids. Once the staring ceased, he would immediately become his usual self. His pediatrician was able to provoke one of the spells by having the boy hyperventilate in the office.

Questions:

1. What is the most likely diagnosis in this patient?
2. What other diagnoses need to be considered?
3. What is the drug of choice in this syndrome?

Case 2. A 27-year-old woman in the second trimester of her first pregnancy was referred to the epilepsy clinic from the high-risk obstetrics clinic. She had her first generalized tonic-clonic seizure when she was 21 years old, while studying for a final exam. She had three more seizures during her early 20s, each beginning with an unpleasant sensation in her abdomen, followed on one occasion by staring and picking at her blouse buttons before progressing into a generalized tonic-clonic seizure. She was the product of a normal pregnancy and delivery with normal developmental milestones. At age 15 months she had experienced two prolonged seizures with high fever, both lasting approximately 25 minutes and associated with transient paralysis of her right arm. She had continued to develop normally and had been successful both athletically and scholastically. Since age 24 years she has been taking phenytoin, 200 mg twice a day, and has had no seizures. Her only other medications are prenatal vitamins and supplemental folate, 1 mg a day.

Questions:

1. What type of seizures does this patient have?
2. What diagnostic tests does this patient need?
3. What are the drugs of choice for this patient?
4. How should this patient be managed:

   a. through the rest of her pregnancy?
   b. thereafter?

Case 3. A 55-year-old woman had a generalized tonic-clonic seizure while grocery shopping one afternoon. She had been experiencing moderately severe headaches early each morning for about a week, but she had been well previously. When the emergency medical service arrived, the patient was having a second generalized tonic-clonic seizure. A witness reported generalized stiffening of all four extremities followed by clonic movements associated with cyanosis, frothing at the mouth, and urinary incontinence. The patient had two more seizures without recovering consciousness before reaching a local emergency room. The emergency room physicians diagnosed convulsive status epilepticus.

Questions:

1. Do you agree with the emergency room doctors' diagnosis?
2. How should this patient be managed in the emergency room?
3. How should this patient be investigated after her seizures are controlled?

II. Approach to Seizures

Four questions must be addressed in a patient who has had a seizure:

1. Is the diagnosis correct?
2. Is urgent treatment necessary?
3. Why did the patient have a seizure?
4. What long-term treatment (if any) is indicated?

Question 1 is addressed in Part IV. The one situation in which treatment of seizure activity is truly urgent is status epilepticus, which is covered in Part VII. Question 3 is addressed in Part V, and Question 4 in Part VI. Part III presents some definitions and necessary background information.

III. Background Information

A. Definitions

epilepsy a brain disorder characterized by an enduring predisposition to generate seizures (and the actual occurrence of at least one seizure)

seizure a transient episode of altered behavior or sensorium caused by excessive and hypersynchronous discharge of neurons

focal seizure a seizure in which the first clinical and electroencephalographic (EEG) changes indicate initial activation of a system of neurons limited to one part of one cerebral hemisphere (synonym: partial seizure)

partial seizure (not currently recommended terminology): synonym for focal seizure

simple partial seizure (not currently recommended terminology): a focal (partial) seizure in which consciousness is not impaired

complex partial seizure (not currently recommended terminology): a focal (partial) seizure in which consciousness is impaired

generalized seizure a seizure in which the first clinical and EEG changes indicate initial involvement of both hemispheres

tonic activity sustained muscular contraction lasting a few seconds to minutes and resulting in rigid extension or flexion

clonic activity rhythmic jerking of muscles

focal (partial) seizure with secondary generalization a partial seizure that evolves into generalized tonic-clonic activity

seizure disorder epilepsy

status epilepticus a state of continuous or frequent seizures with failure to return to a baseline level of alertness between the seizures

B. Clinical Characteristics of Seizures

A seizure is a transient episode of altered behavior or perception caused by a burst of excessive or hypersynchronous neuronal activity. The clinical manifestations of a seizure depend on where the abnormal neuronal activity starts (the seizure focus) and how it spreads.

1. Focal (partial) Seizures:

Any seizure that begins in a localized region in one cerebral hemisphere is called a *focal seizure,* even if the electrical activity subsequently spreads bilaterally and produces bilateral clinical manifestations. "Partial" seizure is an older term for focal seizure. When the focus is in the primary motor area, the seizure typically consists of rhythmic jerking (clonic activity) of the body part represented in that region of the brain, or rigid posturing (tonic activity) of the body part, or alternating tonic and clonic activity. A seizure focus in the prefrontal cortex often produces more complex patterns of motor activity. Seizures that begin in the primary sensory cortex generally consist of localized paresthesias or numbness. A seizure focus in the occipital lobe typically produces visual illusions (distorted perception of real visual stimuli) or hallucinations (visual perception unrelated to actual visual stimuli). As a general rule, seizures produce "positive phenomena" (shaking of a limb, visual, auditory, or olfactory hallucinations, tingling, etc.) as opposed to TIAs, which typically produce "negative phenomena" (inability to move a limb, loss of vision, numbness, etc.). Foci in the medial temporal lobes commonly produce a rising sense of epigastric discomfort or nausea. Other common manifestations of foci in or near the temporal lobe include fear, olfactory symptoms, auditory illusions or hallucinations, and distortions of memory including déjà vu (a strong sense of having had an experience previously) and jamais vu (a sense of unfamiliarity with previous experiences).

Seizures can remain confined to the original focus, or they can spread. One classic (but rare) example of spread is a "jacksonian march" across the motor cortex, with corresponding motor activity that spreads from one body part to an adjacent body part and from there to another, progressively involving one entire side of the body. When the spread of electrical hyperactivity stays in one hemisphere, patients may remain aware of external stimuli and respond normally during a seizure. Traditionally, focal (partial) seizures in which consciousness is maintained are called *simple partial seizures*. Focal (partial) seizures that spread to involve regions in the contralateral hemisphere and result in impaired consciousness have traditionally been called *complex partial seizures*. Recent classification systems eliminate the terms "simple partial" and "complex partial," but the clinical observations are still valid. A common feature of complex partial seizures is a motionless stare during which the patient does not respond to external stimuli. During the period of impaired consciousness, patients often manifest involuntary, automatic motor behaviors known as automatisms. For example, they may smack their lips, make chewing movements, wring their hands, pick at clothes, rearrange objects, walk in circles, or utter short, stereotyped phrases. There may also be forced movement of the head or eyes in one direction. Patients with complex partial seizures generally can not remember them.

2. Generalized Seizures

Some seizures have no apparent focus—from the very beginning, the clinical and EEG manifestations are widespread throughout both cerebral hemispheres. These are called *generalized seizures*. In some cases, generalized seizures can result from a metabolic disturbance (such as hypoxia or hyperglycemia) that affects neurons diffusely. In other cases, generalized seizures can be caused by abnormal activity in some focal region of the brain that can not be readily detected clinically or by EEG, and the abnormal activity spreads rapidly and simultaneously to both cerebral hemispheres.

Generalized seizures usually result in impairment of consciousness, often at the onset, although some generalized seizures (especially myoclonic seizures) may be so brief that impaired consciousness can not be detected. The most common type of generalized seizure is the *generalized tonic-clonic seizure*. There is a sudden, tonic contraction of limb and axial muscles accompanied by upward eye deviation, pupillary dilatation, and loss of consciousness. Contraction of the respiratory muscles and larynx often produces a forced expiration resulting in an "epileptic cry" or gasp, and the patient may become cyanotic. This is followed by jerking (*clonic*) movements that gradually increase in amplitude while the frequency gradually falls to the point where there are discrete pauses between the jerks, and then the jerking stops completely, with relaxation of all muscles. Urinary (and, rarely, fecal) incontinence may occur at this point. Patients may bite their tongue or inner cheek during either the tonic or the clonic phase. The clonic phase usually ends within 60 seconds, and the entire period of involuntary muscle activity usually lasts 90–120 seconds, at which point patients resume breathing but usually remain unresponsive for minutes to hours. On return to consciousness, patients are often confused or sleepy for several hours or longer, and they may have a headache, sore mouth, or generalized aching or stiffness.

Less commonly, generalized seizures can have a tonic phase with no clonic component, or a clonic phase with no tonic component. Some seizures (*atonic seizures*) consist of a sudden decrease in muscle tone leading to a loss of postural control, which can be localized (such as a head drop) or generalized. When the loss of postural control is generalized, patients may fall, usually without loss of consciousness; these are often called drop attacks. The spells typically last 1–2 seconds.

Infantile spasms are characterized by sudden, rapid flexion of the neck and trunk, adduction of the shoulders and outstretched arms, and variable flexion of the lower extremities. Some patients exhibit fragments of the full-fledged movement.

Myoclonic seizures consist of nonrhythmic, rapid, jerking movements that can be local or widespread. Nonepileptic forms of myoclonus also exist; the most common example is the isolated limb jerk that often occurs in normal individuals as they fall asleep. Some patients exhibit diffuse, severe nonepileptic myoclonus after anoxic brain injury.

Absence seizures are characterized by sudden interruption of activity associated with unresponsiveness and a blank stare, sometimes with fluttering of the eyelids. They last less than 10 seconds. They can often be precipitated by hyperventilation.

C. Seizures vs. Epilepsy

Patients with seizures do not necessarily have epilepsy. Even people with a normal brain can have seizures if they are exposed to certain metabolic or physical triggers. For example, hypoxia, hyponatremia, hyperglycemia, hypoglycemia, hypocalcemia, hypomagnesemia, uremia, hepatic failure, fever, and a variety of prescription and recreational drugs can all provoke seizures. As long as the precipitating factor can be identified and treated effectively, these people are no more likely than the general population to have recurrent seizures. Even when a person has a seizure and *no* precipitating trigger can be found, the patient does not necessarily have a brain disorder. In fact, about 50% of patients who have an unprovoked seizure never have another one. It is not clear why this should be the case, but presumably, some rare constellation of metabolic factors (e.g., electrolyte concentrations, glucocorticoid levels, body temperature) and neuronal activation patterns may combine in just the right way to result in a seizure, and that combination may never recur in a patient's lifetime. In contrast, patients who have a *second* seizure have at least a 70% chance of further seizures; thus, a patient who has had two or more unprovoked seizures very likely has a brain abnormality predisposing to recurrent seizures, and will almost certainly require medication.

To reiterate, a patient who has had a single, unprovoked seizure does not necessarily have epilepsy, whereas a patient who has had two or more unprovoked seizures generally does. In fact, the occurrence of two or more unprovoked seizures has traditionally served as an operational definition of epilepsy. Note that the more recent definition (the one listed in Part II) —"a brain disorder characterized by an enduring predisposition to generate seizures (and the actual occurrence of at least one seizure)"—fails to specify what constitutes "an enduring predisposition." As before, the occurrence of two or more unprovoked seizures is a compelling indication that the patient's brain has an inherent predisposition to generate seizures. In some cases, family history or particular EEG features may provide convincing evidence. Certain structural brain abnormalities may, also. In the absence of such evidence, patients who have had a single seizure should not be diagnosed with epilepsy.

D. Epilepsy Syndromes

Epilepsy represents a failure of the protective mechanisms that usually inhibit large groups of neurons from engaging in repetitive, entrained activity. This failure can occur as a result of genetic abnormalities or because a region of brain tissue has sustained structural or metabolic injury. Epilepsy that is due to structural or metabolic injury, either ongoing or in the past, is termed *symptomatic epilepsy*. These patients are identified on the basis of history (for example, a history of neonatal intraventricular hemorrhage, or a history of post-anoxic coma after a cardiac arrest at age 60, or the recent onset of headaches and ataxia), a focal examination, or imaging studies. Epilepsy that conforms to a distinctive, well-defined syndrome with a known—or likely—genetic mechanism is termed *idiopathic epilepsy*. These patients (and their specific syndromes) are identified based on the characteristics of their seizures, age of onset, underlying cause, anatomic substrate, and associated interictal symptoms, signs, and EEG patterns.

Epilepsy syndromes can also be sorted into those that are *localization-related* (focal), in which the predominant seizures are focal and arise from a discrete area of cortical dysfunction, and those that are *generalized,* in which the predominant seizures are generalized and arise from diffuse or multifocal areas of cortical dysfunction. Using this dichotomy as one "axis" and the symptomatic/idiopathic dichotomy as an independent axis, four broad categories of epilepsy syndromes result (see Table 5.1): idiopathic generalized, symptomatic generalized, idiopathic localization-related, and symptomatic localization-related.

Table 5.1. Examples of Epilepsy Syndromes

	Localization-related	Generalized
Symptomatic	Post-stroke Epilepsy Epilepsy due to Mesial Temporal Sclerosis	Lennox-Gastaut Syndrome
Idiopathic	Benign Childhood Epilepsy with Centrotemporal Spikes	Childhood Absence Epilepsy
		Juvenile Myoclonic Epilepsy

E. Electroencephalography

An electroencephalogram (EEG) is a recording of electric activity generated by the brain using electrodes placed at standard positions on the scalp. The electric activity detected by one electrode reflects the summated synaptic and post-synaptic currents of roughly 100 million neurons, particularly the radially oriented pyramidal cells. The EEG, in effect, compares the sum of this activity in the vicinity of one electrode to the sum of activity surrounding an adjacent electrode. I find it somewhat surprising that this provides any useful information—in contrast to an electrocardiogram (EKG), which sums the activity from relatively interchangeable myocardial cells that are all working in concert to produce a coordinated pumping action, each EEG electrode summates the activity of neurons participating in multiple circuits with diverse functions. Not surprisingly, the resulting pattern looks almost random. Nonetheless, the frequency spectrum of this summated activity is relatively consistent across normal individuals. Brain damage can distort the frequency distribution of the electrical activity. During a seizure, in particular, the hypersynchronous activity of large networks of neurons can result in distinctive, abnormal patterns of EEG activity. Thus, an EEG recorded during a clinical spell (referred to as an *ictal* EEG) can be used to determine whether or not the spell is a seizure, if the abnormal electrical activity involves a large enough area of cortex.

Although an EEG recorded between spells (termed an *interictal EEG*) can not be used to determine whether a particular spell was a seizure, an interictal EEG can reveal characteristic "epileptiform" abnormalities that are more common in patients with epilepsy than in the general population. The particular characteristics of the epileptiform activity on EEG may provide clues regarding the nature of the underlying epilepsy syndrome. For example, absence seizures characteristically are associated with a pattern described as regular spike-and-wave activity at a frequency of 3 Hz.

Interictal EEGs are neither completely specific nor completely sensitive. About 2–3% of people with interictal abnormalities on EEG never have any symptoms consistent with a seizure, and about 10–20% of patients with clinically unequivocal epilepsy have consistently normal interictal EEGs. A single interictal EEG will show epileptiform activity in 50–70% of patients with epilepsy. The yield can be increased by obtaining more than one interictal EEG or with activation procedures such as hyperventilation (especially useful for provoking absence seizures) or sleep deprivation. Some EEG abnormalities are more informative than others, and interpretation requires specialized training and expertise.

In some circumstances, it is desirable to characterize seizures as carefully as possible. This requires continuous EEG monitoring and concurrent videotaping of the patient, in the hopes of recording the patient's actual spells (rather than just interictal activity). This approach requires inpatient hospitalization, and is only practical if the patient is known to have spells fairly frequently. For patients in whom long-term monitoring is feasible, the type of EEG abnormality present during a seizure can be very helpful in identifying the nature of a patient's epilepsy syndrome. If a patient has spells during the monitoring and there is no EEG abnormality before, during, or after the spells, they are not seizures (with rare exceptions). Of course, the patient could have *other* spells that *are* seizures—some patients with epilepsy also have nonepileptic spells of psychogenic origin.

F. Pathophysiology of Seizures and Epilepsy

The fundamental mechanisms underlying seizure onset, propagation, and termination remain obscure, and the mechanisms may differ depending on the type of epilepsy. Two key conditions are required for seizures to occur: (1) excessive neuronal excitability and (2) a pattern of synaptic connections between neurons that permits hypersynchrony. Many different cellular processes contribute to these conditions, notably the activity of voltage-gated ion channels (which, in turn, affects the neuron's resting potential and electrical excitability), the distribution and activity of inhibitory (predominantly GABA-ergic) synapses, and the distribution and activity of excitatory (especially glutamatergic) synapses. Glial cells and features of the extracellular space can also affect neuronal excitability and synaptic organization. Experimental manipulation of any of these processes in laboratory animals can cause seizures. It seems likely that in humans, also, seizures can develop as a result of just the right combination of slight perturbations in neuronal excitability and synaptic connections.

The mechanisms underlying epilepsy (as opposed to individual seizures) are also obscure. It is not clear what factors make one region of brain more likely than another to serve as a seizure focus. The formation of positive feedback (recurrent excitatory) circuits is probably important. In one common epileptic condition, mesial temporal sclerosis, the mossy fibers of the hippocampus sprout collateral branches that could serve as the substrate for such circuits. A similar process has been implicated in the formation of neuronal connections during memory storage. Indeed, it could be that one reason the temporal lobe is so commonly involved in localization-related epilepsies is the fact that plasticity and synaptic remodeling occur routinely in the normal hippocampus. There is evidence that seizures themselves may induce collateral sprouting, and thus contribute to recurrent excitatory circuits. This increases the likelihood of further seizures, leading to additional sprouting, and so forth.

Generalized epilepsy syndromes are, if anything, even less well understood than localization-related epilepsy syndromes. Thalamocortical circuits seem to be critical. The normal thalamus enters an oscillatory or "burst" mode during drowsiness or sleep, and these inherent rhythm-generating mechanisms may serve as the substrate for abnormal rhythmic activity when the circuits are damaged. There is evidence for this mechanism in animal models of generalized absence epilepsy.

IV. Diagnosis

When patients present with transient symptoms that might represent a seizure, the diagnostic process involves two steps. The first is to characterize the presenting spell, and to determine if it is likely to be a seizure or some other condition. If a seizure is likely, the second step is to try to identify the cause. Although these two steps are conceptually distinct, they are entwined in practice. Complete and accurate characterization of a seizure often suggests the cause, especially when patients have a recognized epilepsy syndrome. Conversely, identification of a likely cause of epilepsy increases the likelihood that the presenting spell was, in fact, a seizure. Thus, the distinction between these two diagnostic steps is somewhat artificial—information pertinent to one is also relevant to the other. Nonetheless, for purposes of exposition, it is useful to discuss the two diagnostic processes separately. To minimize redundancy, procedures (such as blood tests, MRI, and EEG) that are important in identifying the underlying cause of seizures are discussed in Part V, whereas the current discussion focuses on features of the spells themselves.

A. Characterizing the Presenting Spell

Seizures, like TIAs, are transient. Patients have usually returned to baseline by the time they receive medical attention, so the history is typically more useful than the neurologic examination. Patients with simple partial seizures may be able to provide an accurate description of their spells, but you should also be sure to talk to an independent witness. Patients with complex partial seizures or generalized seizures usually have little or no recollection of the spell, so witnesses' accounts are especially important.

Typical manifestations of seizures were reviewed in Part III. Many of these features can be dramatic and distinctive, but some can be very subtle. Patients and witnesses often overlook important details and misinterpret others (such as generalized tremulousness, which is a very nonspecific phenomenon). You should begin by asking open-ended questions (e.g., "What was the first thing you noticed that seemed abnormal today?"; "Did you have a warning?"; "What's the next thing you remember?"; "How did you feel when you regained consciousness?"; "Were you immediately able to resume what you had been doing before the spell?"), but be prepared to follow up with focused questions (e.g., "Did you smell anything unusual?"; "Was one side of your body different from the other?"; "When you regained consciousness, was there any sign that you had bitten your tongue?"; "Had you wet yourself or soiled yourself?"). Try to obtain as detailed a description as possible of everything the patient experienced and witnesses observed before, during, and after the spell, including the exact sequence of events and how long each stage lasted. Try to determine what the patient was doing just before the episode, and earlier that day, especially anything different from the patient's usual routine. Pay special attention to features that would help determine whether the onset was focal or generalized. Be sure to ask if the patient had any persistent focal deficits after the spell ended, because such deficits are more common with focal seizures. In addition to talking to the patient, you should speak to a witness—telephone this person during the interview if necessary.

B. Identifying Prior Spells

Unless patients spontaneously mention previous spells, you should ask them direct, pointed questions to determine if they have previously experienced characteristic seizure symptoms ("Do you ever smell things that aren't there?"; "Have you ever had the sense that you were outside your body looking down?"). In many cases, you can obtain more useful diagnostic information by concentrating on subtle or minor spells that patients have experienced in the past than you can by trying to characterize the more dramatic spell that brought them to medical attention. If you don't ask about these symptoms explicitly, patients may not volunteer them, because they consider them too insignificant, or too strange, or too embarrassing. Patients may also be too embarrassed to mention incontinence until you ask them about it explicitly.

C. Recognizing Spells that are Not Seizures

In addition to questions regarding typical manifestations of seizures, you should ask about features that might indicate some other disorder. A variety of conditions produce recurrent spells that can be confused with seizures. It is important to keep these conditions in mind and to be aware of the features that help to distinguish seizures from nonepileptic spells.

1. Spells involving loss of consciousness

The most common cause of temporary loss of consciousness is syncope, which occurs when a transient reduction in cardiac output produces generalized cerebral ischemia. Many different conditions can produce syncope, including cardiac arrhythmia, obstructed cardiac outflow (such as occurs with aortic stenosis), sudden cardiac failure from a large myocardial infarction, or impaired autonomic reflexes (e.g., orthostatic hypotension). Excessive parasympathetic tone, often called vasovagal syncope or vasodepressor syncope, is the most common cause. It occurs when there is excessive parasympathetic response to a sudden increase in sympathetic activity, most often in the setting of stress or excitement. Excessive parasympathetic responses may also be responsible for micturition syncope and defecation syncope.

Most episodes of syncope are preceded by a premonitory state known as presyncope, consisting of light-headedness and sometimes nausea, diaphoresis, tinnitus, fading of vision, and change in skin color. These premonitory symptoms may be helpful in distinguishing a syncopal spell from a seizure, but not always—some patients with syncope lose consciousness suddenly, without warning, and others describe presyncopal symptoms that could themselves be confused with complex partial seizures. Another useful distinguishing feature may be the setting in which the spells occur. For example, people who lose consciousness when having their blood drawn probably have vasovagal syncope, and a common setting for orthostatic syncope is during a religious service, when there is venous pooling in the legs due to prolonged sitting or kneeling. Patients are usually only briefly confused, if at all, after syncope, whereas more prolonged post-ictal confusion or focal signs would suggest a seizure. Incontinence is also more common with seizures, though it can occur with syncope. Spells that include rhythmic motor activity are usually seizures, but myoclonic jerks may occur with restitution of blood flow after a syncopal episode, making distinction from a seizure difficult in some cases.

Transient metabolic disturbances, such as hypoglycemia, can produce symptoms that resemble syncope or seizures. Patients with excessive day-time somnolence from any cause can experience "sleep attacks," in which they suddenly fall asleep with hardly any warning. These episodes are not associated with any of the other typical features of seizures, so they are usually not hard to distinguish.

2. Spells without loss of consciousness

Both transient ischemic attacks (TIAs) and migraines may produce transient neurologic symptoms that spread in a manner similar to a focal seizure (see Chapters 4 and 12). Accompanying headache helps to distinguish migraine from seizure, but some patients with otherwise typical migraine never experience headache (so-called migraine equivalents), and some patients who have seizures have severe headaches afterward. The motor or sensory symptoms that occur with migraine tend to evolve more slowly than the symptoms of a seizure, which, in turn, tend to evolve more slowly than the symptoms of a TIA. The sensory and motor manifestations of TIAs tend to be "negative" phenomena, such as numbness or weakness, whereas seizures are more likely to produce "positive" symptoms, such as paresthesias or jerking movements.

Cataplexy—a sudden loss of muscle tone most commonly seen in patients with narcolepsy (see Chapter 9)—is sometimes mistaken for a seizure. A variety of other abnormal movements or behaviors can occur with sleep disorders, and sometimes the only way to distinguish these from seizures is to perform EEG monitoring while the patient sleeps.

3. Spells of psychogenic origin

Psychological conditions can result in spells that resemble seizures. Features that may suggest this possibility include a long period of motionless unresponsiveness, asynchronous limb movements, side-to-side ("no-no") shaking of the head, dramatic bilateral limb movements while talking, and crying shortly after the spell. Spells that vary substantially from one episode to another (such as spells that involve one limb on one day and a different limb the next, or visual symptoms on some occasions and auditory symptoms on other occasions, or spells lasting two minutes at times and two days at other times) would all be atypical of epilepsy and suggestive of a non-neurologic disorder. If the spells occur only when the patient is in a psychologically stressful situation, this may also be a clue that the condition is psychogenic. There are exceptions to all of these generalizations, however. Caution should be exercised before concluding that spells have a psychogenic origin simply because they are unusual or seem inconsistent. All fields of medicine abound with examples of organic conditions that were initially thought to be psychogenic.

V. Determining the Cause of Seizures

Once you have determined that a patient has had a seizure, or that it is at least a realistic consideration, management depends on the underlying cause. Patients who present with seizures can be grouped into three broad categories: (1) those whose seizures are precipitated by clearly identified systemic factors, (2) those with epilepsy, and (3) those who experience a single unprovoked seizure with no evidence of predisposition to recurrent seizures. Patients in the first category are managed by treating whatever precipitating factors are identified. Patients with epilepsy are treated with anti-epileptic drugs or the other modalities discussed in Part VI. Patients with single unprovoked seizures are usually followed conservatively.

A. Provoked Seizures

The most common metabolic causes of seizures are hypoxia, hyponatremia, hyperglycemia, hypoglycemia, hypocalcemia, and hypomagnesemia. Seizures may also occur with acute uremia or hepatic failure. Prescription drugs and recreational drugs are common causes of seizures, especially antidepressants and antipsychotic medications (particularly when doses are increased too rapidly), aminophylline and other methylxanthines, lidocaine, penicillins, narcotic analgesics, cocaine, heroin, methylenedioxymethamphetamine (MDMA, or "ecstasy"), and phencyclidine. Withdrawal from alcohol may produce seizures, which almost always occur after 6–48 hours of abstinence. Withdrawal seizures may also occur in patients who have been abusing barbiturates or benzodiazepines.

Fever is a common precipitating factor in children. About 2–4% of children have a febrile seizure, usually within the first 3 years of life. About a third of children who have a febrile seizure will have one or more recurrences. Febrile seizures typically occur during the rising phase of the temperature curve; they do not correlate with the severity of the fever. They are almost always generalized, and they usually last less than 15 minutes. The incidence of subsequent epilepsy is significantly higher in children who have febrile seizures than in the general population, but the rate is still lower than 5%. Factors associated with a higher likelihood of subsequent epilepsy are seizure duration longer than 15 minutes, seizure recurrence within 24 hours, focal features to the seizure, a history of abnormal neurologic development, an abnormal neurologic examination, and a family history of epilepsy. Children with none of these factors have a <1% risk of developing epilepsy subsequently. Febrile seizures do not require treatment, except prompt administration of anti-pyretic medication and sponge baths to control subsequent fevers.

B. Epilepsy

In order to provide prognostic information and to facilitate management decisions, it is important not just to make the diagnosis of epilepsy, but to characterize the patient's epilepsy syndrome. The four broad categories shown in Table 5.1 and discussed in Part III—idiopathic generalized, idiopathic localization-related, symptomatic generalized, and symptomatic localization-related—provide a useful framework for conceptualizing the epilepsy syndromes, but they are not detailed enough to guide management decisions. More extensive classification syndromes have been proposed, involving more detailed descriptions of the individual seizures and the underlying etiology (when known), but this remains a work in progress. Nonetheless, many individual epilepsy syndromes are well established and well characterized.

One common idiopathic generalized epilepsy syndrome is *childhood absence epilepsy*, characterized by absence seizures that typically begin in children ages 4–8 years old and usually (in two thirds of patients) resolve before adulthood. Another common idiopathic generalized epilepsy syndrome is *juvenile myoclonic epilepsy*. This condition is characterized by myoclonic jerks of the shoulders and arms, usually occurring soon after awakening. More than 90% of patients with this syndrome have generalized tonic-clonic seizures, and about 25% also have absence seizures. The myoclonic jerks precede the generalized tonic-clonic seizures by a year or more in about half the patients. The typical age of onset is 12–18 years. This condition usually responds very well to appropriate medications, but life-long medication is generally necessary.

One example of an idiopathic localization-related epilepsy syndrome is *benign childhood epilepsy with centrotemporal spikes* ("benign rolandic epilepsy"). Patients with this syndrome have simple partial seizures characterized by abnormal movements and sensation of the mouth, and sometimes the hand, with excessive salivation and drooling. The patients are fully conscious, but they may be unable to speak when the focus is in the dominant hemisphere. There may be secondary generalization. The seizures usually occur during sleep. They typically present at ages 5–10 years, and almost always resolve spontaneously by age 18 years.

Symptomatic generalized epilepsies are typically the result of diffuse brain abnormalities, and are commonly associated with more extensive neurologic manifestations, such as spasticity or generalized cognitive impairment. Examples include certain inborn errors of metabolism, diffuse developmental abnormalities and malformations, and prenatal metabolic abnormalities. *Lennox-Gastaut syndrome* is a particularly severe condition that typically manifests between ages 2–8 years. It is characterized by the triad of mental retardation, a diffuse slow spike-and-wave pattern on EEG, and multiple types of generalized seizures, including atonic seizures, tonic seizures, myoclonic seizures, and atypical absence seizures. Status epilepticus is common in patients with this syndrome. A variety of underlying brain disorders can cause this syndrome. In about a third of patients, the underlying cause is not identified.

The vast majority of localization-related epilepsies are symptomatic (i.e., they are caused by focal abnormalities in the brain, such as strokes, trauma, tumors, or vascular malformations). The most common site is the temporal lobe. The older the patient, the more likely the cause is a stroke, even if clinically silent. A common cause in younger patients is a condition known as *mesial temporal sclerosis*.

C. The Diagnostic Evaluation

The process of obtaining a detailed description of the episode (and previous episodes, if any) was discussed in Part IV. Your history should also focus on features that would increase the likelihood of an underlying brain disorder that could predispose to seizures (such as premature birth, developmental delay, a family history of epilepsy, or a history of febrile seizures, head trauma, stroke, meningitis, or encephalitis). You should perform a full neurologic examination—abnormal findings obviously increase the likelihood of underlying brain dysfunction.

You should also take a thorough medical history. Most patients with provoked seizures are already known to have one or more conditions that predispose to seizures. In the absence of such a history, a search for precipitating factors is likely to be unproductive. Nonetheless, when a patient with no prior history of seizures is brought to the emergency department or some other acute care setting for a spell, and the description of the spell is consistent with a possible seizure, serum electrolytes (including calcium and magnesium, which are not routinely included in some screening blood panels), glucose, blood urea nitrogen, creatinine, liver enzymes, and blood counts should be measured. Patients who present acutely with seizures should be evaluated for infection (including a lumbar puncture), and a urine toxin screen should be obtained. The yield of this testing is usually low.

Patients who present with the first seizure of their lives should have an imaging study. An MRI scan performed with and without gadolinium is the imaging procedure of choice. In the acute setting, this is often unavailable, so patients often have a noncontrast head CT scan in the emergency department to exclude lesions that would require urgent treatment, such as intracranial hemorrhage or a tumor producing significant mass effect. They can then be scheduled to have an MRI scan as an outpatient within the next few weeks. Patients should also be scheduled for an outpatient EEG in the same time frame. They will probably not be obliging enough to have a spell during the EEG, so it will most likely be an interictal recording. As discussed in Part III, some interictal EEG abnormalities correlate with a predisposition to generate seizures, and interictal EEG findings can sometimes provide information regarding the specific epilepsy syndrome.

Before these investigations, patients should be advised that the evaluation often fails to identify a specific underlying reason for seizures, so they should not be distressed if the search is unrevealing.

VI. Management of Seizures and Epilepsy

A. Patients with Seizures but No Proven Epilepsy

For patients with provoked seizures, management usually involves correction of the precipitating condition. For example, seizures occurring in the setting of severe hyperglycemia or uremia are best addressed by treating the underlying metabolic abnormality, and seizures related to drug toxicity or alcohol withdrawal require management of the underlying substance abuse problem. Treatment directed at the seizure itself is generally unnecessary. The main exception is status epilepticus due to an underlying toxic/metabolic disorder, for which antiepileptic drugs (AEDs) may be required acutely until the underlying abnormality can be corrected (see Part VII).

For patients who have experienced an isolated, unprovoked seizure, management decisions are complicated. Because only about half of these patients will go on to have further seizures (i.e., they will prove to have epilepsy), the risk of prolonged AED use when it is not necessary must be balanced against the risk of delay in starting an AED in a patient who ultimately proves to need it. Initiation of an AED after a single unprovoked seizure reduces the risk of recurrence but does not affect long-term prognosis. Thus, for patients in whom there is no evidence of a brain disorder predisposing to seizures, it is reasonable to follow the patient conservatively and only prescribe an AED if the patient has a second seizure. In contrast, certain abnormalities on neurologic examination, imaging studies, or EEG can signify an underlying condition that predisposes to seizures and warrants treatment after a single episode.

B. Patients with Epilepsy

1. Antiepileptic Drugs (AEDs)

A few patients have seizures very infrequently, perhaps once every few years, and they would rather live with these rare seizures than take medication on a regular basis. Because there is no proof that such rare seizures produce any long-term adverse consequences, this choice can be reasonable for some patients. This situation is quite rare, however. Most patients with epilepsy have more than one seizure a year. Even patients whose seizures are infrequent often find them so disturbing that they will go to great lengths to avoid them. Thus, almost all patients with epilepsy receive AEDs.

The term "anti-epileptic drug" simply refers to the fact that a drug is useful in treating patients who have epilepsy. These medications suppress seizures—there is no evidence that they affect the underlying epilepsy. All of the medications in this category are known to alter the electrical properties of neurons, typically by affecting membrane ion channels or receptors, but they have not been shown to induce any permanent change in the neuron's electrical properties or in the pattern of neuronal connections. Thus, there is no reason to think that they change the underlying predisposition to have seizures—i.e., the epilepsy. Nonetheless, many patients who have been seizure-free for a number of years while taking AEDs are able to discontinue the medications and their seizures do not return. It is not clear why this is so. Most likely, it is due to spontaneous reorganization of the underlying synaptic connections. Given that spontaneous remission is rare in untreated patients with epilepsy, it seems likely that recurrent seizures reinforce the connections responsible for the seizure circuit, and by suppressing those seizures, AEDs may eliminate that reinforcement. In other words, AEDs may provide an environment that allows the epileptic brain to "heal itself" even though they do not directly heal epilepsy.

Table 5.2 lists the most commonly used AEDs, the seizure types for which they are indicated, typical dosage regimens, and side effects. Choice of the optimum AED for a particular patient depends on an accurate classification of the underlying epilepsy syndrome. When the syndrome includes several types of seizures, the goal is to use a single medication that is effective against all the varieties of seizures the patient experiences.

The Federal Drug Administration (FDA) approves new AEDs either for initial monotherapy of a given seizure type or as adjunctive therapy. This reflects the way that new AEDs are tested clinically. Because effective treatment is available for most seizure types, it would be unethical to conduct a placebo-controlled trial in which some patients receive the new, unproven drug as monotherapy and others receive placebo. Instead, most new AEDs are tested in patients with epilepsy who are already taking an established AED, but continue to have seizures despite this treatment. Some of the patients are assigned to receive the new AED as an "add-on" to their ongoing AED, and others to receive a placebo add-on. If the new AED is more effective than placebo, this evidence can be submitted to the FDA for approval of the new AED as an adjunctive medication. It could well be that the new AED would also be effective as initial monotherapy, but the initial clinical trial did not examine this question. Once the new AED had been shown to be effective as adjunctive therapy, it is ethical to conduct studies in which some patients receive the new AED as monotherapy and others receive an established AED. Such trials have been conducted for some AEDs, and have demonstrated the drug's efficacy as monotherapy, so that the FDA has revised the drug's indication. Other AEDs either have not been studied as initial monotherapy or the results have not been submitted to the FDA (in part because physicians can legally prescribe an approved medication to any patient, whether or not the patient has the condition for which the medication was approved, so if enough physicians are convinced that an AED approved for adjunctive therapy is a reasonable choice for initial monotherapy, the pharmaceutical company has little incentive to seek formal FDA approval). The older AEDs—phenobarbital, phenytoin, carbamazepine, and valproic acid—were released at a time when the FDA applied different standards for efficacy. Table 5.2 lists the official FDA indications for each AED, but some of the medications are used more widely than the table would suggest.

For some types of seizures, Table 5.2 lists several different effective medications. Only a few studies have directly compared one drug to another in specific clinical settings, so the selection of a specific drug from among several effective alternatives is based primarily on issues such as side-effect

Table 5.2. Anti-epileptic Drugs

Generic Name (Trade Names)	FDA-Approved Indications	Routes of Administration	Daily Doses in Adults [mg/kg]	Oral Half-life [Dose Schedule]	Side Effects
Carbamazepine (Tegretol, Carbatrol)	Focal (M, A); Generalized tonic-clonic (M, A)	PO	600–2400 mg [10–20 mg/kg]	7–8 hrs [t.i.d.] (extended release: [daily or b.i.d.]	ataxia, nystagmus, diplopia, hyponatremia, leucopenia, hepatotoxicity, osteopenia, rash
Clonazepam (Klonopin)	Absence (M, A—for patients who have failed ethosuximide); Myoclonic (M, A); Akinetic (M, A)	PO, IV	0.5–20 mg [0.01–0.2 mg/kg]	18–50 hrs [daily or b.i.d.]	sedation, cognitive dysfunction, incoordination
Ethosuximide (Zarontin)	Absence (M, A)	PO	500–1500 mg [15–25 mg/kg]	30–60 hrs [daily or b.i.d.]	nausea, sedation, bone marrow suppression, rash
Gabapentin (Neurontin)	Focal (A)	PO	900–4800 mg [25–60 mg/kg]	5–9 hrs [t.i.d. or q.i.d.]	somnolence, edema, weight gain, fatigue, ataxia, dizziness, nausea, tremor
Lacosamide (Vimpat)	Focal (A)	PO, IV	200–400 mg [3–6 mg/kg]	12–16 hrs [b.i.d.]	dizziness, ataxia, headache, nausea, diplopia, prolonged PR interval

Drug	Seizure type	Route	Dose	Half-life	Side effects
Lamotrigine (Lamictal)	Focal (M – when converting from another AED; A), Generalized tonic-clonic (A), Lenox-Gastaut (A)	PO	*	13 hrs on enzyme-inducers without valproic acid; 60 hrs on valproic acid without enzyme-inducers; 25 hrs otherwise [b.i.d.]	rash (sometimes severe), dizziness, sedation, diplopia, headache, nausea
Levetiracetam (Keppra)	Focal (A), Generalized tonic-clonic (A), Juvenile myoclonic epilepsy (A)	PO, IV	1000–3000 mg [20–40 mg/kg]	6–8 hrs [b.i.d.]	somnolence, dizziness, anxiety, behavioral and psychiatric manifestations
Oxcarbazepine (Trileptal)	Focal (M, A)	PO	900–2400 mg [15–30 mg/kg]	7–12 hrs [b.i.d.]	dizziness, ataxia, diplopia, somnolence, headache, fatigue, hyponatremia, rash
Phenobarbital	Focal ** (M, A), Generalized tonic-clonic ** (M, A)	PO, IV	60–240 mg [1–3 mg/kg]	65–130 hrs [daily]	sedation, dizziness, ataxia, osteopenia, behavior disturbance (in children)

(continued)

Table 5.2. Anti-epileptic Drugs (*cont'd*)

Generic Name (Trade Names)	FDA-Approved Indications	Routes of Administration	Daily Doses in Adults [mg/kg]	Oral Half-life [Dose Schedule]	Side Effects
Phenytoin (Dilantin, Phenytek)	Focal (M, A) Generalized tonic-clonic (M, A)	PO, IV	300–600 mg [5–10 mg/kg]	10–60 hrs [daily]	ataxia, dizziness, sedation, rash, gingival hyperplasia, hirsutism, leucopenia, hepatotoxicity, osteopenia, lymphadenopathy
Pregabalin (Lyrica)	Focal (A)	PO	150–600 mg [2.5–10 mg/kg]	5–7 hrs [b.i.d. or t.i.d.]	weight gain, edema, somnolence, dizziness, ataxia, tremor
Primidone (Mysoline)	Focal ** (M, A) Generalized tonic-clonic ** (M, A)	PO	500–1000 mg [10–25 mg/kg]	primidone: 8–15 hrs; phenobarbital: 65–130 hrs [daily or b.i.d.]	sedation, dizziness, ataxia, osteopenia, behavioral disturbances (in children)
Rufinamide (Banzel)	Lennox-Gastaut (A)	PO	400–3200 mg [10–45 mg/kg]	6–10 hrs [b.i.d.]	dizziness, headache, nausea, ataxia, somnolence, shortened QT interval, anemia, leucopenia

Tiagabine (Gabitril)	Focal (A)	PO	15–32 mg [0.25–0.5 mg/kg]; 30–56 mg in pts taking enzyme-inducers	5–9 hrs (2–4 hrs in pts taking enzyme-inducers) [b.i.d. to q.i.d.]	dizziness, somnolence, cognitive disturbance, irritability, tremor
Topiramate (Topamax)	Focal (M, A) Generalized tonic-clonic (M, A) Lennox-Gastaut (A)	PO	100–500 mg [2–9 mg/kg]	12–30 hrs [b.i.d.]	somnolence, cognitive disturbance, paresthesias, ataxia, dizziness, weight loss, kidney stones, metabolic acidosis, impaired sweating, emotional lability
Valproic acid (Depakote, Depacon, Depakene)	Focal (M, A) Absence (M, A) Others *** (A)	PO, IV	500–4000 mg [15–60 mg/kg]	5–15 hrs [b.i.d. or t.i.d. (for extended release, daily or b.i.d.)	tremor, weight gain, nausea, sedation, hepatotoxicity, hyperammonemia, thrombocytopenia, hair loss, pancreatitis

(continued)

Table 5.2. Anti-epileptic Drugs (cont'd)

Generic Name (Trade Names)	FDA-Approved Indications	Routes of Administration	Daily Doses in Adults [mg/kg]	Oral Half-life [Dose Schedule]	Side Effects
Vigabatrin (Sabril)	Infantile spasms (M)	PO	1000–3000 mg [50–150 mg/kg in infants]	6–8 hrs [b.i.d.]	irreversible visual field constriction, headache, somnolence, dizziness, ataxia, weight gain
Zonisamide (Zonegran)	Focal (A)	PO	200–600 mg [4–8 mg/kg]	50–70 hrs (25–40 hrs in pts taking enzyme inducers) [daily or b.i.d.]	somnolence, cognitive disturbance, kidney stones, weight loss, rash, impaired sweating

M = FDA-approved as monotherapy

A = FDA-approved as adjunctive therapy

* - Lamotrigine dose ranges depend on the other AEDs a patient is taking.

a. For patients taking valproic acid and no drugs that induce glucuronidation (e.g., carbamazepine, phenytoin, phenobarbital, or primidone), lamotrigine dose range is 100–200 mg/day (initial dose 25 mg every other day; after 2 weeks increase to 25 mg/day; increase by 25 mg/day every 1–2 weeks thereafter).

b. For patients taking valproic acid and one or more drugs that induce glucuronidation, lamotrigine dose range is 100–400 mg/day (initial dose 25 mg every other day; after 2 weeks increase to 25 mg/day; increase by 25 mg/day every 1–2 weeks thereafter).

c. For patients taking one or more drugs that induce glucuronidation, but not valproic acid, lamotrigine dose range is 300–600 mg/day (initial dose 50 mg/day; after 2 weeks increase to 50 mg b.i.d.; increase by 100 mg/day every 1–2 weeks thereafter).

For patients not taking valproic acid or drugs that induce glucuronidation, lamotrigine dose range is 200–400 mg/day (initial dose 25 mg/day; after 2 weeks increase to 25 mg b.i.d.; increase by 50 mg/day every 1–2 weeks thereafter).

** - FDA indications for phenobarbital and primidone are vaguely worded.

*** - FDA indications for valproic acid are for (1) monotherapy or adjunctive therapy for focal seizures or absence seizures, and (2) adjunctive therapy for "multiple seizure types that include absence seizures."

profiles, ease of administration, and cost. Taking such factors into consideration, the following general guidelines can be proposed.

a. Focal seizures (simple or complex, with or without generalization). As far as anyone knows, simple partial seizures and complex partial seizures respond equally to any given AED, and focal seizures that generalize respond the same way as those that don't, so all focal seizures are grouped together with respect to AED use. Carbamazepine, phenytoin, oxcarbazepine, topiramate, and valproic acid are approved by the FDA for initial treatment of focal seizures, although valproic acid tends to be less well tolerated than the first four medications. Lamotrigine has FDA approval as monotherapy, but only in patients who have previously been on another AED. There is evidence that levetiracetam and gabapentin are also effective as initial monotherapy, even though they have FDA approval only as adjunctive therapy. Phenobarbital and primidone are probably effective, but they are rarely used in adults due to sedation. The only agent that has *no* role in the treatment of focal seizures – neither as initial monotherapy nor as adjunctive therapy – is ethosuximide.

b. Absence seizures.
Ethosuximide and valproic acid are the two medications approved by the FDA for initial monotherapy. If the patient has other types of seizures in addition to absence, valproic acid is necessary, because valproic acid is effective against a broad range of seizure types whereas ethosuximide has a very narrow range of efficacy. Clonazepam has FDA approval for patients who have failed ethosuximide, but it is very sedating. Lamotrigine is also effective, though not FDA-approved in this setting. In a randomized controlled trial comparing ethosuximide, valproic acid, and lamotrigine, ethosuximide and valproic acid were more effective than lamotrigine for absence seizures, and ethosuximide had less adverse effects on attention than valproic acid did. Thus, ethosuximide is probably the treatment of choice for initial therapy. There is some weaker evidence that topiramate and zonisamide are also effective for absence seizures. In some patients, carbamazepine, oxcarbazepine, phenytoin, and tiagabine may exacerbate absence seizures.

c. Myoclonic seizures.
No randomized trials have examined AEDs for initial monotherapy of myoclonic seizures. Based on extensive open-label experience, valproic acid is almost universally considered the agent of choice for myoclonic

seizures, even though it only has FDA approval as adjunctive therapy. Levetiracetam also has FDA approval as adjunctive therapy for myoclonic seizures in patients with juvenile myoclonic epilepsy. Clonazepam has FDA approval as initial monotherapy, but this is not based on randomized, controlled trials, and clonazepam is highly sedating. Some evidence supports the use of lamotrigine, topiramate, and zonisamide as second-line options.

d. Generalized tonic-clonic seizures.

This is probably the category about which there is the least consensus. Phenytoin, valproic acid, lamotrigine, levetiracetam, and topiramate are all reasonable choices, although of these medications, only phenytoin and topiramate are approved by the FDA as initial monotherapy for this indication. Carbamazepine is also FDA approved in this context, although it can actually exacerbate other types of generalized seizures (absence and myoclonic seizures) in some patients. Phenobarbital and primidone are also effective for generalized tonic-clonic seizures, but typically avoided in adults due to sedation.

e. Infantile spasms.

Vigabatrin is the only AED approved by the FDA for infantile spasms. About a third of patients who receive this drug develop irreversible visual field constriction, so regularly scheduled visual testing is required. Corticotropin (ACTH) is also widely used for infantile spasms.

The following general principles apply to the institution of any AED.

a. Begin at a Low Dose and Increase Slowly

Unless a patient is having frequent and uncontrolled seizures, the drug should be introduced slowly to allow the metabolism to "ramp up" to a steady state and to give the patient time to adjust to the sometimes troubling initial symptoms such as sleepiness and a slight reduction in mental sharpness. The dose should be increased gradually until seizure control is achieved or the patient can't tolerate any further increase because of toxic symptoms. Serum drug levels should not be the principal basis for making dose adjustments. The published "therapeutic range" for any drug is based on a population average. There is considerable variability in individual patients' responses to these drugs. Some patients achieve complete seizure control with levels below the published therapeutic range, whereas others require levels higher than the upper limit of the range. Some patients experience unacceptable toxic effects at the lowest possible doses of a medication, whereas others have no problems at levels above the therapeutic range. Drug levels thus provide only approximate guidelines for therapy. They are useful for monitoring drug compliance, and they may also be helpful in determining why a patient who was previously well controlled has resumed having seizures. If there is a record of the drug level during the period of good control, it can be compared to the current drug level. Superimposed medical illnesses or drug-drug interactions may cause changes in AED levels despite a stable dosing regimen.

b. Use One Drug at a Time

If a patient's seizures remain uncontrolled at the highest dose a patient can tolerate, the medication dosage should be reduced slightly to the highest dose the patient can tolerate, while adding a second medication at a low dose. The dose of this second medication should be gradually increased as necessary for seizure control. If seizures are not controlled even after increasing the dose of the second medication as high as the patient can tolerate, then one of the two medications (whichever one seems to be less effective or harder for the patient to tolerate) should be gradually withdrawn and replaced with a third agent. This maneuver should be repeated (up to a point—see the discussion of surgical resection for refractory epilepsy below) until a medication pair is found that controls the patient's seizures without producing unacceptable side effects. When this has been accomplished, it is usually prudent to leave the patient on both medications for a while, but if the patient remains seizure-free, at some point it is reasonable to consider whether the most recently added medication would be sufficient to control the patient's seizures all by itself—i.e., to withdraw the other medication gradually. If seizures recur, the dose can be increased back to the previously effective dose and the patient can remain on the combination regimen. Only occasionally do patients need to use more than two AEDs at one time.

The same considerations that apply to the initial choice of AED also apply to the selection of subsequent AEDs, but in addition, the potential for drug-drug interactions must be weighed. Levetiracetam, gabapentin, and pregabalin do not affect other AEDs and are not affected by them, so they are the least complicated of the various adjunctive choices. In fact, they have very few interactions with other medications of any type, so they are often prescribed for patients with multiple medical problems who are taking numerous medications. In contrast, carbamazepine, oxcarbazepine, phenobarbital, phenytoin, primidone, and valproic acid affect the plasma levels of many other drugs. The interaction between valproic acid and lamotrigine is particularly important. In patients taking valproic acid, lamotrigine must be started at an extremely low dose and the dose must be advanced very slowly, or the risk of a severe skin reaction is increased.

c. Bone Density

Decreased bone density can occur in patients who take phenytoin, valproic acid, phenobarbital, or primidone on a chronic basis. Carbamazepine may also affect bone metabolism, but the evidence is conflicting. AEDs that do not induce liver enzymes do not appear to affect bone metabolism.

d. Baseline and Follow-up Measurements

Patients must be educated about strict compliance and possible side effects. For certain drugs, periodic laboratory testing is necessary to monitor for potential toxicity (such as bone marrow suppression, liver damage, or osteopenia). These laboratory tests should also be checked before starting the patient on the medication so that a baseline is available for comparison. Some evidence suggests that phenytoin and carbamazepine are associated with elevated cholesterol levels, so patients on these medications should also have lipid profiles checked periodically. For vigabatrin, periodic visual field testing is mandatory.

e. Duration of AED Treatment

When seizure control is achieved, patients should be informed that they must remain on the AED until instructed otherwise by their physician. For patients with some epilepsy syndromes, such as juvenile myoclonic epilepsy, the likelihood of seizure recurrence after AED withdrawal is so high that lifelong medication is usually necessary. For patients with other epilepsy syndromes, it is often reasonable to attempt to withdraw AEDs after the seizures have been completely controlled for 2 years or more, but this should always be performed under the close supervision of a physician. The medication taper should be gradual (over approximately 3–6 months). Seizures are most likely to recur within the first year after drug withdrawal. Factors that favor successful withdrawal from AEDs include a longer period of complete seizure control, a normal neurologic examination, idiopathic seizure type, a low overall number of seizures, and probably a normal EEG or an EEG that is improved over the baseline tracing.

2. Surgical Resection of the Seizure Focus

When seizure control is not achieved after an adequate trial of three AEDs, the likelihood of success with subsequent AEDs is very low. About one fourth of patients with epilepsy have seizures that can not be fully controlled with medications, and about half of these patients are candidates for surgical resection of the seizure focus. To establish that a patient is a surgical candidate, it is necessary to prove that the patient's spells are definitely seizures, that the majority of the seizures originate from a single focus, and that the focus is in a region of brain that can be removed safely. To identify the site of seizure onset as precisely as possible, patients are typically hospitalized for long-term video/EEG recording of ictal activity, sometimes using invasive recording with depth or subdural electrodes. Functional imaging studies of cerebral metabolic activity or blood flow at baseline and immediately after a seizure are also used. Other investigations are aimed at determining whether the portion of brain where the seizures originate may be safely removed without causing serious neurologic deficits (such as severe memory loss, language disturbance, or major motor deficits). In carefully selected groups of patients, resective surgery may produce complete seizure resolution in up to 80% of patients in whom medical therapy has failed.

3. Other Ablative Surgery

In addition to resection of the seizure focus, other surgical approaches are sometimes pursued. Hemispherectomies may be an option in young children with widely distributed epileptic disturbances over one hemisphere, especially when there is a contralateral hemiparesis. Section of the corpus callosum can be of benefit in a small number of patients with refractory seizures characterized by frequent falls and sometimes other seizure types. Such patients may achieve elimination of one seizure type but generally do not become seizure free. Another disconnection procedure that can be effective in select patients is to perform multiple subpial transections.

4. Vagus Nerve Stimulation

Vagus nerve stimulation is another surgical approach that can be tried in patients who are refractory to medical therapy; its mechanism of action is not well understood. Two helical electrode coils are wrapped around the left vagus nerve in the carotid sheath and connected to an infraclavicular pulse generator. The generator is then programmed to deliver pulses of a specified duration, frequency, and amplitude. Patients treated in this way have on average a 25–30% reduction in seizure frequency, and 25–30% of patients have at least a 50% reduction in seizure frequency, which is comparable to the results obtained with most adjunctive medications. Patients also have the option of using an external magnet to activate the device when they start to experience a seizure; for some patients, this can abort the seizure or reduce its severity.

5. Ketogenic Diet

In children with epilepsy whose seizures can not be controlled with medications (or who require such high doses of medication that the side-effects are unacceptable), a high-fat, adequate-protein, low-carbohydrate diet can produce a significant reduction in seizure frequency. The mechanism is not known. The benefit does not appear to depend on seizure type or EEG pattern. Some evidence suggests that this approach (known as the ketogenic diet because it mimics a starvation state and results in increased production of ketone bodies) is also effective in adults, but further study is necessary. Compliance with this diet can be difficult. Constipation and gastro-esophageal reflux are common. Other potential adverse effects include growth retardation, renal stones, and hypercholesterolemia.

C. Patient Education (for Patients with Isolated Seizures or Epilepsy)

Certain issues are such a frequent source of confusion or concern for patients and their family members that physicians should make a point of discussing them explicitly. Good resources can be found online at the websites www.epilepsy.com and www.epilepsyfoundation.org.

1. Reassurance Regarding the Nature of Seizures

Seizures can be very frightening for patients and observers alike. You should reassure patients and their family members that seizures are a common, well-described phenomenon. Explain that if the patient has another seizure, bystanders should try to get the patient into a position that limits the risk of a dangerous fall, but they do not need to intervene in any other way as long as the seizure resolves quickly.

2. Expectations Regarding the Diagnostic Evaluation

Explain that you will be ordering blood tests, urine tests, a brain CT scan, and possibly a lumbar puncture to look for anything that might have provoked the seizure, but that you will not be surprised if all the results are normal–in many patients with seizures, no underlying cause is identified. Similarly, you will be arranging for the patient to have an EEG and MRI at some point in the next few weeks, but it will not be surprising if those results are normal or nonspecific, also.

3. Rationale for Not Starting an AED

Explain to the patient that a single seizure is often an isolated event that never recurs, and for this reason, anti-epileptic medication is not usually recommended after a single seizure. Go into as much detail as the patient requires regarding the relative risks of an unnecessary medication vs. an untreated seizure. When patients insist that they would prefer to be on medication, and you are convinced that they understand the relevant issues and risks, it may be appropriate to prescribe one.

4. Reassurance Regarding Epilepsy

Patients who ultimately prove to have epilepsy often require reassurance that they can still lead normal and productive lives. Many prominent people in the worlds of art, literature, music, politics, and sport have had epilepsy. The stigma that traditionally surrounded epilepsy was misguided.

5. AED Risks and Benefits

When you prescribe an AED, explain how you plan to adjust the dose, and review the potential side effects. Be sure the patient understands that there is no single medication that is effective for all patients with a given type of epilepsy, and that for any given medication the effective dose varies from one person to another, so an element of trial and error is unavoidable. While the medication is being titrated, patients may experience additional seizures, which can cause them and their family members considerable distress, but you should urge them not to overreact. Ultimately, the goal is to eliminate seizures entirely, but some seizures along the way may be unavoidable. Although you should try to avoid unnecessary delays, you should also avoid making changes too quickly. A seizure that occurs shortly after increasing the medication dose may not be a true reflection of the effects of the higher dose. Likewise, it may take several weeks for a side-effect to resolve after reducing the dose. By making sure that patients have realistic expectations and a clear understanding of how they are supposed to take their medications, you can increase the likelihood that they will be compliant.

D. Restrictions (for Patients with Isolated Seizures or Epilepsy)

The laws regarding driving vary considerably from state to state. In twenty-seven states (and the District of Columbia), any person who has experienced a seizure (or any unprovoked episode of altered consciousness in many states) is forbidden to drive for a set period of time that is not subject to modification. The required seizure-free interval is 3 months in seven of these states, 6 months in thirteen states, and 12 months in seven states and the District of Columbia. The other twenty-three states also apply restrictions, but with somewhat greater flexibility, often based on the recommendation of the treating physician. In most states, the physician is required to inform the patient of the law regarding driving and to document in writing in the medical record that the patient has been informed. In six states, physicians are required to notify the Department of Motor Vehicles directly. Individual state driving restrictions are available at the internet sites, epilepsy.com and epilepsyfoundation.org.

Other common-sense restrictions also apply. No epileptic patient should swim alone. Epileptic patients should use a shower rather than a bathtub, as it is possible to drown in just a few inches of water. They should avoid situations that might put them at risk if they were to have a seizure, such as working at heights or using power equipment.

VII. Special Clinical Problems

A. Status Epilepticus

Status epilepticus is defined in Part III. It is a medical emergency with significant mortality (10%) and major morbidity. The prognosis is closely related to the cause. When status epilepticus is due to poor medication compliance in patients previously diagnosed with epilepsy, it usually responds to reinstitution of AEDs and the outlook for the patient is favorable. In patients with no prior history of epilepsy, the most common causes of status epilepticus are stroke, meningitis, encephalitis, and hypoxic-ischemic encephalopathy. The prognosis for these patients is worse. The longer a patient is in status, the worse the outcome. This is partly because the duration is more likely to be prolonged in patients with more severe underlying disease, but there is also considerable experimental evidence that status epilepticus itself damages the brain and that the degree of damage is a function of duration.

The medications that are most commonly used to treat status epilepticus are benzodiazepines, phenytoin (or its prodrug, fosphenytoin), barbiturates, propofol, and valproic acid. Levetiracetam, topiramate, inhalation anesthetics, and electroconvulsive therapy have also been reported to be useful. Zonisamide and lacosamide have also been used. Only a few randomized, controlled trials have directly compared one medication to another in patients with status epilepticus. In one study, use of lorazepam alone was more effective than use of phenytoin alone, so lorazepam is generally considered the initial agent of choice, but its half-life is short, so a second agent is usually necessary.

There is no consensus regarding which agent should be used next, but all experts agree that delay should be avoided. Animal and human studies indicate that the efficacy of treatment decreases the longer the seizures have been present, so in the absence of clear evidence that one AED is superior to another, the physician should simply choose one protocol and commit it to memory so that the treatment of status epilepticus becomes practically a matter of reflex response. This will prevent wasting valuable moments while trying to decide which agent to use or where to find it. Treatment should be initiated whenever seizure activity persists significantly longer than usual for the patient. If the patient's baseline is not known, treatment should be initiated whenever seizure activity persists beyond 5–10 minutes. One such protocol is outlined in Table 5.3.

All of the agents listed in Table 5.3 have the potential to suppress respiration and reduce blood pressure. These parameters must be followed closely, and patients may require intubation with mechanical ventilation or blood pressure support. Arrhythmias can also occur with IV administration of phenytoin, so cardiac monitoring is necessary.

Many of the adverse effects of IV phenytoin occur because it is relatively insoluble in water and the vehicle in which it is administered can cause hypotension. Fosphenytoin, a water-soluble pro-drug that is rapidly and completely converted to phenytoin, was developed to avoid these problems. Compared to phenytoin, fosphenytoin produces less pain at the injection site, has lower risk of serious consequences from extravasation, and causes fewer instances of hypotension or other cardiovascular complications. Doses are expressed in "mg phenytoin equivalents," or "mg PE," which is the amount of phenytoin that will be produced by conversion.

Some experts maintain that the second agent after lorazepam should be midazolam, propofol, or phenobarbital, rather than fosphenytoin. The dosing regimen for midazolam and phenobarbital is indicated in Table 5.3; for propofol, the regimen is 1–2 mg/kg boluses every 3–5 minutes until seizures stop, up to a maximum of 10 mg/kg, then 2 mg/kg/hr. Others advocate valproic acid instead of fosphenytoin as the second agent, especially in patients who are already hypotensive. The dosing regimen for valproic acid is 30 mg/kg over 15–20 minutes. Some experts recommend proceeding as quickly as possible to induced coma with pentobarbital or

Table 5.3. Step-By-Step Management of Generalized Convulsive Status Epilepticus

1.	Ensure adequate cardiorespiratory function, insert an oral airway, give oxygen.
2.	Insert IV line. Measure blood count, electrolytes, blood urea nitrogen, glucose, calcium, magnesium, AED levels where applicable, and toxin screen. Send arterial blood for pH, pO_2, pCO_2, and HCO_3.
3.	Start IV line with normal saline. If hypoglycemia is suspected, confirm by fingerstick, then give 50 mg of 50% glucose and 100 mg of thiamine.
4.	Give IV lorazepam, 0.1–0.2 mg/kg at 2 mg/minute (maximum adult dose 8 mg).
5.*	Give IV fosphenytoin*, 20 mg phenytoin equivalents/kg at 150 mg phenytoin equivalents/minute. (If IV access not available, give IM at same dose. If fosphenytoin unavailable, give IV phenytoin, 20 mg/kg at no more than 50 mg/minute, diluted in 100 ml of normal saline.)
6.*	If seizures persist, give additional IV fosphenytoin*, 10 mg phenytoin equivalents/kg at same rate as before (or IM if no IV access, or phenytoin, 10 mg/kg at same rate as before, if fosphenytoin unavailable).
7.	If seizures persist, give IV midazolam, 0.2 mg/kg load followed by 0.1–0.4 mg/kg/hour infusion.
8.	If seizures persist, give IV phenobarbital, 20 mg/kg at 50–100 mg/minute.
9.	If seizures persist, induce barbiturate coma or initiate very high-dose phenobarbital therapy.

* Many experts prefer valproic acid to fosphenytoin at this stage; some skip this step entirely—see text.

phenobarbital, skipping one or more of the intermediate steps listed in Table 5.3.

If the motor manifestations of status epilepticus resolve, but the patient's mental status does not normalize, an EEG should be obtained to determine if electrographic seizures are still present. Ongoing electrographic seizure activity without any motor manifestation is termed nonconvulsive status epilepticus. If this condition is present, it should be treated as aggressively as if motor activity were still evident (convulsive status epilepticus).

In contrast to the situation in which nonconvulsive status epilepticus evolves from convulsive status epilepticus, some patients present with status epilepticus that is nonconvulsive from the outset. For example, patients with complex partial seizures or absence seizures can develop status epilepticus. Patients with focal seizures can also develop convulsive status epilepticus that only affects one region of the body; this is known as epilepsia partialis continua. In general, these forms of status epilepticus have a better prognosis than generalized convulsive status epilepticus, and a less aggressive management protocol is often applied.

B. Seizures and Pregnancy

Some difficult management issues arise for women with epilepsy who want to have children. Seizures pose a risk to the fetus, and so does AED exposure. Although no controlled trials have directly compared these risks, most experts agree that the risk to the fetus from uncontrolled convulsive seizures outweighs the risk from AED exposure, and that complete AED withdrawal is not a reasonable or safe option for most women. Fortunately, the absolute magnitude of risk is low, and the vast majority of women give birth to perfectly healthy children. The goal should be to identify the medications that pose the lowest risk, and to determine the safest ways to administer them.

Most studies suggest that AEDs taken during the first trimester of pregnancy increase the risk of major congenital malformations in the offspring. Folic acid supplementation before conception and during pregnancy may reduce this risk. The evidence is not conclusive with respect to particular AEDs and specific malformations, and it is difficult to compare the risk of one AED to that of another, but the evidence is most compelling for a link between valproic acid and neural tube defects. The evidence also suggests that the risk of major congenital malformations is lower when patients take a single AED than when they take two or more AEDs, especially when the polypharmacy regimen includes valproic acid. For some AEDs, higher doses during the first trimester are associated with a higher risk of major congenital malformations. Cognitive deficits appear to be more common in children exposed in utero to valproic acid, and possibly in those exposed to phenytoin or phenobarbital. Poor cognitive outcomes are more common in children exposed to polytherapy in utero than in children exposed to monotherapy. Some experts have suggested that pregnant women who are taking AEDs should take oral vitamin K during the month preceding the expected date of delivery to counteract any bleeding diathesis that might result from deficiency of vitamin K-dependent clotting factors, but there is no compelling evidence to support or refute this practice (or the existence of an increased risk of hemorrhagic complications in the newborn period).

Physiologic changes during pregnancy can alter the metabolism, clearance, and protein-binding of AEDs. As a result, total and free drug levels may vary in ways that are difficult to predict.

When taking care of women with epilepsy, you should ask them explicitly if they anticipate getting pregnant in the next few years. If they are planning a pregnancy, and if they have been seizure-free for a number of years, it may be possible to withdraw AEDs. If not, the goal should be to maintain them on a monotherapy regimen, using the lowest effective dose, avoiding valproic acid if at all possible, and perhaps avoiding phenytoin and phenobarbital, also. Before they begin trying to conceive, they should start taking daily folic acid, at least 0.4 mg per day, and you should check baseline free and total serum AED levels. At regular intervals throughout the pregnancy, adjust the medication dosage as necessary to keep the free level the same as the baseline free level. At the time of delivery, the newborns should receive the same dose of vitamin K routinely administered to all newborns.

Women with epilepsy who are not contemplating pregnancy should also be informed of these issues, so that they can seek medical attention promptly if they become pregnant unintentionally. There are many potential interactions between AEDs and oral contraceptive drugs. Clinicians should be sure to review these before starting or stopping any medication.

C. Refractory Seizures

When seizures fail to respond to medications, the treating physician should review the following points: Was the original diagnosis of epilepsy accurate? If so, was the correct type of epilepsy identified and were the appropriate AEDs used? If so, is the patient truly compliant, as determined by adequate AED levels? Does the patient's lifestyle require modification? Were the medications pushed to the highest doses the patient could tolerate? Were combination regimens attempted? Patients who continue to be refractory to medical management should be referred to a major epilepsy center where experimental AEDs or epilepsy surgery may be available.

VIII. Discussion of Case Histories

Case 1: Seven-year-old boy with absence seizures. This history is typical of absence seizures. The provocation of the attacks by hyperventilation is also characteristic. Other entities to be considered in the differential diagnosis would be complex partial seizures (which can also be associated with motionless staring with no other symptoms, but are less readily provoked by hyperventilation), attention deficit disorder, or some other form of behavioral disturbance. The EEG findings were bursts of generalized 3-Hz spike-and-wave activity occurring spontaneously and provoked by hyperventilation. In view of the normal neurologic examination and the generalized nature of the child's EEG discharges, no imaging studies are indicated. This child was treated with ethosuximide, introduced slowly and built up to a dose of 750 mg (25 mg/kg for this 30 kg boy) per day. This drug is well tolerated and eliminates both the seizure activity and the EEG discharges in almost all cases. The outlook for normal neurologic and intellectual development in this patient is excellent.

Case 2: Young woman with localization-related epilepsy. Based on her history, this young woman has seizures that are simple partial at onset, progress to complex partial, and then progress to secondarily generalized tonic-clonic seizures. Of note, she had a higher than average risk of developing epilepsy because the febrile convulsions when she was age 15 months were prolonged and associated with focal abnormalities on neurologic examination, but this was still not sufficient reason to start treatment until she actually experienced seizures later in life. She should have an EEG (if it has not already been done), looking for focal slowing and interictal epileptiform activity that could indicate the site of her seizure focus. She should also have a brain MRI scan looking for a structural abnormality underlying her epilepsy, but it can be delayed until after delivery because the long history excludes a rapidly evolving mass lesion. Similarly, a search for a toxic-metabolic cause of seizures is unnecessary given the long history.

Teratogenic effects of AEDs occur during the first trimester. Because this patient was first seen during her second trimester, it would be prudent to continue drug therapy at the current dose. The patient should be seen frequently during the remainder of her pregnancy. Free levels of phenytoin should be checked regularly, and the dose should be adjusted to maintain a stable free level. She should continue to take daily folate throughout the pregnancy.

She has been seizure-free for 4 years, so she might be a candidate for AED withdrawal, but this should be deferred until she is in a relatively stable physiologic state. She is likely to be sleep deprived for at least several months after delivery, and sleep deprivation is a common precipitant of seizures in predisposed patients.

After delivery, she should return to her pre-pregnancy phenytoin dose by the first month postpartum. An MRI scan should be obtained, as mentioned above, and regular follow-up under the supervision of a neurologist should be arranged. About 6 months after delivery, when her metabolism has returned to baseline and her child's sleep schedule has been established, her physician can discuss the advantages and disadvantages of AED withdrawal with her. She will have to weigh the inconvenience of taking daily medications, and the potential side effects (including teratogenic risk if she becomes pregnant again in the future), against the risk of having a seizure while caring for a young child and the inconvenience of refraining from driving while tapering her medication and for some months thereafter. She must ultimately decide which of these considerations are most important to her; she should be reassured that the physician will support her decision either way. If she chooses to remain on an AED, she should continue to take folic acid, 1 mg daily, to reduce the risk of major teratogenic side effects in the event of future pregnancy.

Case 3: Middle-aged woman in convulsive status epilepticus. The emergency room physicians' diagnosis of convulsive status epilepticus is correct. This patient had four tonic-clonic seizures with failure to return to normal consciousness in between, which certainly satisfies the definition of status epilepticus. Emergency management of the patient should proceed as outlined in Part VII. Even if seizures cease rapidly, all patients who have just been treated for status epilepticus should be admitted to an intensive care unit for at least 24 hours of close observation. An epileptic disorder presenting de novo as status epilepticus requires immediate investigation. In this patient, the likelihood of finding a significant underlying problem is high, especially given the history of headaches for the past week. An MRI scan in this patient revealed multiple areas of signal abnormality that enhanced with contrast. The patient proved to have multiple small cerebral metastases from a primary tumor that was never identified.

Chapter 6

Neuromuscular Disorders

Mark B. Bromberg and Douglas J. Gelb

I. Case Histories

Case 1. A 45-year-old woman reports that about 3 months ago she began having trouble standing up from low chairs, and the problem has progressed to the point that she now must use her arms to push off from any chair. She recently started having difficulty holding up her arms to set her hair. Her weakness is symmetric. Her head and neck muscles are strong, and she has no shortness of breath. She has no pain or sensory disturbance. There is no family history of neurologic disorders. She has no relevant past medical history and is taking no medication.

On examination, she has normal mental status and cranial nerve function. Muscle bulk and tone are normal. Neck flexor strength is grade 4 on the 5-point Medical Research Council scale. Shoulder abduction is grade 4 and hip flexion is grade 3, in a symmetric distribution. She must be helped to a standing position and cannot perform a deep knee bend. Tendon reflexes, plantar responses, and sensory examination are normal.

Questions:

1. Does this localize to the peripheral nervous system? If so, is the problem at the level of nerve, neuromuscular junction, or muscle?

2. What tests would you order to confirm the suspected localization? Is this likely to be a treatable condition?

Case 2. A 55-year-old man has been experiencing double vision, mild limb weakness, and rapid fatigability with routine activities. He first noted double vision 6 months ago. It resolved after several days but reappeared 2 weeks ago, and at the same time he began having trouble climbing stairs. His endurance has decreased markedly, to the point where he now must rest after walking a short distance. He has no pain or sensory loss.

He has no history of previous medical problems, and no family history of neurologic disease. He takes no medications.

On examination, he has normal mental status and cranial nerve function except for weakness in the distribution of the right third and sixth cranial nerves, mild right ptosis, and bilateral eye closure weakness. Shoulder abduction and hip flexion are strong on initial testing, but quickly fatigue after several repetitions of muscle activation. Tendon reflexes, plantar responses, and sensory examination are normal.

Questions:

1. What are the important differences between this and the first case? Is the lesion at the same site?
2. What tests, if any, would distinguish between the two conditions?
3. How should this patient be managed?

Case 3. A 60-year-old man fell one year ago and fractured his left ankle. After the cast was removed, he noted weakness and atrophy of his calf. Prolonged physical therapy did not help. Six months ago he began having trouble unscrewing the tops of jars and turning off the bath faucet completely, and when he tried hard he would get muscle cramps. Currently, he is constantly fatigued and has lost 30 lb. His wife says she "can see his muscles working."

On examination, the patient has normal mental status and cranial nerves. He is thin and has frequent muscle twitching (fasciculations) in his trunk and all four limbs. The intrinsic muscles of both hands are atrophic, and atrophy is also prominent in anterior and posterior muscles in the left leg. A clasp-knife phenomenon (spasticity) is evident with passive manipulation of all limbs. Strength is markedly reduced in distal upper extremity muscles and in his left foot, which he cannot move voluntarily. He has mild weakness in all other muscles. Deep tendon reflexes are hyperactive, and he has a right extensor plantar (Babinski) response. Sensory examination is normal.

Questions:

1. How does this pattern of weakness differ from the patterns in Cases 1 and 2?
2. Where does this localize in the nervous system?
3. How should this patient be managed?

Case 4. A 45-year-old woman has difficulty walking and numbness of her legs. She noted tingling in her toes 6 months ago, and it spread over several weeks to include much of her legs. Her fingers have recently developed a similar tingling. She notes difficulty standing from a chair and complains of unsteadiness when she walks. She had similar problems a year ago, but they were less severe, and they resolved without medical consultation.

On examination, her mental status and cranial nerves are normal. She has mild weakness throughout her lower extremities and in the distal muscles of her upper extremities. Tendon reflexes are absent. Her gait is very unsteady, and she cannot maintain her balance with her eyes closed. Vibratory perception is absent in the feet and reduced at the fingers.

Questions:

1. What components of the nervous system are involved? How do they differ from those in Case 3?

2. How would electrodiagnostic tests help distinguish between Cases 3 and 4?

3. How should this patient be managed?

II. Approach to Neuromuscular Diseases

When a patient's symptoms are limited to limb weakness, sensory symptoms, or both, they could localize to the peripheral nervous system. Diseases of the peripheral nervous system are commonly referred to as neuromuscular diseases. Unlike the central nervous system, where a single structural lesion may produce widespread effects because of disruption of ascending and descending fiber tracts, a single structural lesion in the peripheral nervous system produces symptoms in a narrowly localized region of one limb or the trunk. Many diseases affect the peripheral nervous system diffusely, however, producing multiple lesion sites. For these diseases, it is impossible to speak of localization to a single lesion site. While the localization approach described in Chapter 1 is still valid for multifocal and diffuse diseases, it is generally most useful to characterize these diseases by determining which *components* of the peripheral nervous system are affected. For example, some diseases affect peripheral nerves and not muscles, whereas other diseases do the converse. In managing patients with neuromuscular disease, four questions are fundamental:

1. Which components of the peripheral nervous system are involved?

2. What is the specific disease?

3. Is urgent treatment necessary?

3a. Is the patient's disease one that is associated with *autonomic instability* or *respiratory failure*? (These are the only two complications of neuromuscular disease that represent true emergencies.)

3b. If so, how rapidly is the patient's condition deteriorating?

4. What long-term management is indicated?

Question 1 implies that you have already determined that the patient does not have a lesion in the central nervous system, based on the localization reasoning process discussed in Chapter 1 and the examination features discussed in Chapter 2. Additional features useful in localizing the disorder to specific components of the nervous system are discussed in Part III. Questions 2, 3a, and 4 are covered in Part IV. Question 3b is addressed in Part V, along with other management issues common to neuromuscular diseases in general.

III. Background Information

A. Functional Divisions of the Peripheral Nervous System

The peripheral nervous system can be divided into the autonomic and somatic nervous systems. The somatic system is further subdivided into sensory and motor nerves. Motor nerves activate muscles through the neuromuscular junction. The autonomic, somatic sensory, and somatic motor nerves are physically intermingled at some levels of the nervous system and separated at others, but it is useful to conceptualize them as distinct pathways. Each can be associated with a variety of symptoms.

Lesions of the autonomic system can produce dysfunction of practically any visceral organ. Some of the more prominent symptoms include postural hypotension, sphincter dysfunction, impotence, and sweating abnormalities. Lesions of sensory pathways can produce positive symptoms, such as pain or paresthesias (sensations typically likened to "pins and needles"), or negative symptoms, including hypesthesia (reduced sensation) and anesthesia (absence of sensation). Lesions of the peripheral motor system can also produce both negative symptoms (e.g., weakness and muscle atrophy) and positive symptoms (e.g., fasciculations and muscle cramps).

B. Proximal-to-Distal Organization of the Peripheral Nervous System

Disorders of the neuromuscular system can be viewed in a proximal-to-distal anatomic pattern, with different clinical syndromes corresponding to each level of peripheral nervous system involvement. The peripheral nervous system portion of the motor pathway originates in the *anterior horn cells*. Conditions that affect anterior horn cells are known as *motor neuron diseases*. The principal clues that suggest a motor neuron disease are (1) motor signs and symptoms (both positive and negative) in the absence of sensory abnormalities and (2) a patchy distribution, often asymmetric, with no obvious pattern of proximal versus distal muscle involvement.

Lesions affecting dorsal and ventral *roots*, or the spinal roots that they form, are called *radiculopathies*. If more than one nerve root is involved, the term "*polyradiculopathy*" is often used. Structural abnormalities can impinge on a single unilateral nerve root, bilateral nerve roots at a single level, or nerve roots at several contiguous levels. Metabolic, inflammatory, and neoplastic disorders can also affect one or more roots. Radiculopathies may be mild and asymptomatic, or they may be associated with severe pain in the back or limbs. Patients with radiculopathies usually have both sensory and motor symptoms, though one or the other may predominate. The main clue that a patient has a radiculopathy is that all of the sensory and motor symptoms and signs are consistent with the known distribution of one or several nerve roots.

Before forming peripheral nerves, fibers exiting the nerve roots undergo a complex crossing and regrouping to form the brachial plexus and lumbosacral plexus. When patients have symptoms and signs that would suggest a polyradiculopathy but the pattern does not conform to the distribution of any individual nerve root or combination of nerve roots, or to the distribution of any individual peripheral nerve or combination of peripheral nerves, *plexopathy* is likely.

Moving another step distally, peripheral nerve lesions take the form of *polyneuropathies* when involvement is diffuse or *mononeuropathies* when a single nerve is involved. Polyneuropathies frequently affect both sensory and motor nerves, though there are exceptions that involve only one type of nerve. Sensory nerves have a peripheral and a central axon, and both may be affected. Most polyneuropathies affect the longest nerves in the body earliest, so symptoms and signs occur in the feet first and progress proximally. When signs and symptoms reach approximately knee level, nerves to the fingers become involved. This is referred to as a stocking-glove distribution. Length-dependent polyneuropathies are usually symmetric.

The next step going from proximal to distal is the neuromuscular junction. In *disorders of the neuromuscular junction*, the most prominent weakness typically occurs in proximal muscles. For obvious reasons, there are no sensory symptoms. Fatigue is a prominent symptom in the most common neuromuscular junction disease, myasthenia gravis.

The most distal component of the motor pathway is the *muscle*. As with disorders of the neuromuscular junction, primary muscle disorders produce no sensory symptoms, and usually (but not always) result in a proximal distribution of weakness. With some exceptions, primary muscle diseases usually spare muscles innervated by cranial nerves, so symptoms like diplopia, dysarthria, and dysphagia are rare, in contrast to neuromuscular junction disorders. Some hereditary abnormalities of membrane ion channels produce weakness that is episodic, and some result in a phenomenon known as myotonia, which is a prolonged muscle contraction after voluntary concussion or percussion of the muscle.

C. Electrodiagnostic and Other Laboratory Studies

The tests that are most consistently helpful in the diagnosis of peripheral nervous system disorders are electrodiagnostic studies. These consist of nerve conduction studies, tests of neuromuscular junction transmission, and the needle electromyogram (EMG). These tests can be considered an extension of the clinical neurologic examination. In nerve conduction studies, the examiner applies an electric stimulus to a peripheral nerve and measures the amplitude of the response (which reflects the number of nerve fibers present) and the conduction velocity (which primarily assesses the myelin sheath around nerve fibers). Nerve conduction studies help demonstrate whether peripheral nerve function is impaired. By evaluating several sensory and several motor nerves, the examiner can often determine which nerves are most affected and whether the damage reflects primary axonal loss or demyelination. Nerve conductions studies principally assess large-fiber somatic nerves; they are relatively insensitive for detecting dysfunction of small-fiber nerves.

The integrity of the neuromuscular junction can be assessed by repeated stimulation of the motor nerve: A normal neuromuscular junction has adequate reserve to ensure that each stimulus will result in an action potential in the muscle fiber, whereas synaptic transmission sometimes fails when there is a neuromuscular junction disorder. Characteristic patterns of failure help to differentiate postsynaptic defects, such as myasthenia gravis, from presynaptic defects, such as the Lambert-Eaton myasthenic syndrome.

The third component of an electrodiagnostic evaluation is the needle EMG, which records the electrical activity of muscle fibers preceding muscle contraction. Needle EMG is very sensitive to denervation and can be used to distinguish between *neuropathic* changes in muscle (due to primary nerve damage such as radiculopathy, motor neuron disease, or polyneuropathy) and *myopathic* changes (due to primary muscle disorders). In focal neuropathic conditions, such as a mononeuropathy or radiculopathy, the pattern of muscle involvement is often useful in localizing the lesion. A variant of this technique, known as single fiber EMG, can provide information about the integrity of neuromuscular transmission, but it is a technically involved procedure that requires a great deal of cooperation from the patient.

Supplementary diagnostic tests include nerve, skin, and muscle biopsies. A nerve biopsy can be useful in determining whether the underlying nerve pathology is primary axon damage or primary demyelination, or it may provide evidence of a vasculitis affecting the small arterioles supplying the nerve. The most common biopsy site is the sural nerve at the ankle. Processes that primarily affect small-fiber nerves produce changes in intraepidermal nerve fiber density and morphology on skin biopsy. These small-fiber neuropathies—most common in diabetes—are often extremely painful, and as noted above, they may not be evident on traditional electrodiagnostic studies. Muscle biopsies help distinguish among dystrophies, congenital myopathies, metabolic myopathies, and inflammatory myopathies. Common muscle biopsy sites are vastus lateralis and biceps brachii muscles. Another informative test is determination of the serum creatine kinase (CK) level. This enzyme is found in highest concentration in skeletal muscle, and an elevated serum level can be an indication of muscle damage. For certain neuromuscular diseases, antibody assays and genetic tests are extremely useful, and often definitive. When the clinical evidence suggests a focal process, such as a mononeuropathy, plexopathy, or radiculopathy, imaging studies of the affected structure can be helpful.

IV. Specific Neuromuscular Diseases

A. Motor Neuron Diseases

Although there are some diseases (especially in infants and children) that exclusively involve degeneration of lower motor neurons (LMNs), and other conditions that exclusively involve degeneration of upper motor neurons (UMNs), the most common form of motor neuron disease in adults is amyotrophic lateral sclerosis (ALS), which involves both LMNs and UMNs. Even in ALS, LMN involvement predominates in some patients and UMN involvement predominates in others. In an individual patient, the pattern of involvement may change over time. For example, a patient may initially present with primarily LMN involvement and only later develop UMN symptoms and signs.

ALS may begin at any adult age but it is more common with increasing age. It is generally thought that symptoms only appear after the disease has been present for a considerable length of time, and that as many as 50% of the motor neurons are lost before weakness is detected. The initial symptom is usually weakness in a focal area, which gradually spreads to contiguous muscles in the same region of the body. Most often, the initial weakness is in an arm. It can occasionally be confined to the distribution of a single nerve or nerve root, leading to potential diagnostic confusion, but it usually includes muscles that are innervated by more than one nerve or nerve root. The lack of sensory involvement helps to differentiate early ALS from mononeuropathy or radiculopathy. Typical symptoms of hand weakness include difficulty turning a key, opening a bottle or jar, buttoning, or turning a door knob. Typical symptoms of lower extremity weakness include unstable gait, falling, fatigue when walking, or foot drop. In about 25% of patients, the initial weakness is confined to muscles innervated by cranial nerves, leading to disorders of speech or swallowing. These patients may be difficult to differentiate from patients with myasthenia gravis or from patients with brainstem mass lesions or infiltrative processes (such as tuberculous meningitis or sarcoidosis). All of these conditions can cause dysarthria, hoarseness, or dysphagia; some useful diagnostic features are that patients with ALS may also display emotional incontinence, inappropriate crying or laughing, or excessive forced yawning.

Fasciculations occur in all individuals, including healthy control subjects, but they are especially profuse and continuous in patients with ALS, because of extensive damage to lower motor neurons. Although fasciculations are not prominent when the disease first presents, almost all patients develop fasciculations soon after disease onset. Cramps are also common in denervated muscles. These are often most distressful to the patient when lying in bed, to the point where they may interfere with sleep. As the disease continues to progress, muscle atrophy occurs. This is often exacerbated by generalized cachexia in patients whose dysphagia prevents adequate caloric intake. Symptoms of UMN involvement include muscle spasms and stiffness, and UMN examination findings include spasticity, hyperreflexia, and Babinski signs (see Chapter 2).

The disease characteristically begins in one upper extremity, then spreads to the contralateral upper extremity, then the ipsilateral lower extremity, then the contralateral lower extremity, and then the bulbar muscles. Any pattern is possible, however. For example, the disease sometimes begins in one lower extremity, spreads to the contralateral limb, and then to the upper extremities. When the initial symptoms are in bulbar muscles, they tend to spread to distal upper extremities first, then the thoracic region, and then the lower extremities. For some reason, extraocular muscles are not affected, nor is there bladder or bowel incontinence from sphincter muscle weakness. The disease is relentlessly progressive, but the rate of progression varies significantly between patients. Although many patients rapidly become disabled and die within several years, others may experience much more gradual progression over ten years or more. Bulbar muscles are eventually affected in more than 90% of patients, leading to inadequate airway protection and increased risk of aspiration, and at the same time producing progressive weakness of respiratory muscles. Respiratory failure and pneumonia are the most common causes of death. The mean survival from the time of symptom onset is twenty-seven to forty-three months. About 25% of patients survive five years, and 8–16% survive ten years.

A substantial percentage of patients (20–40%) with ALS have cognitive impairment, with clinical and neuroimaging features that are consistent with frontotemporal dementia (FTD), a condition covered in Chapter 7. A similar percentage of patients presenting with FTD meet clinical criteria for the diagnosis of ALS.

Before making the diagnosis of ALS, all potentially treatable conditions must be excluded. In particular, structural causes of the UMN and LMN abnormalities should be considered. The most common source of confusion is degenerative disease of the cervical spine, which may produce UMN signs in the lower extremities on the basis of spinal cord compression and LMN signs in the upper extremities because of compression of multiple cervical nerve roots. The diagnosis can usually be clarified using the distribution of findings, the presence or absence of sensory abnormalities, and the results of imaging studies and electrodiagnostic tests, but occasionally the situation remains unclear.

The cause of ALS is not known, and there is no known cure. Most cases of ALS are sporadic, but familial forms also exist. Some cases of familial ALS are associated with mutations in the gene for superoxide dismutase (SOD), which is an antioxidant enzyme, suggesting that oxidative stress may contribute to neuronal death even in sporadic forms of the disease. A simple pattern of loss of enzyme function has not been demonstrated in patients with SOD mutations, however, and the level of enzyme activity does not correlate well with the severity of disease. Moreover, SOD-knockout mice do not develop any apparent motor neuron disease. It may be that the mutant SOD *gains* some additional function that is more pertinent to the pathogenesis of ALS than the *loss* of normal SOD function. In transgenic mouse models, the mutant SOD forms conspicuous cytoplasmic inclusions in motor neurons (and sometimes in astrocytes), which develop before the onset of motor dysfunction. Patients with nonfamilial ALS are also known to have ubiquinated cytoplasmic inclusions in many (but not all) motor neurons. These inclusions have been found to contain a protein called TAR (transactivation response region) DNA binding protein, or TDP-43, leading to the proposal that this protein is a factor in the pathogenesis of ALS. TDP-43 is also associated with FTD, which may help to explain why so many patients have clinical features of both. Missense mutations in the gene coding for TDP-43 have been found in some cases of familial and sporadic ALS; curiously, most of the patients with these mutations had no dementia. Mutations in the *fused in sarcoma/translated in liposarcoma (FUS/TLS)* gene have also been identified in some cases of familial ALS. The protein coded by this gene normally resides in the nucleus, but in the mutant forms it accumulates in the cytoplasm. This is analogous to the situation with TDP-43 mutations, suggesting that cytoplasmic protein accumulation may be a factor in the pathogenesis of ALS.

Other factors that may be involved in the pathogenesis of ALS include abnormal processing of tau protein (see Chapter 7), neurofilament dysfunction, mitochondrial dysfunction, altered calcium homeostasis, inflammatory cytokines, reduced neurotrophic support, and glutamate excitotoxicity. Glutamate is the principal excitatory neurotransmitter in the nervous system, including motor neurons, but excess levels of glutamate are toxic to neurons. Riluzole, a drug that modulates glutamatergic neurotransmission, results in a modest prolongation of survival in patients with ALS. The results with other agents with antiglutamate activity have been disappointing. Several trials of other management approaches, including stem cell transplantation, are in progress.

In the meantime, the main focus of treatment is the management of such symptoms as spasticity, cramps, excessive secretions, aspiration, communication difficulty, reduced mobility, and difficulty breathing. There is evidence that the use of bilevel positive airway pressure (BiPAP) may prolong survival and increase quality of life; additional clinical trials are underway. In patients with severe dysphagia, who develop clinically significant weight loss resulting in depletion of fat and protein stores, percutaneous endoscopic gastrostomy (PEG) tubes or other types of feeding tubes may also prolong survival and increase quality of life.

About 10% of patients with motor neuron disease have purely LMN involvement, or *progressive muscular atrophy* (PMA), although the true prevalence of this condition is difficult to establish because many patients initially diagnosed with PMA ultimately develop UMN features—i.e., they prove to have ALS. The term *spinal muscular atrophy* (SMA) refers to patients with genetic disorders affecting LMNs; these diseases usually present in infancy or childhood, but sometimes in adulthood. Some viral infections preferentially target motor neurons. The classic example is poliovirus, but many other enteroviruses can produce the same clinical syndrome: a flu-like illness followed by fulminant focal or multifocal weakness with LMN characteristics. West Nile virus can also produce this syndrome.

B. Nerve Root Disorders (Radiculopathies)

The most common cause of radiculopathy is degenerative disease of the spinal column, involving the vertebral bodies, the facet joints, or the discs. Other structural lesions, including tumors and abscesses, may also compress the nerve roots. The diagnostic and management considerations for these structural causes of radiculopathy are discussed in Chapter 15.

Nerve roots may also be involved by many of the same processes that produce neuropathies, including vasculitis, infections, metabolic abnormalities, and inflammatory demyelination. Usually the radiculopathy and neuropathy coexist; the evaluation and management is discussed in Section D. On occasion, the radiculopathy occurs without a significant neuropathy; this is most often seen in diabetic patients, especially in the thoracic nerve roots. Such patients should be evaluated for a structural cause (especially neoplastic) before concluding that the radiculopathy is due to metabolic disease.

Herpes varicella-zoster virus produces a radiculopathy that may be excruciatingly painful; it is usually straightforward to diagnose because of the accompanying skin lesions in the distribution of the affected root, but they are occasionally absent. Zoster is discussed in further detail in Chapter 10. Lyme disease and cytomegalovirus both may produce a polyradiculopathy; treatment is directed at the underlying infection.

C. Plexus Disorders (Plexopathies)

Common causes of *plexopathies* are cancer, radiation therapy, metabolic disorders such as diabetes mellitus, or trauma. There are also idiopathic plexopathies; although the cause is not known, they are thought to be autoimmune. For some reason, diabetes affects the lumbosacral plexus much more frequently than the brachial plexus, whereas the converse is true of autoimmune plexopathies. Plexus disorders are diagnosed by establishing relevant details of the history (e.g., a history of radiation therapy or recent immunization), performing electrodiagnostic tests to confirm the localization, and—if the cause is not clear from the history—imaging the plexus to exclude a structural lesion. Treatment is directed at the underlying cause; only supportive therapy (mainly pain control and physical therapy) is available for idiopathic plexopathies, but fortunately, the outcome is generally favorable.

D. Peripheral Nerve Disorders (Neuropathies)

Patients with peripheral nerve disorders may have an isolated abnormality of a single peripheral nerve (*mononeuropathy*), a combination of several mononeuropathies (*mononeuropathy multiplex*; Figure 6.1), or a more generalized process involving peripheral nerves (*polyneuropathy*; Figure 6.2). Using the terminology defined in Chapter 3, polyneuropathy is a diffuse process, whereas mononeuropathy multiplex is multifocal. Unless otherwise qualified, the term *neuropathy* is usually used interchangeably with the term *polyneuropathy*.

The most common cause of mononeuropathy is compression, especially at a site where the nerve is particularly confined and subject to trauma (such as the median nerve at the carpal tunnel, the ulnar nerve at the elbow, or the peroneal nerve at the knee). In typical cases, diagnostic testing may be unnecessary; when there are atypical features, electrodiagnostic studies usually clarify the diagnosis. Imaging studies are sometimes helpful. Compression mononeuropathies (also called entrapment mononeuropathies) often respond to stabilization of the joint with a splint or protection with a pad. Local steroid injections can also be helpful. When the response to these treatments is unsatisfactory, or when the compression is already moderately severe by the time the patient seeks medical attention, surgical decompression of the nerve is indicated.

Unlike peripheral nerves elsewhere in the body, cranial nerves are generally well insulated from external pressure, so compression injury to cranial nerves is usually due to pressure from within the nervous system itself. Mass lesions such as tumors or aneurysms or even tortuosities in the vertebral or basilar arteries can compress cranial nerves directly. Cranial nerves may also be compressed as a result of increased intracranial

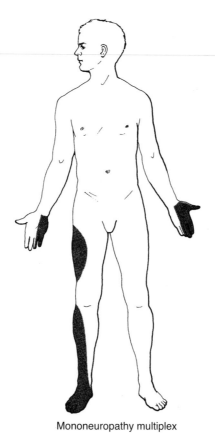

Mononeuropathy multiplex

Fig. 6.1 The regions of sensory involvement in a patient with mononeuropathy multiplex. This is a multifocal process affecting several discrete peripheral nerves (in this case, the left median nerve, right ulnar nerve, right lateral cutaneous nerve of the thigh, and right peroneal nerve). The involved areas are not confluent or symmetric.

pressure caused by distant mass lesions. A lesion of cranial nerve III due to transtentorial herniation is the most notorious example (see Chapter 11). Trauma can damage cranial nerves either directly or by producing shear injury. Cranial nerves I and IV are at particular risk for shear injury. Isolated cranial nerve palsies often result from ischemic disease of penetrating arteries, especially in patients with diabetes or hypertension.

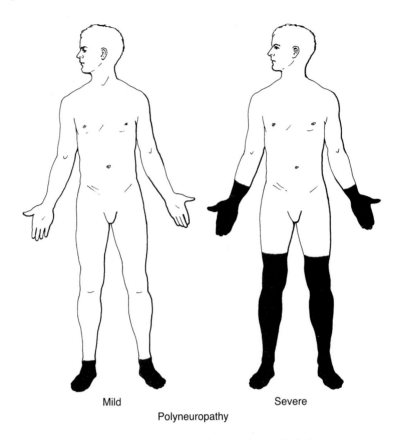

Mild   Severe

Polyneuropathy

Fig. 6.2 "Stocking-glove" distribution of sensory loss typical of polyneuropathy. This is a diffuse process in which involvement is confluent and symmetric. With mild disease (the figure on the left), only the distal lower extremities are involved. With more severe disease (the figure on the right), there is proximal extension in the lower extremities and the distal upper extremities are also involved.

Inflammatory disease, both infectious and noninfectious, can cause cranial neuropathies. Neoplastic spread to the meninges can do the same.

Bell's palsy, or idiopathic facial nerve palsy, deserves special mention because it usually has a benign course, in contrast to stroke (with which it is sometimes confused). There is evidence that herpes simplex or varicella-zoster viruses are responsible for most cases of Bell's palsy. The distinctive feature of Bell's palsy is a LMN pattern of facial weakness, including the forehead muscles (see Chapter 2). There is often associated pain, especially in the ear, and there may be changes in hearing or taste. Patients may also have sensory complaints. Almost all patients recover to some extent within 3 months, and the recovery is complete in 55–85% of patients. Complete facial weakness at the peak of the episode (present in roughly one-half the patients), non-ear pain, and older age are associated with a poorer prognosis. Several well-designed trials have demonstrated that a ten-day course of prednisolone, started within three days of symptom onset, improves outcome. Acyclovir is often used in conjunction with predniso-lone, but the evidence for this practice is much less compelling.

Patients who have multiple cranial neuropathies without involvement of the brainstem parenchyma itself should be evaluated for inflammatory diseases or carcinomatous involvement of the meninges (see Chapter 10). Patients who have multiple mononeuropathies in the limbs may simply have several entrapment mononeuropathies, especially if they engage in activities that involve forceful, repetitive movements. Obese patients have an increased risk of developing compression mononeuropathies, and so do patients with diabetes or thyroid disease. There is also a rare familial condition, hereditary neuropathy with liability to pressure palsies, which should be considered even when there is no apparent family history. When patients have none of these predisposing factors, or when mononeuropa-thies occur at sites where entrapment is unusual, the most likely cause of mononeuropathy multiplex is vasculitis. Vasculitis produces nerve damage by affecting nutrient vessels to the nerve. It can be associated with a more widespread collagen vascular disorder, or it can occur as an isolated pro-cess restricted to the blood vessels supplying peripheral nerves while spar-ing other blood vessels and other organ systems.

When mononeuropathy multiplex is severe, the nerve involvement can become confluent, resembling polyneuropathy. In such cases, the most reliable way to distinguish mononeuropathy multiplex from polyneuropa-thy is to inquire about the onset of the disease. Mononeuropathy multiplex affects first one nerve and then another in an unpredictable sequence, whereas polyneuropathy affects nerves in a systematic pattern that is evident throughout the course of the disease. The typical pattern of poly-neuropathy is that the longest nerves in the body are affected first, and progressively shorter nerves become involved as the condition progresses, resulting in a "stocking-glove" distribution of symptoms. Some polyneu-ropathies may exhibit variations or deviate from this pattern. In some cases, only myelinated nerves are affected; in others, only small, unmyelinated nerves are involved. Some patients report only sensory symptoms. Many of these patients actually have a mild sensorimotor polyneuropathy, and although they are unaware of motor involvement, it is apparent on clinical testing or electrophysiologic testing. Some polyneuropathies really do affect only sensory nerves, however. In one condition (leprosy), it is said that the coldest (i.e., the most exposed) nerves are involved. In general, if the pattern of nerve involvement cannot be expressed in a rule that makes some physiologic sense, a polyneuropathy is unlikely. For example, it is hard to imagine a plausible rule that would result in involvement of the right median nerve but not the left, or of the left median and radial nerves but not the left ulnar nerve. These would be examples of mononeuropathy multiplex, not polyneuropathy. In time, however, patients with either of these patterns of nerve involvement from mononeuropathy multiplex might progress to have involvement of the median, ulnar, and radial nerves bilaterally, as well as nerves throughout the lower extremities, at which point the pattern of nerve involvement would resemble that seen with a polyneuropathy. Only by taking a detailed history of the onset and progression of the symptoms could the distinction be made.

There are many causes of polyneuropathy. A frequently used mnemonic is **DANG THERAPIST**:

D   iabetes

A   lcohol

N   utritional (deficiencies of vitamins B12, B1 [thiamine], B6, and E)

G   uillain-Barré (acute inflammatory demyelinating polyradiculoneuropathy [AIDP])

T   oxic (lead, arsenic, other metals, excessive vitamin B6, many medications)

HE   reditary

R   ecurrent (chronic inflammatory demyelinating polyradiculoneuropathy [CIDP])

A   myloid

P   orphyria

I   nfectious (leprosy, human immunodeficiency virus [HIV], Lyme disease, diphtheria, mononucleosis)

S   ystemic (uremia, hypothyroidism, lupus, Sjögren's, Wegener's)

T   umors (paraneoplastic; also CIDP associated with myeloma)

The first two diagnoses in this list merit special comment. Diabetes is the most common cause of polyneuropathy in the United States, and probably the world. There are several patterns of diabetic polyneuropathy, including a painless loss of sensation with weakness (resulting in unnoticed foot injury and ulcers) and a painful loss of distal leg sensation. Patients with impaired glucose tolerance (i.e., normal fasting glucose and glycosylated hemoglobin levels, but 2-hour glucose tolerance test in the impaired tolerance range) also have an increased incidence of primarily painful sensory neuropathies. This is probably due to a combination of an inherent susceptibility and the episodic spikes in glucose levels that occur in impaired glucose tolerance. Impaired glucose tolerance is frequently a component of the metabolic syndrome that includes hypertension, hyperlipidemia, and increased waist circumference, so there may be a combination of factors contributing to the polyneuropathy.

Alcohol has traditionally been considered to be another common cause of neuropathy, but it appears that the neuropathy associated with alcohol use may be primarily related to malnutrition. Patients with neuropathy who have a history of alcohol use should be evaluated for other potential causes of neuropathy, rather than attributing their condition to alcohol.

A detailed history may help to identify specific conditions from the above list that are particularly likely in an individual patient. The pattern of nerve involvement can also be helpful, since different "rules" are followed by different causes of polyneuropathy, as already mentioned. For example, pure sensory neuropathies may be associated with paraneoplastic syndromes or connective tissue disorders, such as Sjögren's syndrome. Determining whether the process is demyelinating or axonal may also narrow the differential diagnosis of a polyneuropathy. Demyelinating neuropathies primarily affect the myelin sheath, resulting in slowed conduction in myelinated nerves. Axonal neuropathies primarily involve the underlying axons; both myelinated and unmyelinated fibers are affected. Demyelinating and axonal neuropathies can usually be distinguished based on the results of nerve conduction studies: Demyelinating neuropathies result in abnormal nerve conduction velocities with relatively normal amplitudes, whereas axonal neuropathies produce the opposite pattern. Most metabolic and systemic diseases produce axonal polyneuropathies. The most common demyelinating polyneuropathies are the *inflammatory demyelinating polyradiculoneuropathies*. They are characterized by inflammation of the myelin sheath both proximally at the root and distally along peripheral nerves. Examples include *acute* forms (*AIDP*, the most common cause of the clinical condition known as *Guillain-Barré syndrome*) and *chronic* forms (such as CIDP). The weakness peaks within 4 weeks in patients with AIDP, whereas the characteristic course of CIDP is slowly progressive over more than two months or relapsing and remitting. Patients with AIDP and CIDP usually have an elevated spinal fluid protein, with a normal cell count.

Hereditary neuropathies are usually very slowly progressive and may go unnoticed in affected family members. The most common forms of hereditary neuropathy fall into the general category of hereditary motor sensory neuropathy, or Charcot-Marie-Tooth (CMT) disease (based on the names of the first clinical observers). CMT disease encompasses a group of neuropathies that are distinguished, in part, on the basis of clinical and electrodiagnostic criteria (such as whether nerve conduction velocities are slow or normal). Further distinction of different forms of CMT is based on genetic testing. A growing number of mutations have been identified, associated with a variety of functions including formation and compaction of myelin, response to growth factors, mitochondrial processes, protein synthesis and degradation, axonal transport, transfer of ions and small molecules between cells, and signal transduction.

Treatment of neuropathies depends on the underlying cause. Polyneuropathy due to nutritional deficiency, for example, is treated with dietary replacement, and polyneuropathy due to a toxin is treated by removing the causative agent. For diabetic polyneuropathy and the polyneuropathy associated with impaired glucose tolerance, the only available treatment is exercise and tight glucose control. AIDP and CIDP are believed to include a humorally mediated component, and they respond to plasma exchange (also called plasma apheresis, or plasmapheresis). This is a procedure in which units of whole blood are removed from the body and separated into the red cell and plasma fractions. The red cells are reinfused, while the plasma, which contains the antibodies, is discarded. Intravenous immunoglobulin (IVIG) administration is also effective for both AIDP and CIDP. Prednisone is effective for CIDP, but not for AIDP. Other immunosuppressive agents are also used to treat CIDP. There are no specific treatments for hereditary neuropathies.

E. Neuromuscular Junction Disorders

Some disorders of neuromuscular transmission affect the presynaptic terminal and others affect the postsynaptic membrane. Botulism and Lambert-Eaton myasthenic syndrome (LEMS) are examples of presynaptic disorders, and myasthenia gravis is the prototypical postsynaptic disorder. Myasthenia gravis is much more common than LEMS, and other disorders of the neuromuscular junction (including botulism) are extremely rare.

Myasthenia gravis can begin suddenly or gradually. Patients usually present with ptosis, diplopia, or both. Problems with speech, swallowing, or chewing are also common early in the course. In about 25% of patients, the weakness remains restricted to lid, eye, and bulbar muscles, but most patients subsequently develop limb weakness. In many patients, the limb weakness is relatively mild, and it may only be evident on formal testing. It generally affects proximal muscles more than distal muscles. One characteristic feature is fatigability—with repeated muscle use, more neuromuscular junctions fail to transmit impulses, and weakness rapidly becomes apparent as a sense of fatigue. Transmission improves when the muscle is rested. As a result, the symptoms typically get worse as the day progresses or with prolonged activity. For example, jaw weakness tends to get worse when chewing tough meats or chewy candy. Speech can deteriorate markedly after a few sentences, yet recover when the patient pauses to listen to other people speak. The symptoms also fluctuate from day to day.

The peak age of onset is between 20 and 30 years in women and between 50 and 60 years in men. The course of the disease is extremely variable. Even in untreated patients, the weakness may improve spontaneously and may even resolve completely in rare cases, but the improvement is typically followed by a relapse. In treated patients, most relapses are associated with reductions in the dose of medication. As a general rule, patients experience their maximal degree of weakness within two to five years. This means that if their disease is restricted to ocular weakness during the first five years, they are unlikely to experience limb weakness at a later date. Conversely, those who experience weakness of limbs and respiratory muscles early in the course can develop severe exacerbations that may include respiratory failure. Eventually, if left untreated, the weakness becomes progressive. Even optimally treated patients may develop fixed weakness in the muscles of the eyes and face, and rarely in limb muscles. Before the advent of effective treatment for the underlying disease, and before the introduction of intensive care units, mechanical ventilation, and other treatments for respiratory failure, the prognosis for this disease could be grim (hence the name "gravis"). With treatment, most patients do well, and patients with respiratory failure can be treated and weaned.

Several clinical features distinguish the different disorders of neuromuscular transmission. In addition to affecting the neuromuscular junction, LEMS and botulism disrupt transmission in autonomic ganglia, causing symptoms such as dry mouth and impotence. Although the reasons are not clear, neuromuscular junction transmission abnormalities in botulism and myasthenia gravis frequently affect a combination of extraocular and lid levator muscles, while these muscles are less involved in LEMS. In some patients with LEMS, strength improves during brief exercise (and then declines as the exertion is sustained). This can be demonstrated when testing tendon reflexes—they will be depressed or absent in the rest state due to failed transmission, but if the patient activates the tested muscle for about 10 seconds, neuromuscular transmission briefly improves and the tendon reflex can be elicited. Detailed electrodiagnostic testing can also help differentiate between the various neuromuscular junction disorders.

Serologic testing is also helpful in diagnosis. Antibodies to the acetylcholine receptor are present in the serum in 80–85% of patients with generalized myasthenia and in 55% of patients with myasthenia whose clinical manifestations are restricted to the extra-ocular muscles. The role of these antibodies is not completely understood. They could simply occupy the receptors, blocking the binding of acetylcholine, or they could induce cross-linking of receptors, prompting endocytosis and degradation of the receptors. They could also cause injury to the post-synaptic membrane. Certainly, the post-synaptic membrane is simplified and the normal folded pattern is lost in patients with myasthenia, but it is not clear that the antibodies to the receptor are responsible for these morphologic changes. About half of the patients with myasthenia who do not have antibodies to the acetylcholine receptor have antibodies to a protein called muscle-specific kinase, or MuSK. During development, this protein appears to play a key role in aggregation of acetylcholine receptor antibodies at the motor end plate, but the protein's role in adult life is not clear. Low-affinity acetylcholine receptor antibodies are present in many patients who are seronegative for MuSK and acetylcholine receptor antibodies using conventional assays. LEMS is most likely due to an abnormality of the voltage-gated calcium channels on presynaptic motor nerve terminals. In normal subjects, these channels open in response to an action potential, causing calcium to enter the nerve terminal and stimulate the mobilization of acetylcholine. In LEMS, this mobilization is abnormal, so that the number of quanta of acetylcholine released in response to an action potential is smaller than normal. Antibodies to the voltage-gated calcium channels are present in the serum of almost all LEMS patients. Disease severity does not correlate with antibody titers in either myasthenia or LEMS.

Although the exact mechanism is not understood, the thymus plays an important role in the pathogenesis of myasthenia gravis. About 15% of patients with myasthenia have thymomas. In addition, 65–70% of patients with myasthenia have hyperplastic changes in the thymus. All patients with newly diagnosed myasthenia should have a CT scan of the chest to look for thymoma.

About 50% of patients with LEMS have an underlying malignancy, and about 80% of these have small cell lung cancer. The cancer is often subclinical, and may be so small that it can take several years to grow to sufficient size for detection on imaging studies. Those who do not have cancer often have immune-mediated diseases or organ-specific auto-antibodies in their serum, further supporting an immune mechanism. Patients with LEMS should be evaluated for these underlying conditions, and even if the evaluation is unrevealing, they should be monitored for cancer for several years.

There are three approaches to treating myasthenia gravis: acetylcholin-esterase inhibitors, immunomodulation, and thymectomy. Acetylcholin-esterase inhibitors, such as the oral drug pyridostigmine (Mestinon), provide a purely symptomatic benefit. These agents slow the enzymatic degradation of acetylcholine, thereby prolonging its availability at the post-synaptic receptor on the muscle membrane. One traditional test for myasthenia gravis has been to see if weakness briefly improves immedi-ately after administering an intravenous dose of edrophonium (Tensilon), a short-acting acetylcholinesterase inhibitor, although this test can be dif-ficult to standardize and can cause bradycardia.

Although pyridostigmine can be very effective, it does not treat the under-lying pathology, which is thought to be an autoimmune antibody-mediated attack on the postsynaptic receptor or neighboring muscle membrane. For this reason, immunosuppressive medications (such as prednisone, azathio-prine, cyclosporine, or mycophenolate) are used. Alternative treatments include administration of intravenous immunoglobulin or removal of the offending antibodies by plasma exchange. Plasma exchange is often very effective, but it does not address antibody production. In severe myasthenia gravis, a combination of all of these treatment modalities is used.

Retrospective analyses indicate that thymectomy increases the likeli-hood of remission or improvement, although its effectiveness has not been demonstrated in controlled trials. It is commonly recommended for patients whose symptoms begin before age 60 (and it is clearly indicated for patients who have a thymoma, because total resection is possible if the thymoma has not grown to invade surrounding structures).

Patients with LEMS should undergo extensive evaluation for an underly-ing malignancy. They sometimes respond to acetylcholinesterase inhibitors, plasma exchange, or IVIG, but the results are not as consistent as in myasthenia. Symptoms may improve with 3,4-diaminopyridine, which blocks potassium channels and thereby prolongs the presynaptic action potentials, thus increasing the amount of acetylcholine released by motor nerve terminals with each action potential. This medication is not available for general use in the United States., but it can be obtained by application to the FDA, and a related drug, 4-aminopyridine (dalfampridine), is FDA-approved for use in multiple sclerosis. Patients with botulism who receive intensive medical support, especially respiratory support, usually do well, although recovery can be very slow. Antitoxin administration is controversial because of a high incidence of side effects, and a lack of consistent benefit.

F. Muscle Disorders (Myopathies)

As with neuropathies, the differential diagnosis for myopathy is very broad. It includes some disorders that are hereditary and others that are acquired disorders. The *muscular dystrophies* are hereditary diseases caused by mutations that affect structural proteins that maintain muscle membrane stability. These disorders most often present early in life, but some forms only become symptomatic in middle age or later. The progression is gradual. Genetic testing is available for some types of muscular dystrophy.

Other hereditary myopathies result from biochemical defects that interfere with the mobilization of energy sources (typically, abnormalities of glycogen metabolism or of lipid metabolism), resulting in exercise intolerance. Some of these defects, such as myophosphorylase deficiency (McArdle's disease), prevent the rapid breakdown of glycogen to glucose. These patients are often relatively asymptomatic at rest, but they experience pain, cramping, and fatigue within the first few minutes of forceful exertion. They can sometimes experience a "second wind" as their muscles convert to increased utilization of free fatty acids. In contrast, carnitine palmitoyltransferase (CPT) deficiency causes defective utilization of fatty acids, so patients develop pain, cramps, and weakness after prolonged exercise, and they do not experience a second-wind phenomenon. They can perform short, intense exercise without symptoms. Disorders that interfere with the ability of mitochondria to generate usable energy for cellular processes also produce myopathies.

Acquired myopathies can be caused by endocrine disorders, such as hypothyroidism, hyperthyroidism, hyperparathyroidism, and Cushing's syndrome. Some other systemic illnesses, such as sarcoidosis, cysticercosis, and trichinosis, can cause myopathy. A variety of medications can cause myopathy, notably exogenous steroid therapy and statins. Chronic alcohol use can also cause myopathy.

Acquired myopathy can also be due to intrinsic muscle inflammation, not due to infection or systemic inflammation. The three forms of inflammatory myopathy are dermatomyositis, inclusion body myositis (IBM), and polymyositis. Dermatomyositis is the most common form throughout childhood and through middle adult life. IBM is the most common acquired myopathy after age 50. Both dermatomyositis and polymyositis cause symmetric, proximal muscle wasting and weakness. Patients with IBM often have a distinctive pattern of weakness, with prominent involvement of forearm flexor muscles and knee extensor muscles. The muscle involvement is often asymmetric. Dysphagia is also common in IBM, and there is mild involvement of facial muscles more often than in polymyositis or dermatomyositis.

As with other myopathies, the course is gradual, typically progressing over weeks in dermatomyositis, months in polymyositis, and years in IBM. Muscle pain occurs more commonly than with other myopathies, but the pain is usually mild, and the disease is painless in a significant proportion of patients. Dermatomyositis is associated with a characteristic skin rash, typically on the face and hands.

Although serum CK levels and EMG are typically abnormal in dermatomyositis and polymyositis, the results usually do not distinguish between these disorders and other primary muscle diseases. Muscle biopsy is the most reliable diagnostic test for inflammatory myopathy. In rare cases, biopsy can even establish the diagnosis of dermatomyositis in patients who have no rash.

Dermatomyositis is a humorally mediated autoimmune disorder, and polymyositis is cell mediated. The immunologic abnormality in IBM is less clear, but it is thought to be a cell-mediated immune disorder, like polymyositis. Muscle fibers in IBM reveal accumulations of beta amyloid and hyperphosphorylated tau, analogous to that seen in the brains of patients with Alzheimer's disease (see Chapter 7). IBM is also associated with inclusions containing TDP-43, the protein that accumulates in ALS and frontotemporal dementia. About 10–20% of adult patients with dermatomyositis have a systemic malignancy. In contrast, the incidence of systemic malignancy in patients with polymyositis or IBM is no higher than in the general population.

There is no known treatment for IBM. Polymyositis and dermatomyositis respond to prednisone, although relapses sometimes occur when a prednisone taper is attempted, necessitating long-term steroid use that can itself cause myopathy (as well as many other side effects including diabetes mellitus, osteoporosis, high blood pressure, promotion of cataracts, and bleeding gastric ulcers). Steroids also slow the rate of progression in patients with some muscular dystrophies; the mechanism is not known. Metabolic and systemic myopathies are addressed by treating the underlying disease when possible, and toxic myopathies by removing the causative agent.

V. Symptomatic Treatment

Specific treatments are available for some neuromuscular diseases (such as myasthenia gravis, dermatomyositis, and polymyositis) but not for others (such as hereditary neuropathy and IBM). Either way, treatment directed at symptoms rather than at the underlying disease process may be beneficial.

A. Emergency Measures

Any patient who has a rapidly progressive condition with the potential to affect muscles of respiration should be hospitalized for observation until it is clear that the clinical situation is stable. These patients should be monitored with daily (and sometimes more frequent) bedside respiratory testing of forced vital capacity (FVC) and negative inspiratory force. Patients whose FVC falls below 10–12 ml/kg require elective intubation. Patients with a rapidly deteriorating negative inspiratory force or FVC should be intubated even sooner, when the FVC falls to 15 ml/kg.

When a patient has a condition that can produce autonomic insufficiency (particularly AIDP), continuous electrocardiogram monitoring and frequent assessment of vital signs are necessary until the clinical situation has stabilized. Significant hypotension and arrhythmias should be treated with medications as needed; in some cases, temporary or permanent cardiac pacing may be required.

B. Non-Urgent Measures: Motor Symptoms

Whether or not there is a treatment for the underlying cause of a patient's weakness, efforts should be made to prevent unnecessary deterioration and to take full advantage of the strength that remains. Physical therapists can teach patients exercises to this effect, and occupational therapists can recommend facilitative devices and environmental modifications to improve function. A formal swallowing evaluation by a speech pathologist

may be indicated for patients with dysphagia; depending on the results, simple swallowing strategies may be adequate for some patients, whereas others may require a temporary or permanent feeding tube. Strategies are also available for patients with dysarthria.

Patients with progressive, irreversible diseases such as motor neuron disease should be encouraged at a relatively early stage in their illness to consider whether they want to be intubated when their respiratory function fails. They should express their wishes clearly to family members, preferably by taking formal legal measures such as writing a living will or designating a durable power of attorney for medical issues.

C. Non-Urgent Measures: Sensory Symptoms

Neuropathic pain often responds to symptomatic treatment with tricyclic antidepressant medications, duloxetine (a selective serotonin and norepinephrine reuptake inhibitor), or certain anti-epileptic drugs, notably carbamazepine, gabapentin, pregabalin, topiramate, and phenytoin. The necessary doses are often much lower than those required to treat depression or seizures. Because these medications have many potential side effects and the treatment will not change the underlying condition, patients should be started at low doses and titrated up slowly. An alternative treatment is capsaicin cream, a medication that binds to specific receptors on pain-sensitive neurons. It often produces initial irritation, so some advocate applying a topical lidocaine preparation before applying the capsaicin.

There is no reliable treatment for numbness or paresthesias, but if the patient reports significant discomfort, tricyclic antidepressants or gabapentin may be tried.

VI. Discussion of Case Histories

Cases 1 and 2: In Cases 1 and 2, the absence of sensory symptoms suggests a primary muscle disease, a neuromuscular junction disorder, or a disease exclusively of motor neurons. In both patients, the limb weakness appears to involve mainly proximal musculature, which is typical of a primary muscle disease or a neuromuscular junction disease (but not motor neuron disease). The prominence of diplopia in the second patient makes a defect in neuromuscular junction transmission most likely, and the fatigability is characteristic of myasthenia gravis. Case 1 is an example of polymyositis, a primary disorder of muscle.

The course of myasthenia gravis fluctuates, accounting for the initial episode of diplopia in Case 2. Primary muscle disease, such as polymyositis, does not fluctuate in this manner.

In both cases, nerve conduction studies were normal for both sensory and motor nerves. This provided additional evidence that these patients did not have a disorder of the peripheral nerves. In Case 2, tests of neuromuscular transmission showed abnormalities consistent with those seen in myasthenia gravis, and ruled out the other main diagnostic consideration, Lambert-Eaton myasthenic syndrome. The patient was also found to have acetylcholine receptor antibodies in his serum. He was treated with pyridostigmine, with marked improvement. His symptoms did not resolve, however, and prednisone was eventually added. A CT scan of the chest showed no thymoma. A thymectomy was offered to the patient, but he declined it.

In Case 1, the EMG was consistent with myopathic damage, but it is difficult to distinguish by EMG between several of the primary muscle diseases, including inflammatory muscle disease (dermatomyositis, polymyositis, and IBM), muscular dystrophy, and congenital myopathy. The best test to distinguish among the primary muscle diseases is muscle biopsy, which in this case showed characteristic findings of polymyositis. This patient was treated with steroids, and her symptoms gradually resolved. The steroids were successfully tapered.

Cases 3 and 4: In both Case 3 and Case 4 there is evidence of LMN dysfunction: weakness, fasciculations, and atrophy in Case 3, and weakness with areflexia in Case 4. In Case 4, there is also sensory disturbance, so the site of pathology must be at the level of nerve roots, plexus, or peripheral nerves. This patient's sensory symptoms fit a "stocking-glove" distribution, as is typically seen in a peripheral polyneuropathy, but she has both distal and proximal weakness, which would be unusual early in the course of a polyneuropathy. In most neuropathies, the longest nerves in the body are affected first, and the disability progresses from distal to proximal. In contrast, when there is a polyradicular component, roots going to proximal muscles as well as distal muscles are affected, causing proximal and distal weakness. Thus, the pattern of this patient's symptoms suggests a combined polyradiculopathy and polyneuropathy. The patient in Case 3 has no sensory problems, making radiculopathy, plexopathy, and neuropathy less likely. In addition to the LMN involvement, this patient has signs of UMN involvement, with spasticity, brisk reflexes, and an extensor plantar response. This pattern of both UMN and LMN involvement is seen in ALS. Although structural lesions can sometimes affect both UMNs and LMNs, a structural lesion causing LMN findings in the legs (such as this patient's leg muscle atrophy and fasciculations) would have to be located in the lumbosacral spinal cord or distally, and such a lesion could never cause UMN findings in the arms (such as this patient's arm hyperreflexia and spasticity). LMN loss is widespread in ALS, resulting in diffuse atrophy that can explain the weight loss and the general level of fatigue. The initial fall could have been the result of leg weakness unrecognized by the patient at the time.

Electrodiagnostic studies confirmed these impressions. The patient in Case 4 had a nerve conduction study that showed markedly reduced conduction velocities implying an element of demyelination. Based on these results, together with the clinical history, the findings on physical examination, and an elevated spinal fluid protein, the diagnosis of CIDP was made. In this case, an initial episode remitted spontaneously, while the recurrence took place over 6 months. This woman refused a course of steroids but accepted treatment with intravenous immunoglobulin, and her symptoms stabilized.

The patient in Case 3 had normal nerve conduction studies, but needle EMG showed widespread denervation, consistent with the clinical diagnosis of motor neuron disease. He received physical therapy and appropriate counseling and was treated with riluzole and BiPAP. His weakness continued to progress, and he developed an aspiration pneumonia 18 months later. His respiratory status declined precipitously, and in accordance with his previously expressed wishes, he was not intubated or resuscitated.

Chapter 7

Dementing Illnesses

Linda M. Selwa and Douglas J. Gelb

I. Case Histories

Case 1. A 72-year-old woman with a history of hypertension has been brought to the emergency room by her daughter, who says, "She's been getting worse for 6 months, but I hoped it wouldn't come to this." Her decline began with stomach troubles, which prompted her first visit to a doctor in years, and ranitidine (Zantac) was prescribed. She was started on metoprolol (Toprol XL) because her blood pressure was noted to be high, and when her blood pressure failed to normalize, lisinopril (Zestril) was added. She began calling her daughter late at night to complain that she couldn't sleep and that she was scared to be alone. She was given a prescription for flurazepam (Dalmane) to treat her insomnia. Her gait became unsteady, and she fell and hurt her hip one week ago. She has been taking pain medicine ever since. When her daughter went to check on her late this afternoon, she was lying in bed and the sheets were soaked with urine. She did not recognize her daughter at first, and when she did, asked her, "Who are all those little men with you?"

On examination, the patient is alert, but agitated and inattentive. Her speech is fluent, but often tangential or irrelevant. She follows simple commands but becomes irritated with complicated ones. She is disoriented to time and thinks she has been brought to "the precinct house." She states her name correctly, except that she gives her maiden name rather than her married name. She recalls two of four objects after 4 minutes and can spell "world" forward, but not backwards. When asked to name the president, she becomes angry. She can name all five of her siblings but can't remember where they each live. The rest of her examination is normal, except that her reflexes are slightly more brisk on the right than on the left. She has a high serum white blood count, pyuria, normal electrolytes, and normal renal and hepatic function. A head CT scan and lumbar puncture are normal.

Questions:

1. Is this woman likely to have Alzheimer's disease?
2. How would you evaluate her in the emergency room?
3. 3 What underlying illnesses are possible?
4. How would you direct her subsequent evaluation and treatment?

Case 2. An 81-year-old man has come to see his family doctor because his wife "thinks I need to be checked out." The patient reports that nothing is wrong with him and that his wife has always been overly protective. His wife reminds him that he has had trouble driving recently, getting lost on several familiar streets, and that at a recent reunion he had been unable to recognize some old friends. She says that her husband has forgotten to pay several bills over the past year, and they hired an accountant two years ago because her husband said that the finances were "just too complex." She notes that her husband has not been taking his usual care in dressing. The patient responds that she is "making mountains out of anthills." He says that she would do better to worry about the recent burglary in their house. When his wife asks, "What burglary?" the patient says he had not wanted to worry her, but ever since they returned from a recent trip, "things were missing" around the house and new scratches had appeared on their antique furniture. He had concluded that the home was burglarized and might still be "under watch."

Except for a long history of gout and an ulcer many years ago, the patient has no history of medical problems. He takes no medications. His general physical examination is normal. He is very outgoing and speaks fluently, frequently joking about his age. He makes frequent paraphasic errors (i.e., he uses incorrect words) and sometimes makes up his own words. He cannot recall any of three simple objects and says, "That was much too long ago." He is aware of the clinic name but not the town and says it is "fallish" in 1982 or 1992. He cannot name the current president, but when told the answer, he says, "I knew that. I thought you asked if I had ever met him." He is unable to name two of his five children. He has significant difficulty drawing a clock. The remainder of his examination is normal.

Questions:

1. Does this man have Alzheimer's disease?
2. What tests would be appropriate in his evaluation?

3. What other questions about his daily life would be important in management?

4. Would it be appropriate to discuss a durable power of attorney?

Case 3. A 64-year-old woman was brought in for evaluation because she had been "acting strangely" for several months. Six months ago, she lost a significant amount of vision in her right eye and was told she had a "stroke in the eye." Since then, she had complained of headaches and seemed to have a gradually progressive memory problem. She had been intermittently sleepy, was often confused about her location, and did inappropriate things that were "out of character," including urinating in bed and not dressing properly. At times, she appeared to function perfectly normally but at other times seemed delusional.

At the time of evaluation, she had a low-grade fever and complained of headache. Her general physical examination was normal. She was alert at times but at other times tended to doze off. She had fluent speech, with normal comprehension, repetition, and naming abilities. She could spell "world" forward, but had difficulty spelling it backwards. She could only recall two of four objects at 5 minutes. She was disoriented to place, but could readily report all of her seven grandchildren's ages and middle names. She could name the president, mayor, and secretary of state. She demonstrated an appropriate level of abstraction when interpreting similarities and differences, but her judgment seemed impaired. Except for visual acuity of 20/50 in the right eye, the remainder of her neurologic examination was normal. She had a high peripheral white blood count, erythrocyte sedimentation rate (ESR) of 74, and normal electrolytes. Urinalysis revealed a urinary tract infection (UTI). Head CT and lumbar puncture were normal except for minimally elevated cerebrospinal fluid (CSF) protein of 60.

Questions:

1. Is this woman likely to have Alzheimer's disease?

2. What further evaluation is necessary?

3. What is the best plan for follow-up and treatment?

II. Approach to Dementing Illnesses

Patients with symptoms of cognitive impairment should be evaluated systematically by addressing the following questions:

1. Are the patient's symptoms truly abnormal?

2. Does the patient have memory deficits exclusively, or are other cognitive functions impaired also?

3. Is the problem progressive?

4. Does the patient have a potentially reversible cause of progressive dementia?

5. Do the patient's history, examination, and test results suggest a specific primary dementing illness, especially Alzheimer's disease, dementia with Lewy bodies (DLB), frontotemporal dementia (FTD), or vascular dementia?

The following discussion expands on each of these questions and their significance.

A. Is It Abnormal?

As patients age, they or their family members commonly express concern to physicians about declining memory. Even young adults frequently worry about the fact that they have trouble thinking of words or remembering facts. People who have watched close associates or family members struggle with Alzheimer's disease may be especially anxious when they perceive themselves having similar difficulties. They become very self-conscious, as any slight mistake serves to confirm their worst fears. Dementia is an inherently terrifying prospect to most people, because it affects functions that are integral to their personality and sense of self. The physician's task is to identify those patients in whom there is a legitimate suspicion of dementia and reassure the rest.

Most people find themselves unable to recall the name of a casual acquaintance on occasion. They may sometimes misplace items, forget to pay bills, or miss appointments. The more they focus on minor errors, the more anxious and self-conscious they become, and the more mistakes they make—which makes them even more anxious. Reassurance may be all that is required to break this cycle. In contrast, when patients report problems with routine cooking or other chores at home, when they have trouble working the controls of appliances, when they get frustrated by financial decisions that were previously second nature, when they have episodes of disorientation while driving in areas that should be familiar, or when employers or colleagues at work express concern about their job performance, a thorough evaluation is necessary.

Some patients with dementia are oblivious to it, but many recognize that they have a problem and are distressed by it. They typically have trouble providing specific examples of their deficits, however. They may say they have problems remembering names, or trouble at work, or trouble remembering where they left items around the house, but they usually express these concerns in fairly general terms. When patients report specific incidents that happened on specific days—and proceed to describe all the details of exactly what they could do and what they couldn't, and how they felt about it—a dementing illness is unlikely. When the patient acknowledges memory problems but must turn to family members to provide examples, the memory loss is more likely to be significant.

B. Is It Dementia?

Dementia is defined as an *acquired, persistent decline of intellectual function that causes impaired performance of daily activities, without clouding of the sensorium or underlying psychiatric disease.* This definition explicitly excludes some important categories of disease, which must be considered before concluding that a patient has dementia.

Delirium is defined as an *acute, transient, fluctuating confusional state characterized by impairment in maintaining and shifting attention, often associated with sensory misperception or disorganized thinking.* Patients with delirium usually have a toxic or metabolic problem, and their evaluation is described in Chapter 11.

Differentiation between dementia and *depression* may be extremely difficult at times. A "chicken and egg" problem arises: Demented patients often are depressed, partly because they are upset by their decline, and partly because the underlying brain degeneration can affect the circuitry involved in mood. On the other hand, patients with primary depression may have so much slowing of their thought and speech and such limited motivation that they appear demented. This has been called the *pseudodementia* of depression. If a patient has vegetative signs, such as changes in eating or sleeping patterns, or if the cognitive decline began after the death of a spouse or some other emotional trauma, depression is a major consideration. These clues are not always reliable, however. Cognitive symptoms may go unnoticed until the death of a spouse who had previously been "covering for" the patient's deficits. Furthermore, patients with primary dementia can develop changes in eating or sleeping patterns that resemble the vegetative signs of depression. Various diagnostic tests have been suggested for differentiating dementia and depression, but none is completely reliable. At times, an empiric trial of antidepressant medication is necessary.

Recognition of dementia is particularly difficult when the symptoms are mild. As discussed in Section A, most people experience occasional cognitive lapses, and in some cases it is relatively easy to determine that a patient's concerns are within the range of normal experience. In other cases, the patient or family members may describe symptoms that seem a little more severe than usual. The boundary between normal and abnormal is indistinct, and it becomes even more blurred with increasing age. Even in people with no evidence of neurologic disease, cognitive functions decline with age. In fact, as early as the third or fourth decade of life, sophisticated testing reveals slight slowing of some cognitive processes. This deterioration becomes more prominent with increasing age, but the rate of decline varies from person to person. Because of this variable rate of decline, and the wide variation even in baseline cognitive abilities, it is often difficult to define the precise point at which cognitive deficits are severe enough to qualify as dementia. For many patients, even after thorough evaluation, the diagnosis remains indeterminate. In explaining the situation to these patients, it is helpful to have a relatively brief term that means, essentially, "cognitive deficits that are more extensive or more severe than usual, but not severe enough to be considered dementia." A shorthand term is also useful for research—patients in this category have been the subject of extensive investigation, aimed at identifying the subgroup who will eventually prove to have dementia and determining what interventions can prevent, delay, or lessen the severity of dementia in that subgroup. Many terms have been proposed, and the one that has become most prevalent is *mild cognitive impairment* (MCI). MCI is defined as an *acquired, persistent impairment in one or more cognitive domains (typically memory) that is more severe than would be expected with normal aging, but not severe enough to interfere with social and occupational functions; consciousness is preserved.* Patients with MCI can be further subdivided into those with *amnestic* MCI and those with *nonamnestic* MCI based on whether or not their cognitive deficits include memory disturbance. Other terms that mean roughly the same thing as MCI (with some subtle distinctions) include "cognitive impairment/no dementia (CIND)," "pre-dementia," "questionable dementia," "age-associated memory impairment," and "benign senescent forgetfulness." Isolated memory impairment (IMI) is a term that refers to patients with amnestic MCI who have relatively normal cognitive function apart from their memory deficits.

References to MCI in the popular press (and sometimes in the medical literature) often make it seem as if it is a well-defined condition. In fact, it is simply a convenient way to refer to a heterogeneous group of patients. Some patients with MCI eventually progress to the point where they clearly have dementia. Other patients with MCI never reach that level of severity— it may be that they are simply be at one extreme of the normal "bell-shaped curve" with respect to the cognitive decline that occurs with aging. Others may have unrecognized depression, or some other undiagnosed condition. When diagnosing MCI, you should inform patients that the situation is ambiguous, and that you will need to follow them over time to see if they eventually develop dementia. Formal neuropsychological testing is often useful, because it provides quantitative measures that can be monitored for progression.

It might seem reasonable to treat MCI using one of the medications typically prescribed for Alzheimer's disease—after all, at least half of the patients with MCI eventually prove to have dementia; Alzheimer's disease is the most common cause of dementia; and for most diseases, early treatment is better than later. Controlled trials of those medications in patients with MCI have failed to demonstrate a convincing long-term benefit, however.

If you establish that a patient's cognitive symptoms are truly abnormal, severe enough to interfere with daily functions, and not due to delirium or depression, the next step is to try to identify the cause of dementia. Dementia is a syndrome, not a single disease. Most patients with dementia have a primary degenerative disease of the brain, but many other conditions can cause dementia. Some of these conditions are potentially reversible, so it is important to look for them.

C. Is It Progressive?

Striking loss of short- and long-term memory with preserved immediate recall and relatively preserved remote memory occurs in Korsakoff's syndrome, a condition caused by chronic thiamine deficiency, most commonly in chronic alcoholics. Patients who have experienced an episode of brain dysfunction from a wide variety of causes, such as anoxia, encephalitis (especially herpes simplex), head trauma, surgical procedures, electroconvulsive therapy, radiation therapy, meningoencephalitis, status epilepticus, or subarachnoid hemorrhage, may be left with significantly impaired cognitive function that subsequently remains stable or improves. These nonprogressive dementias do not present the same diagnostic or management issues as the progressive dementias and are not considered further here.

D. Is There a Potentially Reversible Cause?

Dementia is sometimes just one component of a more generalized disease process, such as Parkinson's disease, tertiary syphilis, or hypothyroidism.

A careful history and thorough physical examination can identify many of these conditions, but some may be relatively subtle. Hematologic diseases, systemic infections, and disorders of electrolytes, glucose, renal, or hepatic function are unlikely to be the underlying cause of dementia without producing delirium or obvious systemic symptoms. Even so, screening for these conditions is important because dementia from any cause may be exacerbated by systemic illness, and treatment of the systemic disease may result in significant improvement of cognitive function even when the underlying dementing illness is irreversible. Furthermore, a demented patient may fail to report symptoms that would otherwise make a systemic illness obvious. Thus, patients with dementia should be tested for thyroid disease and deficiency of vitamin B12 or folate, as well as renal disease, liver disease, electrolyte abnormalities, diabetes, chronic infections, and common tumors. In patients for whom a history of syphilis exposure is a realistic possibility, serum FTA (fluorescent treponemal antibody) or MHA-TP (microhemagglutination-treponema pallidum) should be tested. VDRL and RPR (rapid plasma reagin) are not sufficient in this context, because they convert back to normal in a substantial fraction of patients with late stages of syphilis.

On rare occasions, dementia is due to structural brain disease, such as hydrocephalus or mass lesions (including primary or metastatic brain tumors, abscesses, or subdural hematomas). This usually produces focal abnormalities on neurologic examination, but not always (especially if the disease affects both hemispheres equally), so patients with progressive dementia should have a brain CT or MRI scan. An imaging study is also helpful in determining the likelihood of a multi-infarct state. If the dementia has progressed rapidly, the evaluation should include HIV testing and spinal fluid analysis for chronic meningitis or other inflammatory conditions. Systemic inflammatory diseases such as systemic lupus erythematosus or giant cell (temporal) arteritis may present with dementia, and a sedimentation rate can be used as a screen.

To summarize, a standard battery of tests to screen for potentially reversible causes of dementia includes the following:

Serum: electrolytes, blood urea nitrogen, creatinine, glucose, calcium, liver enzymes, complete blood cell count, differential, sedimentation rate, vitamin B12, folate, thyroid-stimulating hormone, and (in selected cases) FTA or MHA-TP.

Urine: urinalysis.

Imaging: head CT or MRI.

E. Which Diagnosis Is Most Likely?

In most cases, dementia is due to a primary degenerative disease of the brain. Although it is important to look for other causes, especially systemic diseases or structural brain lesions that might be reversible, patients and families should be warned in advance that the blood, urine, and brain imaging studies discussed in Section D will probably have a low yield. In fact, these tests might be unnecessary except for the fact that there are no completely reliable diagnostic tests for the most common primary dementing illnesses, and systemic or structural causes of dementia can sometimes mimic them fairly closely. Definitive diagnosis of one of the primary dementing illnesses usually requires neuropathologic confirmation, but clinical features permit an accurate diagnosis during life in most patients. The diagnosis is based on how closely a patient's history, examination, and test results match the typical pattern of one of these conditions.

Because the treatment options for the primary dementing illnesses are limited, it might seem unimportant to make the effort to differentiate between them. Most patients and families are eager for a specific diagnosis, however. They appreciate knowing what to expect, and what to watch for, and this differs depending on the underlying disorder. You should be open with patients and families about the diagnosis or potential diagnoses. Some physicians avoid using terms like dementia or Alzheimer's disease because they are reluctant to frighten or depress patients, but they should realize that the possibility will not come as a surprise to most patients and families.

III. Primary Dementing Illnesses

A. Alzheimer's Disease

1. Epidemiology, pathology, and etiology

Alzheimer's disease is the most common cause of progressive dementia in adults, accounting for about 60% of cases of dementia. As a rough guideline, its prevalence is about 1% among 60-year-old people, and doubles every five years thereafter (2% at age 65, 4% at age 70, 8% at age 75, 16% at age 80, and 32% at age 85). In one survey of community residents, Alzheimer's disease affected 47% of individuals aged over 85 years.

Familial Alzheimer's disease (FAD), with an autosomal dominant pattern of inheritance, accounts for about 10% of cases of Alzheimer's disease. There is no straightforward hereditary pattern in the remaining 90% of patients, although susceptibility genes—associated with an increased likelihood of developing the disease, but not a 100% correlation—have been identified. The strongest association is with the gene for apolipoprotein E (ApoE). There are three common alleles of the ApoE gene: E2, E3, and E4. The frequency of the E4 allele in patients with late-onset sporadic Alzheimer's disease is approximately double the frequency found in control groups. Moreover, the age of onset of Alzheimer's disease correlates with the number of E4 alleles, such that the average age of symptom onset is considerably lower in homozygotes for E4 than in heterozygotes, and highest of all in patients with no copies of the E4 allele. Even so, some homozygotes never develop the disease, and a significant fraction of patients with Alzheimer's disease have no E4 allele. Other genes that may be associated with a higher risk of Alzheimer's disease include the HLA-A2 gene and low-density lipoprotein–related protein gene. Genome-wide association studies have identified associations with a gene encoding apolipoprotein J (clusterin; CLU), a gene encoding the complement component (3b/4b) receptor 1 (CR1), and a gene for phosphatidylinositol-binding clathrin assembly protein (PICALM). It remains unclear how ApoE and other genes influence pathogenesis.

The characteristic pathologic features are loss of neurons, loss of synapses, shrinkage of large cortical neurons and their dendritic arbors, amyloid (neuritic) plaques, and neurofibrillary tangles. At autopsy, cell loss is most prominent in the temporal and parietal lobes, although functional imaging studies show abnormalities in the posterior cingulate cortex even before they are evident in the temporal lobes. A number of neurochemical abnormalities have been described, including loss of choline acetyltransferase in neurons with cell bodies in the nucleus basalis of Meynert, the major source of cholinergic input to the cerebral cortex.

Neurofibrillary tangles are cytoplasmic inclusions located in the axon hillock of neurons. They are composed of filaments twisted around each other in a helical structure, called "paired helical filaments." The filaments, in turn, are composed of hyperphosphorylated forms of the microtubule-associated tau protein. In the normal brain, phosphate groups are rapidly removed from tau protein by phosphatases, whereas the tau protein in the paired helical filaments of AD patients is relatively resistant to dephosphorylation. The excess phosphorylation presumably interferes with the function of the microtubule-binding regions, leading to destabilization of microtubules and abnormal cellular transport mechanisms.

Amyloid plaques are extracellular proteinaceous deposits that are composed mainly of a peptide known as beta amyloid, or Aβ-peptide, surrounded by degenerating or dystrophic nerve endings (neurites).

Beta amyloid is a part of a larger protein, called beta amyloid precursor protein (APP), which is a transmembrane protein expressed in both neural and nonneural tissue. Its function is not known. The primary metabolic pathway for APP in normal cells involves an enzyme known as α-secretase, which cleaves the APP just above the surface of the membrane and produces a large fragment, soluble APP. An alternative APP processing pathway, which normal cells use much less often than the primary pathway, involves cleavage further from the membrane by an enzyme known as β-secretase, followed by cleavage at a site in the intra-membranous portion of APP by an enzyme known as γ-secretase. This results in the production of Aβ-peptide (see Figure 7.1). The cleavage site for α-secretase (the primary processing pathway) lies within the Aβ-peptide domain, because it is closer to the cell membrane than the cleavage site for β-secretase. Thus, in normal individuals, α-secretase ensures that only small amounts of

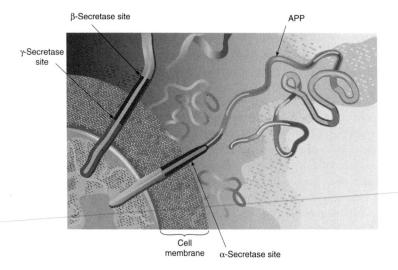

Fig. 7.1 Sites of action of α-secretase, β-secretase, and γ-secretase. The APP protein spans the cell membrane. The β-secretase cleavage site is outside the membrane, and the γ-secretase site is within the membrane; the fragment of APP produced by their combined action is the Aβ-peptide (in the figure, the two dark regions that have one end within the membrane and the other and outside the cell). The α-secretase cleavage site is outside the cell membrane but not as far out as the β-secretase site, so it lies within the Aβ-peptide domain. Thus, α-secretase activity prevents Aβ-peptide formation.

Aβ-peptide are produced. In Alzheimer's disease, however, there is increased production of Aβ-peptide, which aggregates as insoluble β-pleated sheets that form the basis of the neuritic plaque.

For many years, it was unclear whether the increased production of Aβ-peptide was a fundamental step in pathogenesis or whether it was simply a marker or a waste product that appeared in response to the disease. Current evidence indicates that it plays a fundamental role, at least in some cases. All three of the genes implicated in FAD result in increased Aβ-peptide production. One of these genes is the gene for APP itself. A second, known as presenilin-1, has been shown to be a component of the γ-secretase complex. The third gene, presenilin-2, is a protease homologous to presenilin-1 but located on a different chromosome. Transgenic mice that express mutations in APP or presenilin (or both) display behavioral and neuropathologic features that are analogous to human Alzheimer's disease. It is postulated—but not proven—that the abnormal protein products initiate an inflammatory process or trigger release of excitatory amino acids, resulting in a cascade of pathologic events that lead to neuronal death and atrophy. Some evidence suggests that Aβ-peptide exerts its toxic effect before it is sequestered into neuritic plaques, and the plaques may actually represent the brain's attempt to sequester Aβ-peptide and contain the damage.

The severity of dementia correlates more closely with the extent of tangle formation than it does with the extent of plaque formation, suggesting that the tangles also play a role in pathogenesis. Researchers have produced mouse models of Alzheimer's disease by manipulating the expression of tau protein. Mutations affecting tau protein can influence the effects of amyloid mutations, and vice-versa, but the mechanisms are not known.

2. Clinical features

Although patients with Alzheimer's disease have widespread cognitive deficits, not all cognitive functions are affected equally. There is no "typical" pattern of deficits. Some patients have nearly preserved language function and social skills that allow them to compensate for their memory deficits, which are only evident with explicit testing. Others have dramatic word-finding difficulty, but they are still able to handle their finances. Some become irritable and argumentative, while others become placid. There are countless variations. Even so, memory loss is typically the first symptom noted in Alzheimer's disease, and it remains the most prominent symptom throughout the early course of the disease (if not longer). Indeed, if some other cognitive dysfunction (such as a language disturbance, "frontal lobe deficits," or a problem with visuospatial perception) is the principal abnormality, conditions such as FTD or focal cortical degeneration should be considered.

Patients who have typical clinical features of Alzheimer's disease and in whom testing reveals no evidence for any other cause of dementia are classified as having *probable Alzheimer's disease*; this is the highest degree of diagnostic certainty that can be achieved while the patient is alive. When patients meet all the clinical criteria for probable Alzheimer's disease and autopsy findings are typical of Alzheimer's disease, they are classified as having *definite Alzheimer's disease*. Depending on the neuropathologic criteria applied, 64–86% of patients who meet the clinical criteria for probable Alzheimer's disease and who later come to autopsy prove to have definite Alzheimer's disease. Patients who have one or more clinical features that are atypical of Alzheimer's disease (such as an abnormal gait early in the course, or predominance of a focal cognitive deficit) are classified as having *possible Alzheimer's disease*. The classification of possible Alzheimer's disease also applies to patients who demonstrate typical clinical features of Alzheimer's disease but in whom another potential cause of dementia is present.

For most patients with Alzheimer's disease, dementia is the only neurologic abnormality present early in the course of the disease, but additional abnormalities commonly develop over time. About 20–40% of patients with Alzheimer's disease eventually develop bradykinesia and rigidity, which are features that are typical of Parkinson's disease (see Chapter 8). In some patients with Alzheimer's disease, bradykinesia and rigidity are already present at the time of their initial evaluation. This can lead to diagnostic uncertainty, because 25–40% of patients with Parkinson's disease eventually develop dementia, and up to 80% may have some manifestations of dementia by the time of death. DLB (see Section B) is also characterized by a combination of cognitive impairment and parkinsonism. Thus, patients who have both dementia and parkinsonism could have any of the following patterns of neuropathologic abnormalities: (1) typical findings of Alzheimer's disease, but no evidence of Parkinson's disease or DLB; (2) typical findings of Parkinson's disease, but no evidence of Alzheimer's disease or DLB; (3) typical findings of DLB (which include some features of Parkinson's disease), but no evidence of Alzheimer's disease; (4) features of both Alzheimer's disease and Parkinson's disease; or (5) features of both Alzheimer's disease and DLB. Some investigators view Parkinson's disease and DLB, and possibly even Alzheimer's disease, as different manifestations of a single underlying process. Nonetheless, they are distinct enough in most cases to consider them different diseases. In most patients with Alzheimer's disease, the parkinsonian features are less prominent and develop later than the cognitive deficits, but exceptions occur.

Myoclonus is also common in advanced Alzheimer's disease, but it is rarely present at the onset of cognitive impairment. Seizures occur in up to 10% of patients, especially late in the course. Complex partial seizures can be quite subtle in demented patients, so this possibility should be considered whenever episodes of unresponsiveness are reported. Patients with Alzheimer's disease may also develop spasticity, dysarthria, and dysphagia. Incontinence occasionally occurs early in the course but is much more common later, and it is often one of the most difficult issues caretakers confront. Another difficult management problem is posed by psychiatric manifestations. When these are prominent early in the course of the disease, an alternative diagnosis—especially DLB—should be considered, but psychiatric symptoms eventually occur in about 50% of patients with Alzheimer's disease. Delusions, agitation, and depression are common. Hallucinations are less common but also occur. Wandering behavior and sleep disturbances can also present management challenges.

The course of Alzheimer's disease is extremely variable, so it is very difficult to predict exactly when individual patients will lose specific functions or how long they will live. The average length of survival after the onset of symptoms is 8–10 years but can range up to 20 years. Patients with Alzheimer's disease have a shorter life expectancy than age-matched controls. Some studies have indicated that the best guide to prognosis is the rate at which deterioration has occurred to date; other studies indicate that the current degree of severity is the best predictor. In any case, family members should be told that the disease is invariably progressive: At some point, patients will have to restrict their activities, and other people will have to handle finances, cook, or do home repairs. Patients will eventually develop deficits in reading, reasoning, or visual perception that make it unsafe for them to drive. At later stages, they will lose the ability to maintain personal hygiene. They may become progressively more agitated to the point of violence, or progressively more withdrawn to the point of akinesia. They will eventually lose the ability to recognize even spouses and children. Death usually results from infection, most often due to aspiration pneumonia or urosepsis.

3. Diagnostic tests

Alzheimer's disease is associated with many radiologic and laboratory abnormalities, but not consistently enough for any of them to be reliable diagnostic tests. For example, atrophy on a CT or MRI scan is more common in patients with Alzheimer's disease than in age-matched controls, but some patients with Alzheimer's disease have normal brain volume on imaging studies and some normal subjects have substance loss. For that matter, the criteria for identifying atrophy on imaging studies are not standardized. For these reasons, the principal reason to obtain a structural imaging study of the brain is not to identify Alzheimer's disease, but to exclude other potential causes of progressive dementia. Functional imaging studies (positron emission tomography [PET], single photon emission tomography [SPECT]) show a typical pattern of reduced temporo-parietal metabolism and blood flow in patients with probable Alzheimer's disease, but the sensitivity and specificity of these results have not been adequately established, especially in patients with early or equivocal dementia. PET scans using an amyloid-binding agent also show characteristic abnormalities in patients with Alzheimer's disease, as well as some patients with MCI. It appears that these abnormalities may help to identify those patients with MCI who will ultimately develop Alzheimer's disease, but this work is still preliminary.

Cerebrospinal fluid levels of Aβ-peptide and tau protein may also prove to have diagnostic utility. The cerebrospinal fluid of patients with Alzheimer's disease contains lower than normal levels of Aβ-peptide and higher than normal levels of both total tau protein and phosphorylated tau protein. Furthermore, among patients with MCI, high cerebrospinal fluid levels of tau and low levels of Aβ-peptide correlate with an increased likelihood of eventually developing Alzheimer's disease, but the positive and negative predictive values of these results (individually or in combination) are not high enough to make them definitive. In addition, assays differ substantially between laboratories, so further standardization is necessary before widespread clinical use can be considered.

Despite the strong association between ApoE genotype and the risk of developing Alzheimer's disease, at least 35–50% of patients with Alzheimer's disease carry no E4 alleles. It has been suggested that the presence of an E4 allele is specific for Alzheimer's disease in patients who meet clinical criteria for probable Alzheimer's disease, but this result requires verification in a wide range of clinical settings. Elevated cerebrospinal fluid levels of neuronal thread protein, as well as other serologic tests, radiologic tests, skin tests, and pupillary reaction measurements, have also been proposed to have diagnostic utility, but no test has yet been demonstrated to have sufficient sensitivity or specificity to be clinically reliable.

4. Treatment

Four medications have been approved and are currently marketed for use in patients with Alzheimer's disease: donepezil (Aricept), rivastigmine (Exelon), galantamine (Razadyne), and memantine (Namenda). The first three are inhibitors of acetylcholinesterase, and memantine is an antagonist of the NMDA (N-methyl-d-aspartate) subclass of glutamate receptors. All of these agents have been shown to produce a modest, but statistically significant, improvement on neuropsychologic measures and on clinician and family ratings of symptom severity. The amount of improvement is roughly equivalent to the amount an average patient deteriorates in 6 months, so the effect of treatment can be likened to "setting the clock back" by 6 months. Treatment does not stop disease progression or even slow it down. The duration of the beneficial effect is unknown—most of the controlled trials lasted 6 months, but follow-up studies suggest that the cholinesterase inhibitors continue to be beneficial for at least a year. There is no evidence that any one of the cholinesterase inhibitors is more effective than another, so selection of a specific drug is based mainly on side effects or convenience. All three of them are FDA-approved for the treatment of mild to moderate Alzheimer's disease; donepezil is also FDA-approved for patients with severe Alzheimer's disease, but there is no obvious biological basis for thinking that it differs from the other two cholinesterase inhibitors in this regard. All three of these agents are available in pill form, and rivastigmine is also available as a transdermal patch. If a patient's cognitive function continues to decline steadily despite treatment, it might be reasonable to try changing from one cholinesterase inhibitor to another, because it is conceivable that certain patient subgroups have different responses to the different agents.

Memantine and the cholinesterase inhibitors have comparable effects on cognitive function. Simultaneous treatment with both memantine and donepezil results in better cognitive performance than treatment with donepezil alone, but the difference is not dramatic. Memantine is approved for the treatment of patients with moderate-to-severe Alzheimer's disease. A common approach is to begin treatment with one of the cholinesterase inhibitors when Alzheimer's disease is first diagnosed, and to add memantine when the patient's dementia becomes moderately severe. It is not clear whether memantine produces improvement that is purely symptomatic (possibly because of an effect on the function of hippocampal neurons) or whether it slows disease progression (possibly by preventing glutamate-mediated excitotoxicity).

Immunization with Aβ-peptide reduces pathologic features of Alzheimer's disease in a transgenic mouse model, and some promising reports were reported in a human trial, but the trial was terminated because 6% of the patients developed encephalitis. A second-generation vaccine engineered to provoke less of a cellular immune response is currently under investigation. Monoclonal antibodies to various domains of Aβ-peptide are also being studied. There has been considerable interest in developing ways to inhibit the activity of β-secretase or γ-secretase, or to promote the activity of α-secretase, but one difficulty is that these secretases are also involved in the processing of a variety of proteins throughout the body. Clinical trials targeted at amyloid aggregation, amyloid binding to receptors for advanced glycated endproducts, tau protein phosphorylation, and tau protein aggregation are also underway.

Dimebolin ("Dimebon"), an antihistamine with "mitochondria-stabilizing" properties, was found to be beneficial in a randomized, controlled trial conducted in Russia, but it was no better than placebo in a larger trial conducted in Europe, North America, and South America; further studies are in progress. A variety of other classes of agents, including muscarinic and nicotinic agonists, serotonergics, glycinergics, noradrenergics, calcium channel blockers, metabolic enhancers, and nerve growth factors, are still under investigation. Antioxidants may have a beneficial effect in patients with Alzheimer's disease, based on a study in which patients were randomized to receive alpha-tocopherol (vitamin E), selegiline, both, or neither. The placebo group reached the primary outcome states (nursing home placement and death) more quickly than the other three groups. This study had some methodologic flaws, however, and vitamin E may be associated with increased mortality at the doses used in the study (1000 IU twice a day), so the role of vitamin E in the management of Alzheimer's disease remains unclear. Selegiline has no role, because it has more potential side effects and confers no added benefit. Some studies have suggested that ginkgo extracts may be beneficial in Alzheimer's disease, but the evidence to date is not persuasive.

Epidemiologic studies indicate that postmenopausal estrogen replacement therapy may be associated with a reduced risk of developing Alzheimer's disease, and chronic users of nonsteroidal anti-inflammatory drugs may also have a lower risk of developing Alzheimer's disease than other individuals. All of the evidence to date comes from nonrandomized population analyses, so although the findings may signify that these medications have a protective effect, another possibility is that these medications are typically used by patients who for some reason already have a lower than average risk of developing Alzheimer's disease. Whether or not these agents have a protective effect, controlled trials have demonstrated no benefit for estrogen, nonsteroidal anti-inflammatory drugs, or prednisone in patients who already have Alzheimer's disease.

The current standard for managing patients with Alzheimer's disease consists of a cholinesterase inhibitor (with or without vitamin E), eventual addition of memantine, and symptomatic treatment. This includes antipsychotic agents or anti-epileptic drugs in patients with agitation severe enough to be potentially dangerous to themselves or others, and antidepressants and antibiotics as necessary. The newer antipsychotic medications are less likely to exacerbate confusion or cause parkinsonism than the older drugs, but they are also associated with increased cardiac mortality. "Sundowning" and sleep disorders sometimes respond to light therapy. Safety issues are important, and access to stoves, power tools, driving, and even unsupervised walks should be individually discussed and monitored.

Measures to ease the burden on caregivers are also critical. Families should be advised of community resources such as senior apartment complexes, home health aides, day care activities, visiting nurses, temporary respite programs, and (for more debilitated patients) full-time nursing care or nursing home placement. The availability of these resources depends on the community and the family's financial situation and insurance coverage, and families may wish to consult a social worker.

Patients should be encouraged to issue advance directives while they are still competent. Advance directives are documents expressing patients' wishes regarding medical, legal, and financial decisions. The two most common forms of advance directive are the living will and durable power of attorney. In a living will, a patient expresses specific preferences regarding specific situations (such as when the patient would want to be put on mechanical ventilation, if ever). With durable power of attorney, the patient designates an individual who will be responsible for making these decisions for the rest of the patient's life. Neither a living will nor a power of attorney can be issued unless the patient is legally competent, and patients who are legally competent can change or revoke these documents at any time.

B. Dementia with Lewy Bodies (DLB)

Lewy bodies are eosinophilic intracytoplasmic neuronal inclusions that were originally described in the substantia nigra and other subcortical locations in patients with Parkinson's disease (see Chapter 8). It was subsequently discovered that in about 15–25% of patients with dementia, autopsy revealed Lewy bodies distributed throughout the cortex. When researchers retrospectively reviewed the medical records of patients with these neuropathologic findings, they realized that these patients often exhibited clinical features that were not typical of Alzheimer's disease, and concluded that this represented a separate disease. This condition is known as *dementia with Lewy bodies,* or DLB. The principal distinguishing features that can occur in DLB, and would be unusual in Alzheimer's disease, are (1) the appearance of parkinsonian features, especially rigidity and bradykinesia, early in the course; (2) visual hallucinations early in the course; and (3) marked fluctuations in cognition or alertness. Other features that are suggestive of DLB include (1) REM sleep behavior disorder (see Chapter 9); (2) extreme sensitivity to antipsychotic medications; and (3) some specific abnormalities on certain nuclear medicine scans of the brain or heart. Other common, but nonspecific, features include (1) repeated episodes of falling or loss of consciousness; (2) systematized delusions, or tactile or olfactory hallucinations; and (3) prominent depression.

In some cases, the diagnosis can be fairly straightforward, but at times, DLB can be difficult to distinguish from Alzheimer's disease or from Parkinson's disease, especially because many patients with Alzheimer's disease have parkinsonian features and many patients with Parkinson's disease have dementia. Compared to patients with Alzheimer's disease, patients with DLB tend to have less severe memory deficits and more severe impairment of visuospatial and executive functions. Whereas patients with Parkinson's disease usually do not develop dementia until their disease has progressed to moderate or severe stages, patients with DLB either present with dementia or develop it within a year of symptom onset. These distinctions are not always reliable, however. In fact, as mentioned in Section A, some investigators argue that Parkinson's disease and DLB are really just gradations along a spectrum of a single underlying disease process. Because of the uncertainty in diagnosis, it is hard to define the clinical course of DLB very precisely. It appears to progress a little more rapidly than Alzheimer's disease, but the pattern and time course of progression are variable.

The neurochemical abnormalities in DLB resemble a composite of those that occur in Alzheimer's disease and Parkinson's disease. There is a dopaminergic deficit in cortical and subcortical areas due to loss of substantia nigra neurons, and a severe cortical cholinergic deficit related to loss of neurons in the nucleus basalis of Meynert. The cause of DLB is unknown, but Lewy bodies are obvious candidates for investigation. Biological characteristics of Lewy bodies and their principal component, the protein α-synuclein, are discussed in Chapter 8.

Cholinesterase inhibitors can produce some cognitive improvement in patients with DLB. Based on one study, memantine may also be beneficial. Levodopa and dopamine agonists are much less reliably effective in DLB than in Parkinson's disease, and the magnitude of benefit is usually less dramatic, but it is still reasonable to try them when parkinsonian features interfere with the patient's function. The same symptomatic treatment modalities used for Alzheimer's disease also apply to DLB, except that extreme sensitivity to antipsychotic agents has been reported, so these medications should be used with particular caution. If these medications are unavoidable, it is probably best to use one of the agents with fewer extrapyramidal side effects, such as clozapine (Clozaril), quetiapine (Seroquel), or olanzapine (Zyprexa), and to start with very low doses. Sleep disorders should be treated as they would be in other patients.

C. Frontotemporal Dementia (FTD)

In contrast to Alzheimer's disease, which preferentially involves the temporal and parietal lobes, some degenerative disorders have a predilection for the frontal and temporal lobes. These disorders are collectively known as frontotemporal dementia (FTD). The age of onset tends to be younger than for Alzheimer's disease. Only about 5–15% of patients with dementia have FTD, but the percentage is probably about twice that high among patients who develop dementia before age 65.

The clinical presentation generally falls into one of two categories: progressive behavioral disturbance or progressive language difficulty. Patients with the behavioral manifestations typically have involvement of both frontal lobes, and demonstrate prominent changes in personality and behavior. They may have apathy, blunted affect, difficulty sustaining and directing attention, poor planning, impaired reasoning, changes in eating habits, disinhibited conduct, inappropriate sexual behavior, or neglect of personal hygiene.

Patients with FTD and predominant language abnormalities typically manifest either a syndrome known as *progressive nonfluent aphasia* or a syndrome known as *semantic dementia*. Progressive nonfluent aphasia is characterized by nonfluent speech and relatively preserved comprehension, and it is associated with degeneration of the frontal and temporal lobes in the region bordering the Sylvian fissure. Semantic dementia (also known as semantic variant) is characterized by fluent but empty spontaneous speech and early loss of comprehension, usually with profound anomia and difficulty understanding the meaning of individual words; this syndrome is associated with degeneration in the anterior temporal lobe.

Progressive nonfluent aphasia and semantic dementia are both examples of *primary progressive aphasia*. This term refers to a clinical syndrome, independent of underlying pathology. As the name implies, this syndrome is characterized by gradually progressive language impairment with relative sparing of memory and other cognitive functions, at least initially. Although many patients with primary progressive aphasia have FTD, some have other diseases, such as Alzheimer's disease, corticobasal degeneration (CBD; see Chapter 8), or progressive supranuclear palsy (PSP; see Chapter 8). There are three main clinical sub-types of primary progressive aphasia – progressive nonfluent aphasia, semantic dementia, and a syndrome known as *logopenic progressive aphasia* (or "logopenic/phonologic variant"), characterized by slow, hesitant speech, profound word-finding difficulty, impaired repetition, and abnormal comprehension of syntax. This third clinical sub-type is more commonly associated with Alzheimer's disease than with FTD, but it can occur in FTD patients with degeneration of the posterior temporal lobe and inferior parietal lobule. Most patients with semantic dementia have FTD. FTD accounts for only a minority of cases of progressive nonfluent aphasia; most of these patients have CBD or PSP.

Most cases of FTD are sporadic, but as with Alzheimer's disease, hereditary factors can influence susceptibility to FTD. In about 10% of cases, the disorder is inherited in an autosomal dominant pattern. Many of these patients also have parkinsonian features.

FTD also overlaps with motor neuron disease: many patients with motor neuron disease develop cognitive and behavioral symptoms suggestive of frontotemporal dementia, and many patients with FTD (whether sporadic or dominantly inherited) develop features of motor neuron disease.

Just as the clinical syndrome of FTD is heterogeneous, so is the microscopic appearance. One particularly distinctive pattern is that of Pick's disease, marked by the presence of neuronal inclusions known as Pick bodies, which contain tau protein. Pick's disease is also characterized by neuronal loss and swollen neurons in the atrophic regions of brain. The swollen neurons are similar to those seen in CBD, a movement disorder characterized by accumulation of tau protein (discussed in Chapter 8). In most patients with FTD the classic pathologic findings of Pick's disease are absent, but these patients still have inclusions within neurons and glial cells. The inclusions contain either tau protein or ubiquitin, which is a component of the principal cellular mechanism for degrading and eliminating proteins that have become unfolded or misfolded. The ubiquinated inclusions in patients with FTD consist primarily of a protein known as TAR (transactivation response region)-DNA binding protein 43, or TDP-43. Some patients have inclusions that contain neither tau nor TDP-43; most of these patients have accumulations of the "fused in sarcoma" (FUS) protein. As discussed in Chapter 5, TDP-43 inclusions are also present in the motor neurons of many patients with ALS, and mutations in the gene coding for this protein have been found in some patients with ALS (both sporadic and familial forms); mutations in the gene coding for FUS have also been found to cause about 4% of cases of familial ALS. Mutations in the genes for TDP-43 and FUS have also been reported in patients with FTD, but only rarely. Most of the mutations that have been identified as causes of familial FTD have been in either the gene for tau protein or the gene for progranulin, a protein whose biologic function is not well understood, although some evidence suggests that it plays a role in TDP-43 processing. Both the tau gene and the progranulin gene are located on chromosome 17. Other causative genes have also been identified in FTD, but very rarely.

To summarize, most patients with FTD (whether sporadic or familial) have either TDP-43 inclusions or tau inclusions, and most of the rest have FUS inclusions. Mutations in the gene for progranulin are the most common identified causes of familial FTD with TDP-43 inclusions, and mutations in the gene for tau protein are the most common identified causes of familial FTD with tau inclusions. Some clinico-pathological correlations have emerged. Manifestations of ALS occur only in patients with TDP-43 or FUS inclusions, not in patients with tau inclusions. Semantic dementia is also more common in patients with TDP-43 inclusions, whereas progressive nonfluent aphasia is more common in patients with tau inclusions.

The diagnosis of FTD is based primarily on the clinical presentation and the exclusion of other diseases that can produce a similar pattern (such as herpes simplex encephalitis, brain tumors, or chronic subdural hematomas). Neuroimaging studies show a frontotemporal distribution of atrophy and hypometabolism, with a distinct pattern for each of the three major clinical subtypes (behavioral, progressive nonfluent aphasia, and semantic dementia). In contrast, patients with Alzheimer's disease typically show a temporoparietal pattern of hypometabolism. The Centers for

Medicare and Medicaid Services will reimburse PET studies obtained in patients suspected of having FTD.

FTD is steadily progressive. On average, it progresses more rapidly than Alzheimer's disease, but the rate of progression varies. The course is most rapid in patients with associated features of ALS. No specific treatment is available for FTD. There is no indication that cholinesterase inhibitors are beneficial. Behavioral management is often the most prominent practical issue.

D. Vascular Dementia

Dementia can result from any disorder that affects regions of the brain that are critical to cognition. Ischemic disease is a common culprit. Some patients develop cognitive impairment at the time of an unambiguous clinical stroke, and then proceed to have subsequent strokes that are clinically apparent and that clearly correlate with stepwise progression of cognitive impairment. In cases like this, the diagnosis of vascular dementia is straightforward. Other patients abruptly develop cognitive impairment that progresses in a stepwise manner, and although they don't have concurrent focal neurologic symptoms they display focal abnormalities on neurologic examination or brain imaging studies. The diagnosis of vascular dementia is fairly straightforward in these patients, also.

Other patients have a clear history of strokes, but the progression of their dementia does not correspond to the timing of the strokes. The diagnosis of vascular dementia is more problematic in these patients. The strokes may be the cause of the dementia, or they may be coincidental. The strokes could also be exacerbating an underlying (possibly unrecognized) dementia from some other cause, such as Alzheimer's disease. Similar diagnostic uncertainty results when patients with dementia have radiologic findings that suggest chronic ischemic changes, but there is no evidence of clinical strokes on history or neurologic examination. There is general agreement that dementia can result from the accumulated effects of multiple strokes, each of which in isolation might be clinically insignificant. The size, location, and number of strokes necessary to cause dementia are not known, however. Even the terminology is confusing—the terms vascular dementia, ischemic vascular dementia, multi-infarct dementia, leukoaraiosis, and Binswanger's disease are used interchangeably by some authors, whereas other authors impart specific and distinct meaning to some of these terms and discourage the use of some of the other terms altogether. In fact, different consensus groups meeting to clarify the situation each chose different terms for the diagnosis and produced somewhat different diagnostic criteria. Even so, all investigators agree that certain factors increase the likelihood that a patient's dementia is due to vascular disease: a history of recognized strokes, focal abnormalities on the neurologic examination, a history of stroke risk factors, abrupt onset of dementia, stepwise progression, and brain imaging studies that suggest multiple ischemic lesions.

The clinical features of vascular dementia are extremely variable and depend on the timing, location, and size of the strokes. The prevalence of vascular dementia depends on how it is defined, and also on the specific population under consideration. In general, Alzheimer's disease is about four to five times as common as vascular dementia. Some patients have both. In fact, conditions that predispose to vascular disease may also contribute to the pathogenesis of Alzheimer's disease.

The average life expectancy after the onset of symptoms of vascular dementia is six to eight years. In principle, progression can be halted completely if future strokes can be prevented, so these patients are candidates for all of the primary and secondary stroke prevention measures discussed in Chapter 4. One difficult issue that can arise is whether carotid stenosis should be considered symptomatic or asymptomatic in a patient with vascular dementia but no history of discrete episodes of focal neurologic deficits. As discussed in Chapter 4, endarterectomy is an effective treatment for severe stenosis in both symptomatic and asymptomatic patients, but the results are far more compelling for symptomatic patients. Patients who are thought to have vascular dementia on the basis of penetrating artery disease would fall into the category of asymptomatic carotid stenosis. In this situation the patients' overall physical condition and coexisting medical problems may be the most important factors in deciding whether to perform an endarterectomy.

Some studies suggest that cholinesterase inhibitors result in some cognitive improvement in patients with vascular dementia, so it is usually reasonable to try one of these medications. Otherwise, most treatment is symptomatic. The same considerations that apply to Alzheimer's disease in that regard are relevant to patients with vascular dementia.

E. Normal Pressure Hydrocephalus (NPH)

Patients with obstruction to ventricular outflow accumulate CSF at increased pressure in all portions of the ventricular system proximal to the obstruction. This condition, called obstructive hydrocephalus, is associated with cognitive deterioration, gait disturbance, and incontinence, together with symptoms and signs of increased intracranial pressure. Treatment is directed at removing the obstruction, if possible, and draining the enlarged ventricular system.

Normal pressure hydrocephalus (NPH) is an analogous syndrome, except that the ventricular enlargement occurs without an increase in intracranial pressure, and there is no structural obstruction to outflow. Some of these patients have a history of previous meningeal irritation (e.g., from meningitis or subarachnoid hemorrhage), presumably resulting in impaired CSF absorption at the level of the arachnoid granulations. In other patients no cause can be identified. In any event, NPH is a syndrome characterized by the clinical triad of dementia, gait disturbance, and incontinence; enlargement of the ventricular system on brain imaging studies; and clinical improvement in response to ventricular shunting procedures.

Unfortunately, the entire syndrome rarely presents in a clear-cut fashion. Some patients have one or two components of the clinical triad, but not all three. Even when the clinical triad is present, it is not necessarily specific. For example, patients with Alzheimer's disease can develop gait abnormalities because of parkinsonian features or spasticity, and incontinence is common late in the disease. The radiologic features can be ambiguous, also. Many patients have sulcal enlargement that is at least as prominent as the ventricular enlargement, suggesting that the primary problem is brain atrophy, not hydrocephalus.

Even among patients with characteristic clinical and radiologic features, shunting is sometimes unsuccessful. Among patients with atypical features, the failure rate is higher, but some of these patients still respond to shunting. Investigators have proposed a variety of clinical rules to help identify the patients who are most likely to benefit from shunting. For example, some investigators have found that shunting is most likely to be beneficial in patients for whom dementia was not the presenting symptom. Others have found that the longer symptoms have been present, the less likely a shunt will produce improvement. Unfortunately, for every rule that has been proposed, there are also studies finding it to be an unreliable guide to shunt response. This has led to a search for a useful diagnostic test. MRI scans, cisternography, blood flow studies, CSF pressure monitoring, CSF infusion tests, and high-volume lumbar punctures have all been proposed as indicators of likelihood of response to shunting. None of these tests has proved to be consistently reliable.

As a result, when some features suggest NPH but others do not, the clinician ultimately must make a judgment call. In such situations, shunting is often worth a try (assuming the patient and family understand the risks and uncertain benefit, and still wish to proceed). The major complications of shunting are infection and subdural hematoma, but in general, the procedure is fairly benign. Dramatic improvement is uncommon, but many patients and families conclude that even a slight chance of significant functional recovery is worth the risk of the procedure.

F. Creutzfeldt-Jakob Disease (CJD)

Creutzfeldt-Jakob disease (CJD) is an extremely rare condition that is of interest principally because of its public health implications and its novel biological features. It is characterized by a rapidly progressive dementia that leads to death within months to a year (average: seven months). It usually affects people over 50 years of age. During the first few weeks to months, patients typically have discrete neurologic or psychiatric symptoms, such as change in appetite, altered sleep pattern, loss of libido, loss of energy, memory problems, difficulty concentrating, poor problem solving, inappropriate behavior, emotional lability, or self-neglect. Over the next few months, cognitive function deteriorates rapidly, and most patients develop frequent myoclonic jerks. Many patients also demonstrate cerebellar abnormalities (ataxia and dysarthria), and about a third have significant behavioral disturbance or psychosis. In the final stages, patients become progressively more withdrawn and ultimately enter a state of akinetic mutism. In one variant of the disease, cerebellar symptoms are prominent early in the course. In another variant, visual symptoms predominate and may be the only symptoms at first. Another variant is marked by early muscle wasting and fasciculations that can mimic motor neuron disease. The typical neuropathologic findings are widespread neuronal loss and vacuolation, producing a spongy appearance; this condition is also called *subacute spongiform encephalopathy.*

CJD is usually sporadic, but 5–15% of cases are familial. Under certain rare conditions, the disease can be transmitted. The transmissible pathogen is a proteinaceous infectious particle, known as a prion. The unique feature of this pathogen is that unlike a virus or any other previously described infectious agent, it contains no nucleic acid. Disease occurs when the normal cellular prion protein (PrP^C), which is located on the outer surface of the cell, is replaced by the pathogenic form, PrP^{Sc}, which has the same amino acid sequence but a different conformation, resulting in a dramatic change in physical-chemical properties, including increased resistance to proteinases, reduced solubility in water, and increased tendency to polymerize. The physiologic role of the normal cellular prion protein,

PrP^C, is not known. For all three modes of transmission (hereditary, sporadic, and transmitted), a critical feature of disease propagation is that PrP^{Sc} has the ability to bind to PrP^C and induce it to change conformation and convert to PrP^{Sc}.

It is not clear what triggers the sporadic forms of CJD. The hereditary forms are caused by mutations in the gene that encodes the prion protein. Most of the documented cases of human transmission of prion diseases have involved situations in which individuals were exposed to high concentrations of substances derived from the nervous systems of other individuals. Kuru, a prion disease (with clinical manifestations similar to those of CJD) that was once endemic among the Fore tribe of Papua, New Guinea, was ultimately linked to cannibalism. Other cases have been attributed to human growth hormone derived from pooled pituitary tissue from cadavers, corneal transplants, contaminated surgical instruments, implanted EEG electrodes, and dural grafts.

The propagation of PrP^{Sc} involves interactions with prion-associated proteins that differ between species, so transmission between species is even less common than transmission within species. Nonetheless, the species barrier is not insurmountable. In experimental animals, distinct patterns of disease are produced depending on the prion isolate used. A variant form of CJD that was first reported in Great Britain in 1996, affecting younger patients (mean age of onset: 28 years), with more prominent psychiatric manifestations and a longer survival time, is thought to be related to the ingestion of beef derived from cattle infected with bovine spongiform encephalopathy (BSE, so-called mad cow disease), a prion disease of cattle. As of August 2010, only 217 cases of variant CJD had been reported, most of them in the United Kingdom.Only three cases had been reported in the United States—two of them were epidemiologically linked to likely exposure to cattle products contaminated with BSE while living in the United Kingdom, and one while living in Saudi Arabia. Twenty-one cows with BSE had been detected in North America as of August 2010: fourteen since March 2006 (all in Canada), and seven before that (four in Canada and three in the United States—two since the FDA began an enhanced screening program in 2004, and one cow before that; in each case, containment measures were taken immediately). Four cases of likely transmission of variant CJD through blood transfusion have been documented; blood-borne transmission has never been proven for any other form of CJD.

Even though CJD is rare, it should be considered when a patient presents with very rapid progression of dementia, or with prominent myoclonus or ataxia early in the disease course (although myoclonus also occurs in other dementing illnesses). The majority of patients with sporadic CJD demonstrate a characteristic abnormality on EEG, periodic complexes occurring about once a second, but this finding is less common in inherited or transmitted forms of CJD. MRI scans usually show increased signal in the cortex or basal ganglia on diffusion-weighted or FLAIR sequences, but the sensitivity and specificity of these findings remain unclear. Most patients with CJD have elevated CSF levels of 14-3-3 protein, a protein found in the cytoplasm of CNS neurons and thought to have a chaperone function in intracellular signal transduction pathways. Tau protein is also elevated in the CSF of most CJD patients, and so is a protein called neuron-specific enolase. The sensitivity and specificity of these markers remain to be established. Definitive diagnosis usually requires a brain biopsy (or autopsy); special precautions are required in performing these procedures and handling the specimens, to minimize risk of transmission. There is no known treatment for CJD, but if the diagnosis can be established, important prognostic information can be delivered to the family.

G. Other Neurologic Diseases That Produce Dementia

Dementia is common in Parkinson's disease, as discussed earlier. A number of other movement disorders that typically produce dementia are discussed in Chapter 8. In addition to the strong connections between FTD and motor neuron disease, other neuromuscular disorders—including some forms of muscular dystrophy and some myopathies—are sometimes associated with dementia. Dementia can also occur with multiple sclerosis, other inflammatory diseases of the nervous system, and some epileptic syndromes. In most cases, the diagnosis is apparent from the constellation of neurologic abnormalities, and the underlying disease process dictates management.

IV. Discussion of Case Histories

Case 1: This woman's presentation suggests a toxic delirium, rather than dementia. She is irritable, inattentive, and disoriented. She was apparently hallucinating when her daughter found her. Although patients with dementia are at particular risk for delirium, many patients with delirium have no underlying dementia. Until the delirium has been effectively managed, and the patient's sensorium is no longer clouded, it is impossible to determine whether or not the patient has dementia. Patients with delirium most often have a toxic or metabolic problem. Initial evaluation should include electrolytes, a search for underlying infection, and a drug screen to evaluate for narcotics or other contributing agents.

In this case, medications are probably a major component of her delirium. Geriatric patients are very susceptible to the cognitive effects of a number of drugs, including narcotics, H2-blockers, anticholinergics, tricyclic antidepressants, and phenothiazines. They are quite sensitive to benzodiazepines, particularly those with longer half-lives, like flurazepam. Besides taking flurazepam and pain medication, this woman is taking an H2-blocker, a beta blocker, and another anti-hypertensive medication. She also has a urinary tract infection, which can cause fairly severe confusion in the elderly.

If this patient has residual cognitive deficits after simplifying her medication regimen and treating her urinary tract infection, she may need further evaluation for dementia. Vascular dementia is a particular consideration in view of her asymmetric reflexes and history of hypertension, so an MRI scan would be appropriate, in addition to blood tests for thyroid disease and vitamin B12 deficiency. She has already been tested for other potentially reversible causes of dementia. Baseline neuropsychological testing might be helpful in monitoring for future progression.

Comment: All of the patient's medications were stopped and she was managed with calcium channel blockers and nonsteroidals. Her urinary tract infection was treated with a single dose of trimethoprim/sulfamethoxazole. Her mental status cleared completely, and no further tests were performed. She continued to have normal cognitive function at her subsequent clinic visits.

Case 2: This man has a typical history of moderately advanced Alzheimer's disease. He has a prominent memory disturbance with associated language disturbance, visuospatial deficits, and delusions. Social skills remain relatively intact. Formal neuropsychological testing might be useful to demonstrate to him that there is objective evidence of cognitive impairment and that his wife is not just "making mountains out of anthills." Such testing could also identify his areas of relative strength. An imaging study is important to look for structural lesions, but these are unlikely given his history and nonfocal examination. This patient should have the standard laboratory tests to look for a potentially reversible cause of dementia. Hearing should also be assessed to see if it is contributing to problems understanding spoken language. Assuming no other cause of dementia is identified, he meets criteria for the diagnosis of probable Alzheimer's disease, and should begin taking a cholinesterase inhibitor.

Other issues that must be addressed in patients with progressive dementia include safety, behavior problems, and family support. The patient should have a formal assessment of his driving ability. Consideration should be given to whether he should operate tools, cook, or handle any financial matters. The wife's ability to care for the patient and meet her own needs in this situation should be tactfully assessed and support offered. The patient and family should be educated about the illness, and advance directives should be discussed.

Case 3: As with the patient in Case 1, this woman's presentation suggested a subacute delirium rather than dementia. The salient features were intermittent sleepiness, disorientation, and poor processing of new material, with intact higher cognitive functions. Again, a clouded sensorium precludes the diagnosis of dementia. In any patient who has delirium, primary considerations are metabolic abnormalities (especially drug-related) and infectious or inflammatory processes. Of particular concern in this woman was the monocular visual loss. A focal finding makes a metabolic problem less likely and should prompt vigorous evaluation for some other explanation. The lumbar puncture and head CT were thus completely appropriate tests, as chronic meningitis (especially cryptococcal) and abscess were realistic concerns.

Comment: In this woman, symptoms did not resolve after treatment of her urinary tract infection, and repeat ESR 10 days later was 70. Because of her persistent headaches and history of visual loss, a temporal artery biopsy was performed and showed giant cell (temporal) arteritis. After treatment with steroids, mental status and headaches improved and she resumed an entirely independent life. Giant cell arteritis is discussed further in Chapters 12 and 13.

Chapter 8

Movement Disorders

Linda M. Selwa and Douglas J. Gelb

I. Case Histories

Case 1. A 70-year-old woman comes to see you for "shakiness" in one hand that began approximately 6 months ago. She also complains bitterly about "getting older" and losing a lot of her previous energy and motivation. She no longer attends conferences that once occupied much of her time and energy, and she has limited her gardening activities significantly this year. She takes no medications. Her general physical examination is normal. She presents her history clearly and concisely and responds appropriately to questions and instructions. Her cranial nerves are normal except for a rather expressionless face, with no clear facial weakness. She has a slight stoop, but no postural instability. Her stride is normal. She has decreased arm swing on the left, and she turns en bloc in four steps. Her finger movements are slow but normally coordinated. She has a prominent rest tremor in the left arm that improves with volitional movement. There is some cogwheel rigidity on the left. She has normal strength, reflexes, and sensation.

Questions:

1. What would you tell this woman about her diagnosis?
2. What potential complications should be addressed at this stage?
3. What therapy is appropriate?

Case 2 A 59-year-old woman with diabetes presents with complaints of generalized weakness and bilateral upper extremity tremor for the last three months. She has fallen twice, but says that she just tripped. She has been experiencing abdominal bloating and weight loss. Her diabetes has been difficult to manage, and she is also troubled by numbness in her feet. The patient wonders whether her "foot problem" may be causing some of her unsteadiness. Medications include thyroid hormone replacement, insulin, metoclopramide (Reglan), and diltiazem (Cardizem). On examination, she has normal mental status and cranial nerves, though her face is expressionless. Her gait is festinating and slow, with reduced arm swing bilaterally. There is mild postural instability. She has marked bradykinesia, rigidity, and a mild bilateral rest tremor. There is full strength in all muscle groups. Her reflexes are normal in the upper extremities and at the knees but can only be elicited at the ankles with reinforcement. Except for some mild reduction of vibration sense at the toes bilaterally, she has normal sensation throughout.

Questions:

1. How would you proceed with the evaluation?
2. Does she need evaluation for peripheral polyneuropathy?
3. What is the most appropriate treatment for this woman?

II. Approach to Movement Disorders

The term "movement disorder" refers to a heterogeneous group of conditions that result in abnormal form or timing of voluntary movement in individuals with normal strength and sensation. Appropriate management of a patient with a movement disorder depends on the answers to five questions:

1. How can the patient's movements be characterized?
2. Are the movements due to a potentially reversible systemic cause, such as medication toxicity?
3. Do the abnormal movements and accompanying abnormalities conform to a recognized condition?
4. What oral medications are likely to help this condition?
5. If the patient's condition can not be controlled adequately with medications, are injections or surgical interventions feasible?

Question 1 is addressed in Part III. Questions 2, 3, 4, and 5 are addressed in Part IV.

III. Background Information

A. Anatomic Definitions

Basal ganglia: caudate, putamen, globus pallidus, substantia nigra, and subthalamic nucleus

Corpus striatum: caudate, putamen, and globus pallidus

Lentiform nucleus (also called the **lenticular nucleus**): putamen plus globus pallidus

Striatum: caudate plus putamen (synonym: **neostriatum**)

B. Clinical Definitions

action tremor a tremor that is most prominent on voluntary contraction of a muscle; this encompasses both postural tremor and kinetic tremor

akinesia lack of voluntary movements

ataxia incoordination or awkwardness in the performance of a motor task; inability to perform the components of the movement at the right time and/or in the appropriate position

athetosis slow, sinuous writhing of the distal parts of limbs – usually accompanies chorea, and is probably another point on the spectrum of clinical manifestations of the same pathophysiologic mechanism

ballism large-amplitude, involuntary flinging movements of the proximal parts of limbs – probably another point on the spectrum (with chorea and athetosis) of clinical manifestations of a single pathophysiologic mechanism

bradykinesia reduced speed, spontaneity, and amplitude of voluntary movements; sometimes referred to as "hypokinesia"

chorea rapid, jerky involuntary movements appearing irregularly and unpredictably in various body parts, sometimes seeming to "flow" from one region to another. See *athetosis* and *ballism*

cogwheeling ratchet-like, rhythmic interruptions in resistance to passive manipulation.

dyskinesia any abnormal involuntary movement

dystonia involuntary, sustained muscle contractions often having a preferred direction, resulting in maintenance of an abnormal posture or repetitive twisting movements

festination an involuntary tendency for a movement to accelerate and decrease in amplitude; usually applied to gait

intention tremor a kinetic tremor that is most prominent on approaching the target of a goal-directed movement (i.e., a *terminal kinetic tremor*)

kinetic tremor tremor that is accentuated during guided voluntary movement (such as handwriting or touching finger to nose). Kinetic tremor can be subdivided into *initial tremor* (occurring predominantly at the initiation of movement), *transition tremor* (predominantly during the movement), or *terminal tremor* (predominantly at the termination of movement). See *intention tremor*

myoclonus rapid shock-like muscle jerks similar to chorea, but more discrete (less likely to blend into one another) and more likely to be localized

postural tremor a tremor that is most prominent when the body part is maintained in a nonresting posture (such as keeping the arms extended parallel to the floor), less prominent when the body part is completely relaxed

rest tremor tremor that is most prominent when the body part is in complete repose and not working against gravity, less prominent with movement or maintenance of a posture (also called *resting tremor*)

rigidity increased resistance to passive manipulation throughout the range of movement, equal in flexors and extensors, and independent of the velocity of movement

task-specific tremor kinetic tremor that appears or is exacerbated during certain tasks, such as writing, but is absent or attenuated when not engaged in those tasks

tics abrupt, transient, stereotypical, coordinated movements or vocalizations that can often be voluntarily suppressed but at the expense of a buildup of inner tension that is relieved when the suppression is removed

tremor involuntary rhythmic oscillation of a body part, produced by either alternating or synchronous contractions of reciprocally innervated antagonist muscles

C. Classification of Movement Disorders

Movement disorders are closely associated with dysfunction of the basal ganglia, which can be thought of as a brain system devoted to the implementation of motor plans developed in the cortex. The basal ganglia consist of the striatum (the caudate and putamen), the globus pallidus, the substantia nigra, and the subthalamic nucleus. Movement disorders can be grouped into three general categories, *hypokinetic, hyperkinetic,* and *ataxic.*

The hallmark of hypokinetic movement disorders is *parkinsonism,* which is characterized by bradykinesia, rigidity, and rest tremor. It correlates with disruption of striatal dopaminergic transmission, improves with enhancement of dopamine transmission, and worsens in response to dopamine antagonism.

Hyperkinetic movement disorders are characterized by involuntary movements that intrude into the normal flow of motor acts. Chorea, athetosis, and ballism may all represent points on a spectrum of clinical manifestations of the same underlying pathophysiologic mechanism. These movements correlate with dysfunction within the striatum or the subthalamic nucleus. They are suppressed by dopamine antagonism and exacerbated by increased dopaminergic transmission. Postural and kinetic tremors may be due to abnormalities of cerebellar outflow to the thalamus. Dystonia is marked by twisting and repetitive movements or sustained abnormal postures, often with a preferred direction. Dystonia is classified as focal (involving specific, localized muscle groups), segmental (involving two or more contiguous areas of the body), multifocal (involving two or more noncontiguous areas), hemidystonia (involving one side of the body), or generalized (involving the entire body). The neuroanatomic substrate is not known, and different dystonias may originate in different parts of the motor system. No drug consistently improves or exacerbates dystonia. Tics are also classified as hyperkinetic movement disorders.

Ataxic movement disorders are characterized by a lack of speed and skill in performing acts requiring the smoothly coordinated activity of several muscles. Typical features include dysmetria (inaccurate trajectory of a body part during active movements), dysrhythmokinesis (inability to move a body part in a regular rhythm), dysdiadochokinesis (impaired speed, precision, and rhythm when performing rapidly alternating movements), difficulty correcting for perturbations of body position, unstable gait, and dysarthria (characterized by irregular variations in the rate, volume, and pitch of speech). These abnormalities correlate with dysfunction of the cerebellum or its connections. As mentioned above, abnormalities of cerebellar outflow are also associated with tremor.

IV. Specific Movement Disorders

A. Essential Tremor

Essential tremor is a common movement disorder without clearly defined pathophysiology. The characteristic finding is a postural and terminal kinetic tremor most prominent in the upper extremities. The tremor is typically bilateral, but it may be asymmetric, and at onset it may be unilateral. There is often an associated head tremor, and occasionally this is the predominant symptom. There may also be an associated voice tremor, which is less likely to occur in isolation. The frequency of essential tremor ranges from 4–12 Hz, with wide fluctuations in amplitude. Unlike patients with Parkinson's disease, patients with essential tremor have no rigidity, postural instability, or bradykinesia. Many cases are familial. Generally, symptoms are mild and associated with only minor progression over decades, but in some cases the condition is disabling enough to interfere with writing, dressing, and eating. Essential tremor often responds briefly but dramatically to ethanol consumption, which may be a useful diagnostic feature.

The diagnosis of essential tremor is established primarily on the basis of a typical history and examination and the absence of other causes of tremor. Beta-adrenergic agonists, lithium, valproic acid, cyclosporine, tacrolimus, tamoxifen, amiodarone, and thyroxine commonly cause postural or kinetic tremor. Selective serotonin reuptake inhibitors and tricyclic antidepressant medications can also cause tremor. Before making the diagnosis, patients should generally have blood testing to exclude hyperthyroidism.

Once they have been reassured that the condition is not life-threatening (and that they do not have Parkinson's disease), many patients say that the tremor is tolerable and they do not need treatment. When the tremor causes significant embarrassment or interferes with their daily activities, medication should be prescribed. Beta-adrenergic blockers (particularly propranolol) and primidone are the most consistently effective agents. Topiramate and pregabalin were found to be beneficial in controlled trials; the evidence is inconclusive for gabapentin, levetiracetam, zonisamide, anticholinergic medications, benzodiazepines, amantadine, clonidine, acetazolamide, and methazolamide. For severe, refractory essential tremor, surgical implantation of a deep brain stimulator in the ventral intermediate nucleus of the thalamus contralateral to the affected limb produces dramatic improvement in approximately 85% of patients. The mechanism by which high-frequency stimulation reduces tremor is still unclear.

B. Parkinson's Disease

1. Clinical features

The cardinal signs of Parkinson's disease are bradykinesia, rest tremor, rigidity, and (eventually) postural instability. These combine to produce characteristic manifestations. One is *festination*, a tendency toward decreased amplitude and increased frequency when carrying out a sustained motor activity. In the typical parkinsonian gait, for example, the steps get smaller and smaller and faster and faster until the patient is practically walking in place. Another example is *micrographia*, or small handwriting, which gets progressively smaller toward the end of a writing sample. The motor control of speech is also subject to this phenomenon— patients typically speak at low volumes, with their speech growing progressively softer and more rapid the longer they talk. This type of *dysarthria* is classified as hypokinetic. Another typical manifestation is reduced facial expression and blinking rate (a "*masked face*"). As the disease progresses, the postural instability and rigidity may cause patients to *turn en bloc* when walking: rather than pivot 180 degrees in a single step, they make many small angular adjustments while standing in one place. In advanced stages of the disease, patients often have particular difficulty initiating movement, appearing totally "frozen," but after intense effort they set themselves in motion and then proceed to carry out the movement almost normally. Sometimes their initiation of movement can be facilitated by placing an obstacle in their way; it can be quite striking to watch a patient fixed in one spot suddenly begin walking normally when asked to step over the examiner's foot. Before long, however, the steps become smaller and faster, and the patient often gets stuck again. A similar phenomenon is described in a sudden emergency, such as a fire, in which patients have even been observed to run.

The characteristic tremor of Parkinson's disease is a rest tremor, becoming less prominent with voluntary movement. It has a frequency of 4 Hz, and in the hands there is classically a "pill-rolling" character. A low amplitude postural or kinetic tremor of 7–8 Hz also occurs in Parkinson's disease. An individual patient may have either type of tremor or both. Both kinds of tremor may fluctuate dramatically from one moment to the next, independent of medication regimen.

The clinical manifestations of Parkinson's disease often begin in a single limb, gradually progressing to involve the other limb on the same side, and eventually to the other side of the body. A commonly used scale for grading the severity of motor dysfunction is the one developed by Hoehn and Yahr: stage 1 = unilateral disease, stage 2 = bilateral disease without impairment of balance, stage 3 = bilateral disease with some postural instability but physically independent, stage 4 = severe disability but able to walk or stand unassisted, stage 5 = wheelchair-bound or bedridden without assistance.

As discussed in Chapter 7, many patients with Parkinson's disease develop dementia, so it is sometimes difficult to distinguish patients who have Parkinson's disease from those who have dementia with Lewy bodies (DLB) or even from patients with Alzheimer's disease, many of whom have parkinsonian features. Patients with Parkinson's disease may also experience delusions or hallucinations. These are often related to drug therapy. Hallucinations can also occur independently, but this should prompt consideration of DLB. Depression is also common in patients with Parkinson's disease. It appears to be a direct manifestation of the underlying neuropathologic changes, rather than a purely reactive depression, but debate continues on the subject. Pain is often an early feature of Parkinson's disease, and so is olfactory dysfunction. Sleep disorders and some degree of autonomic dysfunction are very common. In fact, REM sleep behavior disorder (see Chapter 9) may precede other manifestations of Parkinson's disease by many years, and constipation is frequently present in the years prior to diagnosis.

2. Epidemiology, pathology, and etiology

Parkinson's disease is uncommon below the age of 50 years, but it affects about 1% of individuals above that age, about 2% of individuals above the age of 65 years, and more than 3% of individuals above the age of 85 years. The incidence is slightly higher in men than in women (1.5:1), and higher in whites than in other racial groups.

Pathologically, Parkinson's disease is characterized by diffuse loss of pigmented neurons in the pars compacta of the substantia nigra, associated with a deficit of dopamine production in the nigrostriatal pathway. Surviving neurons often contain characteristic inclusions known as Lewy bodies, which are also present in the locus ceruleus and several other discrete nuclei. The principal component of Lewy bodies is α-synuclein, a protein that helps to maintain the integrity of neurotransmitter-bearing vesicles and facilitates their transport. Several other proteins are present in Lewy bodies, including ubiquitin. As explained in Chapter 7 (in the discussion of frontotemporal dementia), the ubiquitin-proteasome system is the principal cellular mechanism for degrading and eliminating proteins that have become unfolded or misfolded.

Genetic transmission is rare, but a few pedigrees have been described with familial Parkinson's disease or parkinsonism. Mutations in the gene for α-synuclein have been identified in about 2% of families with dominantly inherited Parkinson's disease, suggesting that this protein plays a role in pathogenesis. Other cases of familial parkinsonism are associated with mutations in genes involved in the ubiquitin-proteasome system, including one known as *parkin*, which encodes ubiquitin E3 ligase.

Mutations in the *parkin* gene account for up to 50% of familial cases of juvenile parkinsonism; the pattern of transmission is autosomal recessive. *Parkin* mutations are present in 18% of patients with sporadic Parkinson's disease of early onset (before age 40 years). Mutations in other genes have also been found to cause familial forms of parkinsonism. The most common is the *leucine rich repeat kinase 2 (LRRK2)* gene, which is expressed in an autosomal dominant pattern and resembles idiopathic Parkinson's disease with respect to the age of onset, severity, and clinical course. Mutations in this gene account for about 5–8% of cases of familial Parkinson's disease, and about 1.5% of sporadic cases. The prevalence is much higher in certain ethnic groups—for example, as many as 40% of patients with Parkinson's disease who are of Arab descent and about 20% patients of Ashkenazi Jewish descent have mutations in this gene, even in the absence of a clear family history of Parkinson's disease. Other genes in which causative mutations have been identified include the gene *DJ-1*, which codes for an antioxidant protein, the *PTEN-induced putative kinase-1 (PINK1)* gene, which codes for a mitochondrial kinase, the gene *ATP13A2*, which codes for a lysosomal ATPase, the *Nurr1* gene, which codes for a nuclear receptor critical to the development and survival of dopaminergic cells, and the gene for ubiquitin carboxy-terminal hydrolase L1 (UCH-L1).

All of these causative mutations are extremely rare. Even the most widespread mutation, affecting the *LRRK2* gene, is absent in the majority of patients with Parkinson's disease. Recent evidence suggests that certain polymorphisms are associated with increased likelihood of Parkinson's disease, even though they are not causative. Some of these polymorphisms are in the gene and promoter for α-synuclein, some in the *LRRK2* gene, others in a gene for a component of the cytochrome P450 system, and others in a gene for glutathione S-transferase pi. Patients with Parkinson's disease also have a much higher than average incidence of mutations in the gene for glucocerebrosidase; mutations in this gene have long been known to be responsible for Gaucher disease, a lysosomal storage disorder.

Environmental factors could also play a role in pathogenesis. Cigarette smoking is associated with a reduced risk of developing Parkinson's disease—one of the few health benefits ever attributed to that habit by anyone outside the tobacco industry. The risk of Parkinson's disease also appears to be lower in coffee drinkers, although the evidence is less consistent. Elevated plasma levels of uric acid are associated with lower rates of Parkinson's disease. In contrast, some studies have suggested increased rates of Parkinson's disease in association with a variety of factors, including rural living, lifetime exposure to well water, head trauma, manganese, lead, pesticides, and herbicides. After chronic exposure to rotenone, a widely used pesticide that is a potent inhibitor of mitochondrial complex I, rats develop a syndrome similar to Parkinson's disease. Some intravenous drug users in the early 1980s developed a parkinsonian syndrome that was ultimately attributed to a synthetic compound, MPTP, a metabolite of which inhibits mitochondrial complex I.

Based on these environmental associations, together with the products encoded by the causative genes and susceptibility genes, several factors appear to be important in the pathogenesis of Parkinson's disease: impaired clearance of unwanted proteins (especially α-synuclein) by the ubiquitin-proteasome system, mitochondrial dysfunction, oxidative stress, and excitotoxicity. Each of these factors could precipitate or exacerbate any of the others, and it is not clear if any one factor is more fundamental than the others.

3. Differential diagnosis

There is no consistently reliable diagnostic test for Parkinson's disease. Even when experienced clinicians make the diagnosis, it is confirmed at autopsy in only 75% of patients. Nonetheless, when patients with typical clinical features experience a substantial and sustained response to dopaminergic therapy, and several "Parkinson's mimics" have been eliminated, the diagnosis is usually straightforward.

Drug-induced parkinsonism is the condition that most closely mimics Parkinson's disease. It must be carefully considered in all cases, particularly when symptom onset is acute or subacute. Early withdrawal of the offending agent is important. Parkinsonism is a frequent side effect of antipsychotic medications (including phenothiazines and butyrophenones) and anti-emetic medications (such as metoclopramide, prochlorperazine, and promethazine). Reserpine and related antihypertensive medications, some calcium channel blockers, amiodarone, and some immunosuppressants may produce parkinsonism; it can also occur after manganese poisoning or exposure to carbon monoxide.

Patients who have had multiple strokes may develop clinical features that resemble Parkinson's disease, and occasionally this can occur after a single subcortical stroke. There are also several syndromes in which parkinsonism accompanies other neurologic abnormalities. The clinical and neuropathologic findings that distinguish these illnesses are reviewed in Section C. Many of the distinctive clinical features may not appear until later in the course of the disease, making it hard to differentiate them from

Parkinson's disease initially. In general, patients with other parkinsonian syndromes are less likely than patients with Parkinson's disease to respond to dopaminergic therapy, and in those who do respond the benefit may be only partial and temporary.

The most common diagnostic question that arises in the context of Parkinson's disease is whether a patient simply has essential tremor. Classically, essential tremor has different characteristics from the tremor of Parkinson's disease, but patients with Parkinson's disease do not always exhibit the "classic" tremor, so differentiation from essential tremor on this basis is sometimes difficult. The most reliable way to distinguish the two disorders is on the basis of accompanying rigidity or bradykinesia, but these may be quite subtle, especially early in the course. At times, a patient must be observed for months to years before the diagnosis is clear.

4. Treatment of motor manifestations

Dopaminergic medication is the cornerstone of therapy. Dopamine itself does not cross the blood-brain barrier and causes systemic side-effects, but two alternative approaches are available. The first is to administer L-dopa (L-dihydroxyphenylalanine, also called levodopa), which crosses the blood-brain barrier and is converted to dopamine within neurons by the enzyme dopa decarboxylase. L-dopa is typically administered in combination with a drug called carbidopa, which blocks peripheral dopa decarboxylase, resulting in reduced conversion to dopamine peripherally and thereby minimizing systemic side effects and increasing the amount of L-dopa entering the brain. The combination of L-dopa and carbidopa is marketed as Sinemet; a long-acting preparation is also available. The second approach to enhancing activity in dopaminergic pathways is to administer dopamine receptor agonists. These have the advantage of acting directly on the post-synaptic receptors, so they do not require processing by the pre-synaptic cells (which are gradually depleted as the disease progresses). The advantage of L-dopa, conversely, is that it is released by the pre-synaptic cells in a manner that is presumably coordinated with motor activity, so it is modulated in a physiologic way rather than according to a fixed dosing schedule.

The currently used dopamine receptor agonists—bromocriptine (Parlodel), pramipexole (Mirapex), and ropinirole (Requip)—have different affinity profiles for the five known dopamine receptors, but it is not clear how these differences influence their relative efficacy and toxicity. Another dopamine agonist, apomorphine, has been approved for subcutaneous administration in patients with an acute episode of bradykinesia; it can also be administered rectally or as a nasal aerosol. Cabergoline (Dostinex), another dopamine agonist, has the potential advantage of a very long half-life, but it is currently approved only for hyperprolactinemia. The FDA approved the dopamine agonist, rotigotine (Neupro), as a transdermal patch. The manufacturer recalled it from the U.S. market in 2008 due to reports of crystallization of the compound on the patch, but hopes to make it available again in the future.

Dopaminergic treatment is generally started once symptoms interfere with a patient's activities. A reasonable approach is to begin with L-dopa. Most patients improve substantially even on very low doses of medication, and almost all patients with Parkinson's disease experience improvement if high enough doses are used. In fact, dopaminergic medication is so consistently effective that a failure to respond should prompt the clinician to re-consider the diagnosis. As the disease progresses, the initially effective dose gradually becomes inadequate. At first, this can be addressed by increasing the L-dopa dose or shortening the time interval between doses, but eventually, many patients develop unpredictable fluctuations between an "on" state in which the medication is effective and an "off" state in which they may be nearly immobile. In addition, some patients develop frequent or continuous involuntary movements, or dyskinesia, to the point where they spend the bulk of their time unable to function because they are either in the "off" state or severely dyskinetic. In an attempt to minimize the development of these adverse motor phenomena, some clinicians introduce a dopamine agonist either before or soon after starting L-dopa, rather than the traditional approach of gradually advancing the L-dopa dose as necessary until limited by side effects. Some clinicians also advocate early treatment with dopamine agonists because of theoretical concerns that L-dopa might actually have negative long-term consequences. This theoretical toxicity has never been convincingly demonstrated in practice, and must be balanced against the high rate of side effects associated with the dopamine agonists. In controlled trials, patients who were started on dopamine agonists early had fewer dyskinesias and motor fluctuations than patients on L-dopa alone, but their parkinsonism was not as well controlled. Thus, the timing of initiation of dopamine agonists relative to L-dopa remains controversial.

Regardless of whether or not dopamine agonists should be prescribed early in the course, their eventual use may modify motor fluctuations and reduce the required L-dopa dose after dyskinesias become prominent. Another strategy for reducing the required L-dopa dose and prolonging the response to each dose (thereby possibly modulating motor fluctuations) is to add entacapone (Comtan). This medication inhibits peripheral L-dopa breakdown by the enzyme catechol O-methyltransferase (COMT). A similar medication, tolcapone (Tasmar), has the advantage of penetrating the blood-brain barrier, but it is rarely used because of hepatotoxicity. Anticholinergic medications are mainly valuable for treatment of rest tremor. All of these drugs (dopamine agonists, COMT inhibitors, and anticholinergic agents) can produce hallucinations and excessive daytime somnolence. Amantadine (Symmetrel) is a useful adjunct to dopaminergic agents, especially when patients develop dyskinesia. Its mechanism of action is poorly understood, but it may relate to antiglutamatergic properties.

Two monoamine oxidase type B (MAO-B) inhibitors, selegiline (Deprenyl) and rasagiline (Azilect), are approved and marketed for Parkinson's disease. Both of these medications improve symptoms; it has been suggested that they might also slow disease progression, but this remains unproven. When selegiline is used in early stages of Parkinson's disease, it postpones the need to initiate dopamine therapy, but this could be explained purely on the basis of selegiline's symptomatic benefit. In a trial employing a novel study design, patients were randomized to receive rasagiline either upon study entry or after a delay of 36 weeks; when assessed 72 weeks after study entry, the early-start group showed less evidence of disease progression than the delayed-start group. This trial provided the best evidence to date of a possible disease-modifying effect, although other interpretations are feasible, and the end-point was achieved with only one of the two doses studied. Preliminary evidence suggests that coenzyme Q10 may be beneficial in patients with early Parkinson's disease, but further study is necessary.

For some severely affected patients who can no longer be managed effectively with medications, several surgical options are available. Ablative procedures, including pallidotomy and thalamotomy, are intended to counteract an imbalance in the circuit connecting basal ganglia, thalamus, and cortex. These procedures are effective, but they have been largely supplanted by the technique of stereotactic implantation of a stimulating electrode in the subthalamic nucleus or the internal segment of the globus pallidus. Although the precise mechanism is debated, deep brain stimulation disrupts the basal ganglia circuitry without producing a permanent anatomic lesion. It produces enduring improvement in bradykinesia, rigidity, tremor, and gait disturbance, but only in patients whose symptoms respond to L-dopa. The degree of improvement is generally comparable to the level of improvement the patient experiences when in the best L-dopa "on" state. The major exception to this rule is tremor, which may respond to deep brain stimulation even when it is refractory to medication. Also, tremor differs from the other features of Parkinson's disease in that it responds not only to stimulator placement in the subthalamic nucleus or the internal segment of the globus pallidus, but also to stimulation of the ventral intermediate nucleus of the thalamus (the same site typically targeted in patients with essential tremor), which is not effective for the other parkinsonian features. Note that deep brain stimulation should not be considered in patients who have dementia. A final surgical option—transplantation of fetal adrenal tissue—is still experimental.

5. Treatment of nonmotor manifestations

Hallucinations are uncommon in patients with untreated Parkinson's disease, but may occur in up to 30% of patients on chronic treatment. Unfortunately, many antipsychotic medications can exacerbate the motor features of Parkinson's disease. When the hallucinations are nonthreatening and nondisruptive, it may not be necessary to treat them at all. When they are severe enough to require treatment, quetiapine and clozapine are the antipsychotic medications least likely to exacerbate the motor symptoms. Clozapine requires routine blood tests to monitor for agranulocytosis, so quetiapine is the medication of choice. Depression affects up to 50% of patients with Parkinson's disease, and responds to standard treatment. Rivastigmine is FDA-approved for patients with Parkinson's disease and dementia; there is no compelling reason to think that it would be more effective than the other cholinesterase inhibitors in this population. The cholinesterase inhibitors are sometimes used instead of antipsychotic medications to treat hallucinations, also. Sleep disorders are very common in patients with Parkinson's disease, and should be evaluated and managed in the standard fashion (see Chapter 9). Dopamine agonists can cause severe daytime somnolence, and may need to be stopped in patients who have this problem. Orthostatic hypotension can also occur in Parkinson's disease. In some cases, it is medication-induced, and manipulation of the medication regimen can be helpful. In other cases, it is due to the underlying disease process, and the same management approaches used in patients with multiple system atrophy may be useful in patients with Parkinson's disease (See Section C).

C. Other Parkinsonian Syndromes

Several diseases are characterized by parkinsonism in association with additional neurologic abnormalities. These conditions share many clinical and pathologic features, leading to considerable diagnostic confusion. Advances in molecular genetics are demonstrating unexpected relationships between some of these conditions that were previously thought to be distinct, while suggesting that other conditions might be more heterogeneous than previously suspected. Many of these diagnostic categories are still in flux.

The accumulation of abnormal protein is a common feature of many conditions that result in progressive dementia, parkinsonism, or both. It is thought that the particular proteins involved, and the specific abnormalities those proteins contain, may determine the nature and distribution of pathology. Thus, these conditions can be roughly categorized into three groups, based on whether the most prominent protein abnormality involves amyloid (Alzheimer's disease), tau protein (progressive supranuclear palsy, corticobasal degeneration, Alzheimer's disease, and sometimes frontotemporal dementia), or α-synuclein (Parkinson's disease, DLB, multiple system atrophy).

1. Dementia with Lewy bodies (DLB)

DLB is discussed in greater detail in Chapter 7. This condition results in cognitive deficits, behavioral abnormalities, and parkinsonism. These symptoms can develop in any order, but the dementia usually appears relatively early in the course, so the standard convention is to diagnose DLB only when the dementia precedes the parkinsonism or develops within a year of the onset of the parkinsonism. Patients who have motor manifestations of parkinsonism for more than a year before developing any symptoms of dementia are classified as having Parkinson's disease with dementia.

2. Progressive supranuclear palsy (PSP)

The earliest symptoms of progressive supranuclear palsy (PSP) often resemble typical Parkinson's disease, but patients eventually develop characteristic eye movement abnormalities. Downgaze palsy is often the initial abnormality. Patients next develop an upgaze palsy and then difficulty with voluntary horizontal gaze. The vestibulo-ocular reflex is intact, indicating that the gaze palsy is supranuclear (see Chapter 2). Other features that help distinguish PSP from Parkinson's disease are that in PSP, prominent gait disturbances and falls occur earlier in the illness, tremor is less common, and response to L-dopa is less consistent. Neck dystonia and axial (trunk and head) rigidity are often present in PSP. Dysphagia develops early in the course and can be a severely limiting feature, and dysarthria is also prominent. Cognitive deficits are often quite subtle and consist primarily of "executive" or "frontal lobe" features such as personality changes, poor judgment, impulsiveness, concrete thinking, and difficulty maintaining or focusing attention. Communication is generally disrupted much more by the dysarthria than by the dementia. Neurofibrillary tangles and other deposits of tau protein are characteristic histopathologic features of PSP, but the specific isoforms differ from those that are present in the neurofibrillary tangles of Alzheimer's disease.

A trial of L-dopa is usually warranted, because some patients experience significant benefit, at least transiently. Positive results have been reported in occasional patients with dopamine agonists, tricyclic antidepressant agents, or methysergide, but most patients do not respond to these medications. Although cholinergic systems show widespread degeneration in PSP, results with cholinesterase inhibitors have been disappointing. Regardless of treatment, patients usually continue to deteriorate; about 50% of patients need assistance walking by the fourth year of the illness, and the median interval from onset to wheelchair dependence is about eight years. Most patients eventually require a feeding tube to prevent aspiration and provide adequate nutrition.

3. Corticobasal degeneration

Corticobasal degeneration (also called corticobasal ganglionic degeneration) usually presents after age 50 with clumsiness, stiffness, or jerking of one arm (or, less often, one leg). It usually spreads to involve the ipsilateral limb before it affects the other side of the body. Patients often have dystonic posturing and apraxia on one side of their body, leading at times to an "alien limb" phenomenon in which patients report that the limb seems to float about their body independent of voluntary control. Some patients develop progressive aphasia or sensory neglect of one side of the body. The primary parkinsonian features are rigidity and bradykinesia. Myoclonic jerks are often prominent, especially in response to external stimuli. Global cognitive deficits are usually mild to moderate, but impaired executive function is common. Dysarthria and dysphagia are also common later in the course. As mentioned in Chapter 7, histopathologic characteristics of this condition overlap those seen in patients with frontotemporal dementia; tau-positive deposits and distinctive swollen neurons occur in both. Dopaminergic treatment helps some of these patients. There is no evidence that cholinesterase inhibitors are helpful.

4. Multiple system atrophy (MSA)

Multiple system atrophy (MSA) is characterized by any combination of parkinsonism, cerebellar dysfunction, and autonomic impairment. Patients may also have spasticity, cranial nerve abnormalities, anterior horn cell dysfunction, or peripheral polyneuropathy in any combination. At least two thirds of patients have REM sleep behavior disorder (discussed in Chapter 9) at some point in the course. The clinical findings and presentation vary widely, but the course is gradually progressive. When cerebellar dysfunction predominates, the disorder is termed MSA-C (for MSA-cerebellar predominant). This category encompasses patients who used to be classified as having olivopontocerebellar atrophy. When the predominant clinical feature is parkinsonism—which is the case for 80% of patients with MSA—the disorder is termed MSA-P (for MSA-parkinsonism predominant). Early in the clinical course, patients with MSA-P are often hard to distinguish from patients with Parkinson's disease, except that they may be more refractory to treatment. Eventually, they develop one or more symptoms of autonomic insufficiency (orthostatic hypotension, urinary retention or incontinence, impotence, constipation, or thermoregulatory abnormalities), or ataxia of limbs, gait, or speech. Dopaminergic medication itself can cause orthostatic hypotension, so if a patient previously diagnosed with Parkinson's disease begins to develop severe orthostatic hypotension, MSA should only be diagnosed if the orthostatic hypotension persists after withdrawing the medication or if the patient develops other signs of autonomic dysfunction. Patients with primarily parkinsonism and autonomic insufficiency have a form of MSA-P that is sometimes called Shy-Drager syndrome.

Pathologic changes include widespread but variable neuronal loss in the striatum, brainstem, cerebellum, and spinal cord nuclei, with special stains revealing prominent glial cytoplasmic inclusions and less prominent neuronal cytoplasmic and nuclear inclusions, all of which contain α-synuclein. At least half of the patients with parkinsonism respond to dopaminergic medication, but the response is usually only partial and transient, and medication-induced dyskinesias are common. Otherwise, treatment is symptomatic. Supportive therapy for gait disturbance or dysphagia may be helpful. Orthostatic hypotension is generally treated with support stockings, increased salt intake, elevation of the head of the bed, and mineralocorticoids such as fludrocortisone (Florinef). Indomethacin is sometimes helpful. Beta-adrenergic antagonists (e.g., propranolol, pindolol), α-adrenergic agonists (e.g., clonidine, midodrine), and cholinesterase inhibitors (pyridostigmine) may also be tried. Syncope is often difficult to treat and is a factor in the relatively poor prognosis; mean survival is 6–8 years.

D. Hereditary Ataxias

1. Friedreich's ataxia

Friedreich's ataxia is the most common inherited ataxia. It has autosomal recessive inheritance. It usually presents early in adolescence with progressive gait difficulty, and it eventually affects coordination of the arms. Neurologic examination typically reveals profound loss of position and vibration sense in the lower extremities, absent tendon reflexes in the lower extremities and often in the upper extremities, ataxic gait, ataxic speech, and extensor plantar responses. About 50% of patients have skeletal deformities such as scoliosis or pes cavus, and about 60% have a hypertrophic cardiomyopathy. Less frequent complications include optic atrophy, deafness, and diabetes mellitus. Pathologic hallmarks are demyelination and degeneration in the posterior column, pyramidal and spinocerebellar tracts of the spinal cord, and cell loss and demyelination in the cerebellar dentate nuclei, Clarke's column, dorsal root ganglia, and peripheral nerves. Disability usually occurs within 15 years. Life expectancy after onset is 35–40 years.

Friedreich's ataxia is caused by an unstable expansion of a GAA trinucleotide repeat in a gene coding for a mitochondrial protein that has been named frataxin. Frataxin appears to be involved in making iron available for several mitochondrial processes. Homozygotes for this mutation have partial deficiency of frataxin, leading to mitochondrial overload, impaired utilization of iron for synthesis of iron-sulfur clusters, decline of mitochondrial respiratory activity, and increased production of free radicals.

The diagnosis of Friedreich's ataxia is established by demonstration of the causative mutation. The genetic test is commercially available. Therapy is supportive.

2. Ataxia telangiectasia

Ataxia telangiectasia usually becomes symptomatic in the first decade of life, within a few years of learning to walk. The child develops an ataxic gait, followed by upper extremity ataxia and ataxic speech. Many patients also develop choreoathetosis or dystonia, and they have a characteristic difficulty initiating saccadic eye movements ("oculomotor apraxia") that requires them to thrust their heads in the intended direction of gaze. Mild intellectual decline may occur by the end of the first decade of life, and most patients are wheelchair-bound by 12 years of age. Patients usually have hyporeflexia and hypotonia on examination. Telangiectasias appear after the onset of ataxia, usually in the second half of the first decade of life. They most frequently occur in the conjunctivae, ears, bridge of the nose, and antecubital fossa. About 60% of patients have immunodeficiency and experience recurrent sinopulmonary infections. Patients also have an increased risk of malignancies, particularly lymphoma.

Ataxia telangiectasia is caused by mutations in a gene of the phosphoinositol 3-kinase family, which is involved in multiple aspects of cell cycle control and DNA damage surveillance. Mutations in this gene result in increased sensitivity to radiation. More than 300 mutations have been associated with ataxia telangiectasia, so genetic testing is usually not practical. The clinical features are diagnostic, once telangiectasias are visualized. In addition, patients consistently have elevated levels of α-fetoprotein. Other than treatment of infections and malignancies, therapy is supportive.

3. Spinocerebellar ataxias (SCAs)

Nearly thirty different forms of spinocerebellar ataxia (SCA) have been reported. They are all dominantly inherited and characterized by progressive ataxia, but beyond this, their clinical presentations are diverse. The clinical syndromes show considerable overlap, so differentiation usually requires genetic testing. In general, symptoms begin in adolescence or later, with ataxia of gait, limb movements, and speech. Progression is usually slow. Neurologic abnormalities that can coexist with the ataxia in some of the SCAs include restricted eye movements, visual loss, hyporeflexia, spasticity and hyperreflexia, choreoathetosis, parkinsonism, dystonia, myoclonus, sensory loss, seizures, developmental delay, mental retardation, and dementia. Therapy is supportive.

The mutations that cause SCA can be classified into three broad categories. The first consists of mutations that are expanded regions of CAG (or CAA in one case) trinucleotide repeats coding for elongated polyglutamine chains. The mutations in this category include the most common causes of dominantly inherited ataxia. It is thought that the polyglutamine chains code for proteins that have abnormal folding patterns and form aggregates that produce deleterious effects that may be independent of the specific gene where the repeats appear. This is consistent with the fact that disease occurs with a single copy of the mutated allele. Larger repeat chains are associated with earlier onset of disease, more rapid progression, or both. In one case (SCA6), the CAG repeat occurs in the gene for a voltage-dependent calcium channel subunit. Interestingly, some hereditary diseases characterized by transient episodes of ataxia have been associated with point mutations (not triplet repeats) in genes for calcium and potassium channels. The second category of SCA-related mutations consists of repeat expansions that are located outside of the protein-coding region of genes. It is thought that the RNA transcribed from these mutations may disrupt gene expression or some other cellular process. The third category consists of conventional mutations (deletions, mis-sense, nonsense, and splice site mutations). The affected genes have diverse functions – for example, one codes for spectrin (a cytoskeletal component), one codes for a voltage-gated potassium channel, one codes for a protein kinase, and one codes for a fibroblast growth factor. It has been speculated that even some of the mutations that do not involve genes for ion channels may still cause secondary ion channel dysfunction.

The development of progressive ataxia in a patient with a clear family history establishes the diagnosis of SCA. Identification of the specific variant of SCA requires genetic testing. This is commercially available for some of the SCAs, but not all.

4. Fragile X-associated tremor/ataxia syndrome (FXTAS)

The maternal grandfathers of boys with fragile X syndrome sometimes develop a syndrome that begins after the age of 55 years and is characterized by slowly progressive ataxia, kinetic tremor, parkinsonism, and polyneuropathy. This has been labeled the fragile X-associated tremor/ataxia syndrome (FXTAS). Whereas the mutation that causes fragile X syndrome produces a triplet repeat expansion greater than 200 repeats in a certain gene on the X chromosome, patients with FXTAS have an expansion of 50–200 repeats in the same region of the same gene. The protein coded by that gene is absent or nearly absent in patients with fragile X syndrome, but it is present at normal or mildly reduced levels in patients with FXTAS. Thus, whereas very long expansions result in a loss of gene function and lead to fragile X syndrome, intermediate-length expansions are thought to exert a neurotoxic effect by sequestering and perturbing the function of nuclear proteins. Female carriers have an additional, normal X chromosome, which is probably why the condition is more common in men. No specific treatment is available.

E. Huntington's Disease

Huntington's disease is an autosomal dominant condition characterized by progressive chorea and dementia, typically beginning in the late third or fourth decade of life. The cognitive disturbances begin as personality changes and evolve to severe memory dysfunction and global intellectual decline. The chorea is often difficult to detect early in the illness. When it is relatively infrequent, patients may appear to incorporate the chorea into normal voluntary actions; for example, they may quickly reach up to smooth their hair as soon as an involuntary twitch begins. The chorea grows progressively more severe over time, and patients often manifest varying degrees of athetosis, dystonia, or parkinsonism. Slowed saccadic eye movements and slowed distal fine finger movements can usually be detected on examination even before the involuntary movements become apparent. Dysarthria and dysphagia are prominent throughout the course. Gait abnormalities are extremely common and eventually become disabling. Depression is very common, and a variety of other psychiatric disorders may also occur. The diagnosis of Huntington's disease is based on the presence of the characteristic movement disorder in an individual with a positive family history. The psychiatric and behavioral manifestations of Huntington's disease are not specific, and in the absence of the movement disorder they are not sufficient for diagnosing Huntington's disease even in individuals with a positive family history. For patients who have the typical clinical manifestations of Huntington's disease but no family history, the diagnosis can be established by testing for the Huntington's mutation.

In approximately 10% of patients with Huntington's disease, clinical symptoms begin before age 20 years; this juvenile form is often characterized by prominent parkinsonism rather than chorea. Juvenile onset is more common in patients who inherited the disease from their father.

Huntington's disease is caused by an expanded, unstable CAG trinucleotide repeat coding for an elongated polyglutamine chain in the tail of a protein that has been named huntingtin. Huntingtin is widely expressed both within the nervous system and outside it. Its function is unknown, but it is thought to be important in embryogenesis. As is the case with the polyglutamine SCAs, the pathology in Huntington's disease is thought to result from a gain of function in the elongated mutant protein (as opposed to a loss of the normal protein's function, which is the situation in most recessively inherited conditions). The mutant huntingtin protein undergoes ubiquitinization and cleavage in the cytoplasm, and aggregates in both the cytoplasm and nucleus. Huntingtin fragments interact with several proteins that function in gene transcription and regulation, glycolysis, and stabilization of glutamate receptors. Mitochondrial dysfunction, free radical toxicity, glutamate excitotoxicity, and caspase-mediated programmed cell death are all thought to play a role in the resultant pathologic process.

Pathologic examination reveals marked atrophy with loss of selective subsets of cells in the striatum, particularly at the head of the caudate. Some neuronal loss is also described in the globus pallidus and thalamus. Characteristic changes in neurotransmitters and receptors (especially GABA [gamma-aminobutyric acid], enkephalin, benzodiazepine, acetylcholine, and excitatory amino acids) have been described.

Therapy is primarily supportive. When the chorea is mild and doesn't impair function, it may not require treatment. Tetrabenazine (Xenazine), a catecholamine depleter, can lessen chorea, but it can cause or exacerbate depression, so it must be used cautiously. Phenothiazines and atypical antipsychotic agents (especially olanzapine) are also used to modify chorea, as well as behavioral disorders. Other mood-stabilizing agents can be helpful. Swallowing problems and gait difficulty should be addressed with education and therapy. Dysphagia, immobility, and dementia usually lead to death in 15–25 years.

Difficult psychosocial and ethical issues arise from the ability to screen for a genetic condition that does not produce clinical manifestations until midlife and for which only limited symptomatic treatment is available. Individuals at risk for Huntington's disease should receive extensive counseling to ensure that they understand how the disease is transmitted and to help them decide whether to be tested.

F. Tardive Dyskinesia

About 20% of patients chronically taking antipsychotic or anti-emetic medications develop hyperkinetic movement disorders, especially dyskinetic movements or dystonic postures. These often appear late in the course of therapy, especially after reducing the medication dose or stopping it entirely. The incidence increases in proportion to the duration of exposure and is highest in the elderly. The most common dyskinesias are repetitive, stereotyped oro-bucco-lingual movements, but in many patients, the trunk and distal extremities are involved as well. The pathophysiologic mechanism is uncertain. Proposed mechanisms include supersensitivity of postsynaptic striatal dopamine receptors, GABA-ergic striatal dysfunction, and excess glutamatergic activity. Even though dose reduction may be the initial precipitating or exacerbating factor, and resuming the drug or increasing the dose may produce short-term improvement, it compounds the problem in the long term. Treatment consists of titrating to the lowest doses of medication needed to control psychotic symptoms (or nausea), and ideally, eliminating the offending medication entirely (if necessary, substituting one of the atypical antipsychotic medications clozapine, risperidone, quetiapine, or olanzapine). Dyskinesias may or may not resolve after discontinuation of the offending agents; improvement may take weeks to months. For disabling persistent movements, benzodiazepines, reserpine, tetrabenazine, clonidine, propranolol, vitamin E, donepezil, levetiracetam, gabapentin, or valproic acid can be tried, though the response is often disappointing. Positive results have also been reported with pallidotomy or pallidal deep brain stimulation, but the evidence is limited.

G. Dystonias

Many different movement disorders (as well as a number of other neurologic diseases and systemic problems) can produce dystonia. Dystonia can also occur as an isolated problem. Although any pattern of muscle activity may be seen, the most common examples of dystonia in adults are the focal syndromes of torticollis, blepharospasm, and writer's cramp. In torticollis (cervical dystonia), the patient's head may be turned to one side, flexed, extended, or tilted; the resultant posture depends on which muscle or muscles are most active. The head may be maintained in a fixed position, or there may be superimposed jerking movements or tremor. In blepharospasm, there is involuntary, bilateral eye closure, often exacerbated by bright light or other environmental stimuli. In writer's cramp, the hand assumes an involuntary, often twisted posture when the patient attempts to write. Many analogous task-specific dystonias also exist. In addition to the inconvenience and embarrassment resulting from these conditions, the sustained muscle contractions often cause considerable pain. The severity of focal dystonia typically fluctuates widely and can be influenced both by the patient's emotional state and by environmental stimuli. The underlying pathogenesis of focal dystonia is not known. In the past, focal dystonias were often assumed to be psychogenic, and the differentiation between an organic focal dystonia and a psychiatric condition is still difficult at times—especially since many psychiatric patients are treated with neuroleptic medications, which can themselves produce dystonia. Hemidystonia implies structural damage in the contralateral basal ganglia.

Dystonia that begins in adulthood is usually focal or segmental, whereas approximately 50% of cases of childhood-onset dystonia are generalized.

The most common form of early-onset generalized dystonia, DYT1 dystonia (formerly termed dystonia musculorum deformans), is inherited as an autosomal dominant trait with relatively low penetrance. It presents in the first decade of life in about 50% of patients. It usually begins in one limb and spreads to the rest of the body over one to ten years. DYT1 dystonia is caused by a deletion in the gene for a protein that has been named torsin A; the test for this mutation is now commercially available. The function of torsin A is unknown, but it is homologous to the adenosine triphosphatases and heat-shock proteins, and it is thought that mutant forms may interfere with endoplasmic reticulum function, intracellular trafficking, vesicular release, or processing of misfolded protein.

Dopa-responsive dystonia, or DYT5, is a rare form of childhood-onset generalized dystonia that is notable for marked diurnal variation. These patients may be almost normal in the morning, but over the course of the day they have progressively increasing dystonia, parkinsonism, and hyperreflexia. Patients with this condition have a dramatic and sustained response to relatively low doses of L-dopa. They do not develop hallucinations, autonomic dysfunction, motor fluctuations, or dyskinesias, even after prolonged L-dopa use, presumably related to the fact that this condition (unlike Parkinson's disease) only affects dopamine synthesis, not the integrity of the dopaminergic neurons themselves. Anticholinergic drugs may also be helpful. More than 75 mutations in the gene for guanosine triphosphate cyclohydrolase-1 (GCH1)—an enzyme involved in the synthesis of tetrahydrobiopterin, which is a cofactor in dopamine synthesis – have been implicated in this condition. It is usually dominantly inherited with incomplete penetrance, and girls are preferentially affected.

Many classes of pharmacotherapy have been used to treat dystonia, most often anticholinergic agents but also baclofen, dopamine agonists, dopamine antagonists, benzodiazepines, catecholamine agonists, and catecholamine antagonists. Except in the case of dopa-responsive dystonia, none of these agents has been effective for more than a handful of patients. Focal dystonias can be treated with local injections of minute quantities of botulinum toxin to weaken the overactive muscles. Although this approach does not directly address the abnormal motor programming responsible for the disorder, it can produce significant symptomatic relief. The effect is temporary, so the injections must be repeated every few months. Botulinum toxin injections can at best provide regional relief to patients with DYT1 dystonia, who eventually develop severe disability in most cases. DYT1 dystonia often responds to a deep brain stimulator placed in the internal segment of the globus pallidus, so this is an option in patients who are refractory to medications. The response is less predictable than in patients with essential tremor or Parkinson's disease, and may not be apparent until several months have elapsed. This treatment can also be effective for patients with torticollis refractory to other management approaches.

H. Wilson's Disease

Wilson's disease is an autosomal recessive disorder of copper metabolism characterized by progressive, but often reversible, dysarthria, dystonia, gait disturbance, tremor, parkinsonism, choreoathetosis, dysphagia, psychiatric symptoms, and cognitive deterioration. These manifestations may occur in any combination and in any temporal sequence. The dystonia can be focal, segmental, multifocal, or generalized. The tremor can be a rest tremor, a postural tremor, or a kinetic tremor. Clinically significant hepatic involvement is common, and other organ systems may also be affected. In general, patients who present with liver abnormalities usually do so between the ages of 8 and 16 years, whereas those who present with neurologic symptoms usually do so after puberty.

Histopathologic examination reveals excess copper deposition in the liver and throughout the brain, with prominent degeneration of the putamen, globus pallidus, brainstem nuclei, and even white matter. Copper deposition in the cornea leads to the characteristic Kayser-Fleischer ring of hyperpigmentation around the limbus; this physical finding is present in practically all patients with neurologic manifestations, but it may be subtle and only evident on slit-lamp examination in early cases.

Wilson's disease is caused by mutations in the gene for ATP7B, an ATPase involved in the excretion of copper into the bile. Normal copper intake is approximately 1 mg per day, but the normal copper requirement is only about 0.75 mg per day. In normal individuals, copper is absorbed in the upper intestine and transported to the liver, where it is taken up with high affinity. In hepatocytes, the ATP7B directs the incorporation of copper into a glycoprotein called apo-ceruloplasmin, which transports the copper into various enzymes and into the plasma. The ATP7B also helps direct the excess copper into a vesicular compartment near the canalicular membrane, and from here the copper is eliminated from the body by excretion into the bile. Mutations in ATP7B are thought to interfere with its ability to direct the copper to the vesicular compartment, resulting in abnormal accumulation of copper in the hepatocyte. This eventually spills over into the blood and affects other organs, including the brain. The mechanism by which excess copper produces organ damage is not clear. Serum levels of ceruloplasmin are low in most patients with Wilson's disease, and the reasons for this are also unclear. It may be that the ATP7B mutations result in reduced incorporation of copper into apo-ceruloplasmin, and without a full complement of bound copper the ceruloplasmin is subject to rapid intracellular and extracellular degradation.

A percutaneous liver biopsy to determine hepatic copper content is the single most reliable test for Wilson's disease, but the diagnosis can usually be made in other ways. A slit-lamp examination will reveal Kayser-Fleischer rings in 98% of patients with neurologic manifestations, but in only 50% of patients with exclusively hepatic manifestations. A serum ceruloplasmin level is a fairly good screening test for Wilson's disease, but ceruloplasmin levels are at the low end of the normal range in up to 15% of patients with the disease and low in 10–20% of asymptomatic carriers. Patients with Wilson's disease almost always have increased copper in a 24-hour urine collection, but other cholestatic disorders can also cause increased urine copper excretion, so unless the level is extremely high this test can be misleading. Total levels of serum copper are of little value, but elevated levels of free serum copper can be helpful.

Without treatment, the disease was once uniformly fatal. Patients are now treated with zinc, trientine, penicillamine, or tetrathiomolybdate. Zinc blocks intestinal absorption of copper, but takes 4–8 months to achieve its effect. Trientine, a chelating agent, promotes urinary excretion of copper. Penicillamine, another chelating agent, has traditionally been the mainstay of treatment, but it is associated with a high incidence of adverse effects, including neurologic deterioration at the onset of treatment in 25–50% of patients. Trientine, like penicillamine, can result in neurologic deterioration initially, but it has fewer overall side-effects. Tetrathiomolybdate impairs intestinal absorption of copper and also forms complexes with copper in the blood. It is generally well tolerated, and the therapeutic results have been impressive, but it is still an experimental agent. Therapy must be continued permanently. Zinc is often used as maintenance therapy, but supplementing it with trientine (or tetrathiomolybdate if available) at the outset may help to achieve a more rapid clinical response. Orthotopic liver transplantation is currently reserved for patients with severe hepatic failure.

I. Gilles de la Tourette's Syndrome

Tourette's syndrome is the most flagrant of a spectrum of tic disorders. Evidence suggests that it is much more common than previously appreciated, but most cases are mild and do not come to medical attention. It is inherited in an autosomal dominant pattern with incomplete and sex-specific penetrance (males more commonly affected than females). Polygenic factors may play a role. The onset is usually between the ages of 3 and 8 years, and almost all patients manifest tics before adolescence. In addition to recurrent motor tics involving multiple muscle groups, there are frequent vocal tics such as grunting, barking, humming, or clearing of the throat. The most dramatic symptom is coprolalia, the involuntary utterance of obscenities, but this is by no means a universal feature. A patient may manifest different tics over the years, with certain tics predominating for months at a time, only to fade gradually and be replaced by other tics. Obsessive-compulsive disorder and attention deficit-hyperactivity disorder each occur in approximately 50% of patients; they can occur together or separately. These associated behavioral problems are usually more disabling than the tics themselves.

The cause of Tourette's syndrome is not known. Most patients with mild tics require no treatment. Tics tend to become less severe over time, and may resolve. For moderate or severe tics, haloperidol, pimozide, fluphenazine, or other neuroleptic medications are often very effective, but this must be balanced against the potential for side-effects with long-term use. Atypical antipsychotics (olanzapine, quetiapine, or risperidone) may also be effective, with fewer side-effects. Clonidine, guanfacine, clonazepam, and tetrabenazine have also been effective in some patients. Obsessive-compulsive disorder responds to selective serotonin reuptake inhibitors or cognitive-behavioral therapy. Attention deficit-hyperactivity disorder is typically treated with methylphenidate or clonidine. Bupropion and tricyclic antidepressants may also be helpful. Deep brain stimulation (targeting either the centromedian/parafascicular nuclei of the thalamus or the internal segment of the globus pallidus) has been reported to reduce tics, depression, and obsessive-compulsive disorder, and may occasionally be an option in very refractory patients.

V. Discussion of Case Histories

Case 1: This patient has typical stage 1 Parkinson's disease. She may be frightened by this diagnosis, especially since Parkinson's disease was essentially untreatable when she was younger. It is important to make sure she understands that the disease is readily treatable but that it will require continuing attention. In stage 1 disease, treatment with selegiline or rasagiline alone would be reasonable, adding L-dopa/carbidopa when her symptoms have progressed to the point where they are interfering with her daily activities.

She also relates symptoms that suggest she may be depressed. Her eating and sleeping habits, as well as her mood, need to be assessed. Depression is a common complication of Parkinson's disease, and it is often inadequately addressed because so many of the features could potentially be due to the Parkinson's disease itself. It is also important to perform at least some preliminary evaluation of memory function. If a mental status examination indicates any problems, formal evaluation of intellectual function and affect might provide a baseline to help assess any future decline.

Comment: This patient did very well on rasagiline.

Case 2: Note that although this patient's complaint was "generalized weakness," she actually has full strength, and what she was really experiencing was parkinsonism. It is not uncommon for patients to perceive or report parkinsonian features as "weakness"—you must ask pointed questions about what they can and can't do to clarify what they mean. The neurologic examination is also critical. In this patient, the progression has been fairly rapid, and the patient already has bilateral parkinsonian findings on examination after only three months of symptoms. These atypical features suggest that the patient may not have idiopathic Parkinson's disease. This case illustrates the common phenomenon of drug-induced parkinsonism. The patient's bradykinesia and tremor began almost immediately after starting metoclopramide (Reglan). All the usual symptoms of Parkinson's disease can be induced by even relatively brief exposure to this medication, and a careful history is critical in diagnosis. The first diagnostic maneuver is to stop the metoclopramide. Treating with anticholinergics or dopamine without stopping the metoclopramide would be inappropriate. Symptoms may take several weeks or more to subside, so follow-up evaluations will be necessary.

Regarding the patient's complaint of foot numbness, the examination findings of hyporeflexia at the ankles and reduced vibration sense at the toes are consistent with peripheral polyneuropathy, a common complication of diabetes. Because her feet are not painful, the findings are mild, and there is a likely explanation, there is no need for further evaluation at this point. It is unlikely that the polyneuropathy is contributing significantly to her gait disturbance, as she has normal distal strength and joint position sense.

Comment: This patient's motor symptoms disappeared within three weeks of stopping metoclopramide. She continued to have numbness in her feet, but this symptom did not bother her once it was explained to her.

Chapter 9

Sleep Disorders

I. Case Histories

Case 1. During one of his routine follow-up visits in the hypertension clinic, a 55-year-old man mentions to you that he was in an accident last week, but, luckily, nobody got hurt. He says he must have "fallen asleep at the wheel"—it happens to him every so often. He doesn't understand why he should be sleepy, because he goes to bed at 10 pm every night and sleeps through the night until he gets up at 7 am the next morning. His wife confirms this but adds that she really couldn't say whether he is asleep that entire time because she sleeps in a different room to avoid his snoring.

The patient's general examination is notable for his hypertension, mild obesity, and a large neck circumference (19 inches). His neurologic examination is normal.

Questions:

1. What diagnoses should be considered?

2. What investigations are necessary?

3. How should this patient be managed?

Case 2. A 45-year-old man asks his family doctor to give him a prescription for fluoxetine (Prozac). He believes he is depressed, and he has heard good things about this medicine. He explains that he has no energy, can't concentrate, and is tired all the time. He can never seem to fall asleep at night. In fact, he can hardly even lie in bed for any length of time, because of a constant unpleasant sensation in his legs, "like worms are crawling over them," causing an almost irresistible urge to move the legs. This feeling only goes away when he is moving his legs or walking. He prefers standing, anyway, because he often gets epigastric pain when he lies down. He wonders if he is going crazy. His examination is normal.

Questions:

1. What diagnoses should be considered?
2. What investigations are necessary?
3. Should fluoxetine be prescribed?
4. What other treatment options are available?

Case 3. A 4-year-old girl has been brought to the pediatric emergency room at 2 a.m. by her parents, who say that at 1 a.m. they were awakened by her frantic screaming. They rushed to her room and saw that she was agitated, sweating profusely, and breathing rapidly. They noted that her pulse was racing. They were unable to calm her, but over the next few minutes she gradually calmed down on her own and drifted back to sleep. In the emergency room, she seems to be normal, except that she is sleepy. She has no memory of the event. Two similar episodes occurred a month ago, but the family had just moved to a new city at the time and the girl's parents had attributed the episodes to the unfamiliar surroundings and the stress of adjusting to a new day care situation. The girl's examination is normal.

Questions:

1. What diagnoses should be considered?
2. What investigations are necessary?
3. What treatment should be given?

II. Approach to Sleep Disorders

In evaluating and managing patients with sleep disorders, three questions are fundamental:

1. Does the patient have trouble staying awake during the day?
2. Does the patient have trouble falling asleep or staying asleep at night?
3. Does the patient have abnormal sensations or behavior during sleep?

These symptoms often go together. For example, people who have trouble staying awake in the daytime may nap excessively during the day and then have trouble falling asleep at night. Some people who have trouble falling asleep at bedtime are not fully rested the following day, so they have trouble staying awake. People who have abnormal behavior during sleep—or, more often, their bed partners—may fail to get the required amount of normal sleep and have trouble staying awake the following day.

Despite the interconnections between these symptoms, it is helpful to consider them separately. Part IV of this chapter addresses Question 1, Part V addresses Question 2, and Part VI addresses Question 3. Part III presents some background information.

III. Background Information

A. Definitions

dyssomnia a disorder resulting in insomnia or excessive daytime sleepiness (or both)

hypersomnia excessive daytime somnolence

insomnia the subjective impression of inadequate sleep

parasomnia an abnormal movement or behavior that occurs during sleep or is brought on by sleep

sleep Definition #1 (conceptual) – a reversible behavioral state of perceptual disengagement from and unresponsiveness to the environment

sleep Definition #2 (operational) – a physiologic state defined by behavioral and physiologic criteria. The behavioral criteria include (1) minimal mobility, (2) closed eyes, (3) increased arousal threshold and reduced response to external stimulation, (4) increased reaction time, (5) reduced cognition, (6) characteristic sleeping posture, and (7) reversibility. The physiologic criteria are based on findings from electroencephalography (EEG), electromyography (EMG), and electrooculography (EOG)

B. Sleep Physiology

Sleep consists of a highly patterned sequence of cyclical activity in various regions of the brain; it is not simply a state of temporary unconsciousness. Although the brain is less responsive than normal during sleep, it is not totally unresponsive. In fact, during sleep the brain responds more readily to meaningful stimuli, such as a crying baby, than to other stimuli.

There are two principal states of sleep that alternate at about 90-minute intervals in the normal adult. *Rapid eye movement* (REM) sleep can be characterized as a period when the brain is active and the body is paralyzed, whereas in *nonrapid eye movement* (NREM) sleep, the brain is less active but the body can move. Most elaborate dreams occur during REM sleep. REM sleep is characterized by EMG suppression, irregular low-voltage activity on EEG, and rapid eye movements. The eye movements sometimes correspond to dream content. The characteristic features of NREM sleep are normal resting EMG, progressive slowing of EEG activity, and the absence of rapid eye movements.

When normal subjects first fall asleep, they progress through three stages of NREM sleep (N1, N2, and N3) that are differentiated on the basis of EEG characteristics. The third stage (N3) is often called *slow-wave sleep* or *delta sleep* because it is characterized by high-amplitude slow waves (also called delta waves) on EEG. Delta sleep may last from a few minutes to an hour, depending on the subject's age, and the subject then reverts to stage N2 sleep. Shortly after this, the first REM sleep period begins. This lasts approximately 15–20 minutes and is followed by another NREM cycle. This alternation between REM and NREM repeats throughout the night, with a total of four to six cycles in all (Figure 9.1). The first two cycles are dominated by stage N3, but after the first third of the night this stage is less apparent, so NREM sleep later in the night consists primarily of N2 sleep, with brief periods of N1 sleep. Conversely, the periods of REM sleep grow longer as the night continues. Thus, the first third of the night is dominated by slow-wave sleep, and the final third is dominated by REM sleep. In normal young adults, about 75% of total sleep time is spent in NREM sleep, and 25% in REM sleep. This cyclical activity is governed by several different neuronal systems.

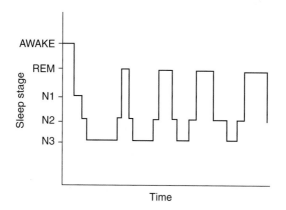

Fig. 9.1 Normal cycling of sleep stages; details explained in text. Note that delta sleep (stage N3) predominates early in the night, but as the night progresses, the amount of time spent in N3 sleep gradually shrinks while the amount of time spent in REM sleep grows.

In the awake state, ongoing thalamic input to the cortex results in stimulus-dependent—and thus, nonrhythmic—cortical activity. The EEG in normal wakefulness is therefore desynchronized and appears nearly random. The thalamus, in turn, receives input from a network of pathways originating in the brainstem, especially the midbrain. These pathways are collectively known as the ascending reticular activating system (ARAS). In experimental animals, ARAS stimulation excites the thalamocortical projections, resulting in EEG desynchronization and behavioral arousal. This is associated with elevated ARAS levels of the neurotransmitters norepinephrine, acetylcholine, serotonin, and histamine. ARAS activity is modulated by input from sensory pathways, cortex, and hypothalamus.

At the onset of sleep, a group of GABA-ergic, "hypnogenic neurons" in the basal forebrain, anterior hypothalamus, and medulla inhibit the ARAS, suppressing thalamocortical activity. This is the beginning of NREM sleep. Progressive inhibition causes slower, more synchronized electrical activity, eventually resulting in the typical appearance of slow-wave (delta wave) sleep. In this state, the cortex is effectively deafferented, or "closed off" from most sensory stimuli. At some point during slow-wave sleep, "REM-on cells," a population of cholinergic cells located in several different brainstem nuclei, begin to fire, stimulating the thalamus and basal forebrain, which results in renewed EEG desynchronization. During this stage (REM sleep), the EEG resembles that in awake subjects. In addition to activating the thalamus and basal forebrain, the REM-on cells have a number of other brain and spinal cord projections that result in saccadic eye movements, suppression of other skeletal muscle activity, preserved respiratory and cardiovascular function, and (probably) increased activity in visual pathways. REM-on cells have a reciprocal inhibitory relationship with REM-off cells, a population of neurons that contain serotonin, norepinephrine, and histamine, and that are scattered across several locations in the brainstem and hypothalamus. During REM sleep, the cholinergic REM-on cells are active and the REM-off cells are silent, but at some point during REM sleep, the REM-off cells become active, and the brain's activity returns to the pattern that characterizes non-REM sleep.

One component of the system regulating REM, NREM, and wakefulness is hypocretin (also called orexin), a peptide located in certain hypothalamic neurons near the fornix. These neurons project widely throughout the central nervous system, including projections to all the ARAS nuclei. Hypocretin functions as a neurotransmitter. The hypocretin system inhibits REM sleep, promotes wakefulness, and stimulates feeding and motor activity. It also appears to be involved in the balance of motor excitation and inhibition during emotionally charged activities.

The trigger for this entire process derives from the interplay of two processes. First, the brain contains a circadian rhythm generator, an "internal clock" in the paired suprachiasmatic nuclei (SCN) of the hypothalamus. The rhythm is generated by feedback loops of transcription and translation in several "clock" genes, which cycle at a very regular frequency. In patients who have been removed from environmental stimuli, the SCN cycles with a period of 24.2 hours, but it can be reset by external stimuli, primarily light. The SCN has reciprocal connections with the pineal gland, which releases melatonin at levels that fluctuate in a regular diurnal pattern.

The second process influencing the timing of sleep onset is the duration of prior wakefulness. The longer a person has been awake, the greater the tendency to sleep. Adenosine appears to be one of the major factors mediating this effect. Caffeine blocks adenosine receptors, which could explain the mechanism by which caffeine helps ward off sleepiness.

In summary, the sleep-wake cycle represents a complex interaction between many systems including cholinergic and monoaminergic (serotonergic, norepinephrine-containing, and histaminergic) cells in the ARAS that maintain wakefulness, GABA-ergic neurons that promote sleep, cholinergic REM-on cells, monoaminergic REM-off cells, and the hypocretin/orexin system (which inhibits REM sleep and promotes wakefulness, in part through its effects on REM-off cells). The timing of the cycle is a function of the circadian process of the SCN, mediated at least in part by melatonin, and the sleep debt process, possibly mediated by adenosine.

C. Diagnostic Tests

Two types of diagnostic test are commonly used to supplement the clinical diagnosis of sleep disorders. A *polysomnogram* is an all-night recording of eye movements, EEG (frontal, central and occipital leads), electrocardiogram, EMG (chin and anterior tibialis surface leads), oximetry, airflow at the nose and mouth, and thoracic and abdominal wall motion. The testing sometimes includes video and additional EEG monitoring, or other physiologic assessments such as snoring sounds, position, esophageal pH, end-tidal pCO_2, or intrathoracic pressure. A *Multiple Sleep Latency Test* (MSLT) is a measure of daytime sleepiness. A subject is asked to take four or five brief naps at 2-hour intervals on the day after an adequate night's sleep (as confirmed by a polysomnogram). The EEG, EMG, and eye movements are monitored to determine the mean time the subject takes to fall asleep.

D. Classification of Sleep Disorders

In this chapter, sleep disorders are grouped into three general categories, based on whether patients have trouble staying awake (Part IV), trouble sleeping (Part V), or abnormal behaviors during sleep (Part VI)—but as noted in Part II, these categories often overlap. The classification system preferred by the American Academy of Sleep Medicine divides sleep disorders into eight general categories: (1) insomnias, (2) sleep-related breathing disorders, (3) hypersomnias not due to a sleep-related breathing disorder, (4) circadian rhythm disorders, (5) parasomnias, (6) sleep-related movement disorders, (7) other sleep disorders, and (8) isolated symptoms, apparently normal variants, and unresolved issues. Although this classification system permits a more precise delineation of the various disorders, I prefer the broader categories for the purpose of exposition.

IV. Trouble Staying Awake

Excessive daytime somnolence (hypersomnia) can be obvious or subtle. At one extreme, patients with chronic, severe hypersomnia can have "sleep attacks," in which they fall asleep even during activities where a nap is clearly inappropriate. The sleep attacks usually last about 15 minutes, at which point patients awaken feeling refreshed. They are not overwhelmed by sleepiness again for 1 or 2 hours. At the other extreme, patients may not even appreciate that they are sleepy. They may be more aware of the consequences of hypersomnia, including loss of energy, fatigue, headaches, lack of initiative, memory lapses, difficulty concentrating, and short temper. Indeed, in many instances, the barrier to diagnosis results from a failure to recognize that there is a problem with sleep in the first place. Patients with symptoms that could be manifestations of hypersomnia should be asked directed questions to determine if they have an underlying sleep disturbance. Once hypersomnia has been identified, the most common causes—insufficient sleep, sleep apnea, and narcolepsy—are often easily recognized based on features of the history.

A. Insufficient Sleep

The demands of modern life lead many people to allot themselves inadequate time for sleep at night. As a consequence, they suffer from unrecognized, self-imposed sleep deprivation. This problem is so common that many people consider it normal to be drowsy or even fall asleep during the day, especially in unstimulating situations or after a big lunch. This is not normal behavior for fully rested individuals, however. Be sure to ask patients what time they wake up on days when they don't set an alarm. If it is substantially later than their usual wake-up time, they probably are not allotting themselves sufficient time for sleep during the week. This problem is managed by educating the patient about healthy sleep habits ("sleep hygiene").

B. Sleep Apnea

Sleep apnea is a condition in which patients periodically stop breathing while asleep. Central sleep apnea results from abnormal central nervous system control of respiration, which can be caused by a variety of processes. Much more commonly, sleep apnea is caused by temporary obstruction of the upper airway; in fact, obstructive sleep apnea is the most common medical cause of excessive daytime somnolence.

Even in normal subjects, the pharyngeal muscles that maintain airway patency relax during sleep. There is normally enough residual volume in the airway to permit airflow, but in patients with obstructive sleep apnea, the muscle relaxation results in partial or complete occlusion of the airway. This leads to reduced inspiratory airflow and increased respiratory effort, which culminates in partial awakening. Sleep cannot be fully restorative when it is disrupted repeatedly throughout the night by these episodes of partial arousal, and the result is excessive somnolence during the day.

The cornerstone of clinical diagnosis is a history of apneic episodes during sleep. Patients are not aware of the episodes because they are brief and arousal is only partial, so the history usually must be obtained from the bed partner. Patients characteristically snore loudly, punctuated with bouts of interrupted breathing that often terminate with snorts or gasps. The diagnosis is also supported by the presence of any conditions that can predispose to obstructive sleep apnea by causing upper airway narrowing. These include obesity (causing fat deposition around the upper airway), facial or mandibular deformities, malignant infiltration of the soft tissue of the neck, laryngeal muscle weakness, and enlarged tonsils, adenoids, soft palate, uvula, or tongue. Polysomnography is used to confirm the diagnosis of sleep apnea and to quantify the severity in terms of the number of episodes of respiratory disturbance per hour, the degree of blood oxygen desaturation, and the presence of any significant cardiac arrhythmias.

Sleep apnea can result in hypersomnia not only for the patient but also for the bed partner and sometimes other family members who suffer disrupted sleep because of the loud snoring. In addition, chronic obstructive sleep apnea is associated with an increased risk of pulmonary hypertension, systemic hypertension, cardiac arrhythmias, sudden death, myocardial infarction, stroke, and motor vehicle accidents. Some evidence suggests that it may contribute to the metabolic syndrome and its components, such as diabetes and hyperlipidemia. Successful treatment of the sleep apnea can reduce the risk of at least some of those conditions. In children, sleep apnea is associated with hyperactivity and poor performance in school.

The most effective treatment of obstructive sleep apnea (short of tracheostomy) is nasal continuous positive airway pressure (CPAP). This raises the pressure in the oropharynx, and thus in the upper airway, reversing the pressure gradient across the wall of the airway and propping it open. This treatment is beneficial in 80–90% of patients; the main reasons for treatment failure are poor compliance (because the patient finds the nightly use of a mask over the nose uncomfortable or unappealing) and nasal obstruction. Other treatment options include weight loss for overweight patients (usually easier said than done), dental appliances that pull the lower jaw forward and widen the upper airway (primarily helpful for mild cases), uvulopalatopharyngoplasty (which is helpful in about one-half the patients, but it is difficult to predict which half), and surgical correction of other abnormalities that obstruct the airway (e.g., tonsillectomy or correction of facial and mandibular deformities). Medications that have been used for obstructive sleep apnea include protriptyline (Vivactil), acetazolamide (Diamox), and mirtazapine (Remeron), but most studies have revealed either no benefit or unacceptable side effects. In patients with residual sleepiness despite effective treatment of their upper airway obstruction, modafinil and armodafinil (initially developed for narcolepsy–see section C) may be beneficial.

C. Narcolepsy

Narcolepsy is a syndrome consisting of excessive daytime somnolence and disordered regulation of REM sleep, resulting in intrusion of components of REM sleep into NREM sleep and the waking state. It usually begins in teenage years. There are four cardinal symptoms:

1. *Chronic excessive daytime somnolence* Unlike somnolence from other causes, the sleepiness that occurs in narcolepsy cannot be relieved by any amount of normal sleep.

2. *Cataplexy* is a sudden loss of postural tone that occurs while the patient is awake but is otherwise identical to the atonia that occurs during

REM sleep. The atonia may involve only a single muscle group, resulting in subtle manifestations such as slight buckling of the knees, drooping of the head or jaw, ptosis, or even just a subjective feeling of weakness, or it may be generalized and lead to complete bodily collapse and paralysis. Auditory function and consciousness are preserved before, during, and after the attack, although some patients pass directly from the attack into sleep. Attacks are precipitated by sudden, strong emotion, particularly laughter, and they typically last several minutes.

3. *Sleep paralysis*, like cataplexy, consists of atonia identical to that of REM sleep. It occurs at the onset of sleep or on awakening. The patient is conscious or half-awake but unable to move. This is often accompanied by intense fear and a sense of being unable to breathe.

4. *Hypnagogic* (or *hypnopompic*) *hallucinations* are vivid auditory or visual dream-like experiences that occur at *the onset of sleep* (or *on awakening*).

Only half of all narcoleptic patients manifest all four of these cardinal symptoms. Excessive daytime somnolence is a universal feature, but only about one third to one half of patients with narcolepsy experience sleep paralysis, and roughly the same proportion has hypnagogic/hypnopompic hallucinations. Each of these three symptoms can occur with any condition that causes sleep deprivation or disruption, so they are not specific for narcolepsy. Cataplexy is the most specific of the four cardinal symptoms—it almost never occurs outside the setting of narcolepsy—but it is present in only about 70% of narcoleptic patients.

The MSLT is used to support the diagnosis: a narcoleptic patient characteristically has a mean sleep latency of 5 minutes or less, whereas rested normal individuals require an average of more than 10 minutes to fall asleep. The MSLT also provides a measure of the tendency to enter REM sleep prematurely, without the normal progression through stages 1–4 of NREM sleep. Any period of REM sleep that occurs in the first 15 minutes of sleep is noted and referred to as a sleep-onset REM period. Two or more sleep-onset REM periods, together with a mean sleep latency of eight minutes or less, are considered diagnostic of narcolepsy.

In 90% of narcoleptic patients with cataplexy, cerebrospinal fluid levels of hypocretin are undetectable or extremely low. Autopsy studies reveal dramatic depletion of hypocretin-containing neurons in patients with narcolepsy. Some animal models of narcolepsy are associated with mutations in a gene coding for a hypocretin receptor, and others with mutations in the gene for a hypocretin precursor, but most patients with narcolepsy do not have these mutations. The precise role of hypocretin in the pathogenesis of narcolepsy is not known.

More than 95% of Asian and Caucasian patients with narcolepsy have the HLA-DR1501 and HLA-DQB1-0602 antigens. This association is not sensitive or specific enough to be useful as a diagnostic test, but it suggests that an autoimmune process could be the underlying cause of narcolepsy. Alternatively, the HLA locus may simply lie near a susceptibility gene for narcolepsy. Patients with narcolepsy have not been found to have antibodies to hypocretin or hypocretin receptors.

Narcolepsy is treated primarily with stimulant medications, especially modafinil (Provigil), armodafinil (Nuvigil), dextroamphetamine (Dexedrine), or methylphenidate (Ritalin). Modafinil is generally considered the first-line agent, because it has low abuse potential and it is not associated with rebound hypersomnolence. Armodafinil is a newer agent marketed as longer-acting, but it has not been demonstrated to be superior to modafinil. Cataplectic attacks respond to tricyclic antidepressants such as imipramine (Tofranil) and protriptyline (Vivactil). Selective serotonin reuptake inhibitors (SSRIs), selegiline, and dextroamphetamine can also help to reduce cataplexy, whereas modafinil does not. Night-time doses of sodium oxybate, or γ-hydroxybutyrate, also improve cataplexy and daytime somnolence. It is classified as a controlled substance because of concerns about its potential for abuse; it has achieved notoriety as a "date-rape" drug. Nonpharmacologic therapy of narcolepsy includes improved sleep hygiene and scheduled therapeutic naps.

D. Other Causes of Hypersomnolence

Excessive sleepiness may be caused by many medications, including sedative-hypnotics, anti-epileptic drugs, antihypertensives, antidepressants, and antihistamines. Withdrawal from stimulants may also result in hypersomnolence. Many metabolic abnormalities can also cause sleepiness, or even obtundation or stupor. These include hepatic encephalopathy, uremic encephalopathy, hyperglycemia, hypoglycemia, hypercalcemia, and (severe) hypothyroidism. Other causes of hypersomnia include meningitis, encephalitis, chronic subdural hematoma, and post-concussion syndrome.

V. Trouble Sleeping

Many different physiologic and psychologic factors can interfere with sleep, and many patients with insomnia have more than one of these factors. The goal is to identify the contributing factors and treat the ones for which therapy is available. There are three main patterns of insomnia: sleep-onset delay (trouble falling asleep), early morning awakening (trouble staying asleep), and sleep fragmentation (repeated awakenings).

A. Sleep-Onset Delay

1. Psychophysiologic insomnia

People who are trying to fall asleep sometimes focus on unpleasant thoughts, emotions, or sensations that they are currently experiencing or that they have experienced recently. This makes it difficult for them to relax and fall asleep, which, in turn, makes them anxious, making it even more difficult for them to initiate and maintain sleep. On subsequent nights, their anxiety about falling asleep (and a heightened concern about the need for sleep) may be enough to provoke this cycle, even after the original unpleasant stimuli have resolved. Over time, patients may develop a conditioned association between their bed and unsuccessful sleep; they often find that they sleep better outside the bedroom. Psychophysiologic insomnia is the term used for this cycle of conditioned behavior, regardless of the original cause (and even when no specific cause can be identified).

Psychophysiologic insomnia can be exacerbated by other causes of insomnia, such as depression, anxiety related to life stressors, or conditions that are associated with physical discomfort. One example is *restless legs syndrome*, a condition characterized by deep paresthesias and crawling sensations in the calves and legs with a compulsion to move the legs. The unpleasant sensations are relieved by stretching the legs or walking. These symptoms are worse in the evening and at night than during the day, and they occur primarily when lying down or sitting. Paresthesias resulting from carpal tunnel syndrome, other mononeuropathies, and polyneuropathy can be equally disruptive.

Other physical symptoms can also trigger or exacerbate psychophysiologic insomnia. Dyspnea and orthopnea can interfere with sleep onset or lead to frequent arousals. Patients with significant mobility problems often have difficulty falling asleep or staying asleep because of minor discomfort that would ordinarily be overcome by slight shifts in position. Hyperthyroidism and Cushing's disease can compromise the initiation of sleep, and so can medications such as steroids, dopaminergic agents, xanthine derivatives (including caffeine and theophylline), and adrenergic agonists.

In treating patients with insomnia, you should try to eliminate—as much as possible—any medications that might be interfering with sleep, and you should treat any medical conditions that might be contributing to the problem. Restless legs syndrome can be associated with iron-deficiency anemia, and sometimes resolves with iron replacement, so you should check iron and ferritin levels in patients with restless legs. Restless legs syndrome commonly responds to dopamine agonists. L-dopa, gabapentin, benzodiazepines, and opiates are also effective.

Most patients with psychophysiologic insomnia can be treated with behavioral interventions (together with treatment of any underlying conditions that are identified). Patients should be instructed to set a fixed time for retiring and awakening, eliminate daytime naps, refrain from caffeine after noon, avoid exercise or anxiety-provoking activities after dinner, and sleep in a dark, quiet, comfortable room. Patients should also be encouraged to associate the bed primarily with sleep; they should read, watch TV, and eat elsewhere. If they are lying in bed unable to fall asleep, they should leave the room and do something relaxing, returning to bed when they feel sleepy. In fact, it may be useful to restrict the total length of time they spend in bed (and prohibit any naps). This will make them sleepier, increasing the likelihood that when they do go to bed they will fall asleep readily and sleep continuously. Once this goal is achieved, the duration of time allowed for sleep can be gradually lengthened. For patients whose insomnia fails to respond to these simple interventions, a variety of structured techniques, known collectively as cognitive-behavioral therapy, are available.

In some situations, sedative-hypnotic medications are an appropriate adjunct to therapy, but there is some potential for drug dependence, especially with benzodiazepines. These agents are typically most helpful when applied for a limited number of nights. Benzodiazepines bind to the GABA receptor complex. Three nonbenzodiazepine drugs that bind to the GABA receptor complex—zaleplon (Sonata), zolpidem (Ambien), and eszopiclone (Lunesta)—and one melatonin agonist—ramelteon (Rozerem)—have been approved by the FDA for treatment of insomnia, and they are less likely than benzodiazepines to be associated with tolerance or withdrawal effects, although the benefits of cognitive-behavioral therapy are more enduring.

2. Delayed sleep phase syndrome

Some people are able to fall asleep readily and sleep for normal periods of time but do so at the "wrong times." These people have sleep-wake schedule disturbances. The most common example is delayed sleep phase syndrome. Patients with this condition do not feel sleepy at bedtime, so they stay up until 3 am or later. They then sleep for a normal interval if allowed to do so, but if the demands of work or school require them to awaken at

8 am or earlier they become chronically sleepy, especially in the mornings. These patients usually compensate by sleeping late on weekends. In some cases, they can adjust their work schedules to accommodate their sleep patterns, but this is not practical for most patients. One approach to treatment is to awaken patients early in the morning and expose them to bright light for at least an hour. This leads them to fall asleep earlier in the night, so that on subsequent mornings being awakened early eventually becomes less onerous. Sustained benefit requires continued strict adherence to a regular sleep schedule. An alternative approach is to postpone bedtime and the time for rising by two or three hours each day until the patient's sleep schedule matches the desired schedule. This approach also requires strict adherence to a sleep schedule, and patients tend to become less compliant after several months. Evening administration of melatonin may be effective in some patients, although most patients relapse after stopping the medication.

B. Early Morning Awakening

1. Psychiatric and psychologic causes

Depression is the most common cause of early morning awakening in older patients. Depression is also associated with a shortened REM sleep latency, reduced slow-wave NREM sleep, and variable disturbance of sleep onset. Alcohol also disrupts sleep in the latter part of the night. This can result in a cycle whereby depressed patients treat their own insomnia with alcohol (because it helps induce drowsiness); they then experience early morning awakening, resulting in more daytime sleepiness, so they take more alcohol on subsequent nights.

2. Psychophysiologic factors

Just as psychophysiologic factors can result in a cycle exacerbating sleep-onset delay, they can also increase the tendency to awaken early, producing greater daytime sleepiness, leading to more anxiety, resulting in even greater tendency to awaken early, and so forth. The behavioral interventions used to treat psychophysiologic insomnia are the same whether it manifests as sleep-onset delay or early morning awakening.

3. Advanced sleep phase syndrome

The advanced sleep phase syndrome is a sleep-wake schedule disturbance analogous to the delayed sleep phase syndrome, except that these patients fall asleep and wake up too early. This condition is sometimes familial, and in two families the causative mutations have been identified. Both of these mutations were in circadian clock genes. Treatment is analogous to the approaches used for delayed sleep phase syndrome.

C. Sleep Fragmentation

Sleep that is frequently interrupted is not sufficiently restorative. Interruptions may result from sleep apnea (see Part IV of this chapter) or from other medical conditions such as nocturia, orthopnea, or gastroesophageal reflux. Cluster headaches and other parasomnias (see Part VI) may awaken patients and fragment their sleep. Sleep fragmentation may even result from the need to awaken to take prescribed medications. Endocrine disorders and medications (especially corticosteroids and dopaminergic agents) can also produce this problem.

Any of these conditions may initiate the same kind of psychophysiologic cycle that leads to delayed sleep onset or early morning awakening. The same behavioral interventions are indicated, together with treatment directed at the underlying conditions.

D. Sleep State Misperception

Occasional patients complain of unrelenting insomnia but are found to have no objective abnormalities on sleep studies. This uncommon condition is called paradoxical insomnia, or sleep state misperception. It may be caused by a failure to perceive sleep, or it may represent hypochondriasis or another psychiatric disturbance. Of course, it is always possible that existing techniques are simply not adequate to demonstrate the underlying abnormality.

VI. Abnormal Behavior During Sleep

Most of the undesirable movements or behaviors that occur during sleep are associated with NREM sleep, probably because the atonia of REM sleep prevents most movements and behaviors of any kind, desirable or undesirable. When parasomnias occur during REM sleep, they are usually associated with disruption of the normal atonia.

A. Nonrapid Eye Movement (NREM) Sleep Parasomnias

1. Night terrors

Night terrors occur primarily in children but occasionally in adults. The child suddenly arouses from slow-wave sleep, screams, and manifests intense anxiety and autonomic activation (e.g., dilated pupils, perspiration, tachycardia, tachypnea, and piloerection). The child cannot be awakened or consoled but calms down after several minutes and returns to sleep. There is usually amnesia for the event, although there may be a vague recollection of a frightful image or mood. In contrast to typical dreams or nightmares, there is no sense of a coherent theme or "plot." Reassurance is often the only treatment necessary, but imipramine, paroxetine, clonazepam, or diazepam can be used for particularly frequent events.

2. Sleepwalking and sleep talking

Almost all people talk in their sleep at some point in their lives, so it is often considered a normal phenomenon. Sleepwalking and night terrors are also very common, but not to the same degree. They sometimes signify underlying sleep disorders such as sleep apnea. Although any of these disorders may be exacerbated by anxiety and psychosocial stress, they are usually not associated with severe psychopathology.

Sleepwalking and night terrors both arise in deep NREM sleep. Sleep talking can occur in any stage, but it usually occurs in light NREM sleep. In sleep talking, speech is often incoherent or elementary. Sleepwalking (somnambulism) involves complex behaviors that can include sitting up in bed, walking, dressing, eating, cooking, voiding, and even driving a car. Sleepwalkers have their eyes open and react partially to their environment; they can avoid objects, but their coordination is poor. Most episodes last a few seconds to a few minutes. Most children who exhibit sleepwalking outgrow it between ages 7 and 14 years. In most cases, no treatment is necessary except for reassurance. Safety restraints on doors, windows, and stairways may be required. When episodes are frequent, patients should be evaluated for sleep-related breathing disorders, and managed accordingly. When no underlying disorder is identified, patients with frequent and disruptive episodes may be treated with diazepam or a tricyclic antidepressant at bedtime.

3. Confusional arousals

Confusional arousals are characterized by confusion, slow responses, inappropriate behavior, and poor coordination following arousal from slow-wave sleep. The episodes typically last a few minutes. They are almost universal in children less than 5 years of age, but most children outgrow them. They are present in about 4% of the adult population. A variety of medications, especially sedative-hypnotics, antihistamines, and antidepressants, can precipitate or exacerbate them. Conservative management is usually sufficient.

4. Enuresis

Enuresis (bedwetting) is involuntary micturition during sleep in an individual who has control of the bladder while awake. Enuresis is usually idiopathic, but it may be a symptom of underlying urogenital disease or another medical problem, or even sleep apnea. In many patients, it probably represents delayed maturation; at age 5 years, about 15% of boys and 10% of girls have episodes of enuresis, which usually disappear by late childhood or adolescence. Psychologic factors or family dynamics sometimes play a role. For frequent episodes, children may be treated with behavioral techniques, tricyclic antidepressants at low doses, oxybutynin, or (rarely) deamino-8-d-arginine vasopressin (DDAVP, Desmopressin). Carbamazepine has also been reported to be helpful.

5. Periodic limb movements of sleep

Periodic limb movements of sleep usually involve the legs, typically resulting in dorsiflexion of the ankle and small toes, with flexion of the knee and hip, sometimes producing a "kicking" movement. These are the same muscles involved in the "triple flexion" response (see Chapter 2), but the movement is slower. These movements occur in "trains" during sleep. Similar movements may accompany arousals from sleep apnea, so it is important to exclude that diagnosis. Some patients with periodic movements of sleep have restless legs syndrome (see Part V of this chapter) when awake, but most do not. In contrast, 80–90% of all patients with restless legs syndrome also have periodic limb movements of sleep. The same medications that are effective for restless legs syndrome are effective for periodic limb movements of sleep.

6. Miscellaneous

About 60–70% of people have *hypnic jerks*—occasional isolated myoclonic jerks that occur at the onset of the first sleep interval of the night. Reassurance is the only treatment necessary. Some patients have conditions that produce more extensive myoclonus, which can sometimes disrupt their sleep or that of their bed partner. Most people grind their teeth at times, but in 5–15% of the population *bruxism* (tooth grinding) is severe or frequent enough to result in jaw discomfort or significant tooth wear. It may contribute to periodontal disease and temporomandibular joint dysfunction. *Sleep-related rhythmic movement disorder* is the label given to a group of uncommon parasomnias in which patients have stereotyped, repetitive movements such as banging of the head, side-to-side head movements, or rocking of the body, sometimes with rhythmic chanting or humming, just before sleep onset and continuing into light sleep. This typically occurs in normal infants or toddlers and usually resolves in the second or third year of life, but sometimes persists into older childhood or adulthood. Some patients with epilepsy have seizures primarily or exclusively during sleep; these can be associated with REM sleep in some patients and non-REM sleep in others.

B. Rapid Eye Movement (REM) Sleep Parasomnias

1. REM sleep behavior disorder

REM sleep behavior disorder is a condition in which the atonia that normally accompanies REM sleep breaks down and patients "act out" parts of dreams. Motor activity is often vigorous enough to cause injury to patients or their bed partners. Most patients are elderly, and the condition is usually idiopathic, but there may be an underlying neurologic disorder in up to one third of patients. REM sleep behavior disorder is particularly common in disorders associated with α-synuclein accumulation, suggesting that it may be due to an abnormality in dopaminergic systems. REM sleep behavior disorder is common enough in patients with dementia with Lewy bodies (DLB) that it is included as a suggestive feature in the diagnostic criteria for that disease. It occurs in at least two thirds of patients with multiple system atrophy (MSA), and up to a quarter of patients with Parkinson's disease. The sleep disturbance sometimes precedes other neurologic manifestations by a decade or more. It is sometimes difficult to distinguish REM sleep behavior disorder from nocturnal seizures on the basis of the history, and polysomnography is very helpful in this regard. Patients are usually treated successfully with clonazepam. Melatonin, L-dopa, dopamine agonists, donepezil, or sodium oxybate are second-line agents that may also be helpful.

2. Nightmares

Nightmares are particularly vivid and disturbing dreams that often are associated with arousal from REM sleep. In contrast to night terrors, there is hardly any autonomic arousal, patients are readily awakened, and the patients can remember the dream, which usually has a story element. Chronic nightmares are often psychiatric in origin. Post-traumatic stress disorder is a common cause. Some medications, such as L-dopa, beta-adrenergic blockers, and antidepressants, can precipitate nightmares, and abrupt withdrawal of some medications can, also. Most patients and families need no treatment other than reassurance, but cognitive-behavioral therapy is sometimes necessary. A REM-suppressing agent, such as a tricyclic antidepressant or a selective serotonin reuptake inhibitor, is occasionally needed.

3. Miscellaneous

Cluster headaches typically occur during REM sleep and are sometimes included in discussions of parasomnias. Further details are presented in Chapter 12. Penile erections are normal in REM sleep; very rarely they are painful enough to disrupt sleep. Catathrenia refers to expiratory groaning that typically begins 2–6 hours after sleep onset and occurs intermittently during the night; it is most common in REM sleep and the lighter stages of NREM sleep. It is not well understood, and no effective treatment is available.

VII. Discussion of Case Histories

Case 1. This patient has hypersomnia. Falling asleep at the wheel outside the setting of sleep deprivation is never normal. It is unlikely that this man is suffering from insufficient sleep, since he allocates nine hours for sleep each night. One important consideration would be a medication effect, as antihypertensive agents can be associated with hypersomnia. The most likely diagnosis, however, is obstructive sleep apnea. The history of snoring, severe enough to prompt his wife to sleep in another room, is the strongest reason to suspect the diagnosis. His obesity and big neck both could contribute to upper airway narrowing. Hypertension is present in about 40% of patients at the time of diagnosis of obstructive sleep apnea. You should ask the patient when he developed his hypersomnia, when he began snoring, and when he started gaining weight. He does not report any of the features that might suggest narcolepsy, although it would be important to inquire about them explicitly.

You should refer this man for polysomnography (especially because his wife cannot reliably say whether he is experiencing apneic episodes during sleep). If frequent episodes of apnea are documented, the study should be repeated with a trial of CPAP to see if the patient is likely to respond to this treatment. You should also encourage him to lose weight, and review his antihypertensive regimen to be sure it is not contributing to his problem. You should warn him not to drive alone until his hypersomnia has been adequately diagnosed and treated.

Case 2. This man is correct that many of his symptoms can be features of depression, but they could also be manifestations of sleep disorders. Depression and sleep disorders have many common features, and it is often difficult to determine which problem is primary and which is secondary. In this case, the biggest clue that the delayed sleep onset might have a cause other than depression is the patient's report that he is unable to lie down for a prolonged period of time. The specific symptoms he describes are characteristic of restless legs syndrome. In addition, he notes epigastric discomfort when he is lying down, suggesting that he may also have gastroesophageal reflux. Both of these conditions can interfere with sleep onset, setting up a cycle of anxiety and insomnia as described in Part V.

The diagnosis of restless legs syndrome is based on the history. Patients should be evaluated for iron deficiency and uremia, both of which are associated with this disorder. This patient should be treated with a dopamine agonist such as pramipexole (Mirapex) or ropinirole (Requip). He should also receive appropriate treatment for gastroesophageal reflux; diagnostic studies are necessary only if his symptoms fail to respond.

This patient may also have established a pattern of psychophysiologic insomnia that will persist even after treatment of his reflux and restless legs syndrome. If so, he will need education about proper sleep hygiene, and he may require the kinds of behavioral interventions described in Part V. Only if depressive symptoms persist despite all these measures should treatment of depression be considered. Even then, fluoxetine (Prozac) would probably not be the optimal medication because it can cause insomnia.

Case 3. The description of this girl's episode is classic for night terrors. The previous episodes may indeed have been exacerbated by the stress of a new home and day care environment, but the family should be informed that there is no evidence that this condition is caused by underlying psychiatric disease. If she has frequent recurrent episodes in the future, she will need to be evaluated for obstructive sleep apnea, but at this point, no additional investigations are necessary and no treatment is indicated other than good sleep hygiene and safety measures to prevent injury. The girl and her parents should be reassured that she does not have a serious disease, and she will probably outgrow these episodes, but they may recur during times of stress.

Chapter 10

Multifocal Central Nervous System Disorders

I. Case Histories

Case 1. A 29-year-old right-handed woman with a history of IV drug abuse has come to the emergency department because of the acute onset of inability to speak. Two days earlier, she had noticed weakness of the left arm after injecting heroin there, and concluded that she must have "hit a nerve." She has been experiencing fevers, chills, and sweats for the past week, and feels tired all the time. Her general examination is notable for a temperature of 39°C and petechiae on both legs. Neurologic examination reveals almost no verbal output, nearly normal comprehension, and left hemiparesis and sensory loss to all modalities (face worse than arm worse than leg). Reflexes are increased throughout the left arm and leg, and a Babinski sign is present on the left.

Questions:

1. Where's the lesion?
2. What diagnoses should be considered?
3. What diagnostic tests would be helpful?
4. How should this patient be managed?

Case 2. A 35-year-old man has made an appointment with his family doctor because for the past three weeks, his left foot has had a tendency to drag after the 3rd mile of his daily 5-mile run. Two years ago, he had a similar problem with the right foot, but he had twisted that ankle a week earlier, and when the symptoms resolved over the next month, he thought nothing more of them. His only other neurologic symptom has been an episode of partial loss of vision in the left eye that happened 8 months ago. It had developed gradually over 5 days and resolved at almost the same rate; he had attributed it to the stress of a divorce and a new job.

His general physical examination is normal. He has normal mental status. He has an afferent pupillary defect on the left, and his cranial nerves are otherwise normal. He has moderate weakness of left ankle dorsiflexion and walks with a mild foot drop on the left, but his motor examination is otherwise normal. Reflexes are increased at the left knee and ankle, and he has a Babinski sign on the left. Sensation is intact to all modalities.

Questions:

1. Where's the lesion?
2. What diagnoses should be considered?
3. What diagnostic tests would be helpful?
4. How should this patient be managed?

Case 3. A 67-year-old woman has come to the emergency department because of the second episode of Bell's palsy within six months. The first episode resulted in only mild weakness of the right side of her face, so she was not treated. She has improved only minimally in the interim. The second episode began yesterday morning when she noted a tendency to drool out of the left side of her mouth, and she awoke this morning with complete inability to move the left side of her face. She has also noted that her voice is hoarser than it used to be, and she thinks the hearing in her right ear is deteriorating. In addition, she reports that two weeks ago, she developed pain in her lower back on the right; for the last week, it has radiated into her right posterior thigh, leg, and little toe.

Her general physical examination is unremarkable. Neurologic examination confirms bilateral facial weakness (including forehead muscles), worse on the left, hearing loss in the right ear, reduced movement of the left side of the palate, and absent gag reflex on the left side. She has slight weakness of right ankle plantar flexion, but the motor examination is otherwise normal. She has no right ankle jerk, but all other reflexes are normal and symmetric. The sensory examination is normal.

Questions:

1. Where's the lesion?
2. What diagnoses should be considered?
3. What diagnostic tests would be helpful?
4. How should this patient be managed?

II. Approach to Multifocal Disorders

There is something elegant about localizing all of a patient's symptoms and signs to a single lesion site. Nature is not always elegant, however. Most systemic illnesses, neuromuscular diseases, dementing illnesses, movement disorders, and sleep disorders affect the nervous system diffusely. Still, even these diffuse conditions possess some pattern and symmetry. The particular pattern of involvement is generally the basis for making a diagnosis.

This chapter addresses multifocal conditions. Unlike focal lesions and diffuse processes, multifocal conditions are characterized primarily by the lack of a consistent pattern. Fortunately, there are only a few conditions like this, so the diagnosis is often straightforward. In other words, the lack of pattern is itself a revealing pattern. The classic multifocal disease is multiple sclerosis (MS). Other inflammatory diseases and neoplastic processes can also produce multifocal manifestations. The time course and epidemiologic factors help to distinguish among these possibilities (see Chapter 3).

There are two broad categories of multifocal disorders. Some diseases propagate in random directions from a single focus. This is typical of infections and neoplastic diseases. Other processes are intrinsically multifocal. Most diseases in this category (including MS) are inflammatory but not infectious.

III. Focal Diseases with Multifocal Propagation

A. Metastatic Cancer

Central nervous system (CNS) metastases occur in 20–40% of patients with systemic cancer, and in more than two thirds of these patients, the metastases are symptomatic. The spinal cord may be involved by direct metastasis, or, more commonly, by epidural compression from a bony metastasis, as discussed in Chapter 15. Brain metastasis is particularly likely in patients with melanoma or testicular cancer, about half of whom have an intracranial tumor found at autopsy. The likelihood of developing brain metastases is 18–63% for patients with lung cancer and 15–30% for patients with breast or kidney cancer. Because lung cancer and breast cancer are common, they are the most likely sites of primary tumor in patients with brain metastases. Lung cancer accounts for 30–50% of all patients with brain metastases, and breast cancer for 10–20%. The next most common primary tumors are malignant melanoma, gastrointestinal tumors, and genitourinary tract tumors, each accounting for 5–10% of cases.

When patients with known cancer elsewhere in their body develop symptoms that localize to the brain and progress over a time course suggestive of a neoplasm (see Chapter 3), metastasis is the prime consideration. The preferred diagnostic test is an MRI scan of the brain. A metastasis typically appears on MRI or CT scans as a well-demarcated, contrast-enhancing, spherical lesion with surrounding edema. This appearance is not specific, however, and a biopsy is sometimes necessary to establish the diagnosis, even in patients with a known primary cancer. The presence of multiple lesions with characteristic features (as opposed to a solitary lesion) increases the likelihood of metastases.

When the systemic cancer is controlled and only a single brain metastasis exists, it should be surgically resected, if possible. When the metastasis is in a surgically inaccessible location, or when the patient is not a surgical candidate, stereotactic radiosurgery is an alternative. This technique uses multiple convergent beams of external irradiation to deliver a high single dose of radiation to a well-circumscribed region. Uncontrolled trials suggest that stereotactic radiosurgery is as effective as surgical resection of brain metastases in selected patients (such as those with a metastasis smaller than 3 cm in diameter), but randomized trials are necessary. Even when two or three metastatic lesions are present, resection may be appropriate if the lesions are surgically accessible, but the more lesions there are, the less feasible surgical resection becomes. Uncontrolled trials suggest that stereotactic radiosurgery may be effective in such cases, also.

The role of whole brain radiation therapy after surgical resection (or after stereotactic radiosurgery) is somewhat controversial. Radiation lowers the risk of recurrence both locally and distantly in the brain, and reduces the death rate from neurologic causes, but does not affect overall survival. In some cases, this benefit may not be worth the risk of long-term toxicity from radiation. If there is any suspicion that the resection was not complete, it should definitely be followed by whole brain radiation.

Patients who have widespread intracranial metastases and patients with a poor overall prognosis (based on their performance status, age, or the extent of systemic spread of their primary tumor) are generally treated with whole brain radiation therapy alone. This can have palliative effects and prolong survival, but it is rarely curative. Chemotherapy may be effective in treating some brain metastases (such as metastases from testicular germ cell tumors), but the response is disappointing for most types of tumor.

Approximately 15% of patients with brain metastases have no known primary cancer and no other symptoms of malignancy at the time their CNS lesions are discovered. These patients require a thorough search for the primary neoplasm so that it can be treated appropriately. Furthermore, if the primary cancer can be found, and multiple brain lesions with typical characteristics of metastasis are present, there is no need for biopsy or surgical resection of the brain lesions. The evaluation should focus on the lungs, because bronchogenic carcinoma is the most common primary tumor in patients with brain metastases, and other primary tumors often metastasize to the lung before spreading to the rest of the body. The evaluation should therefore include a chest x-ray, sputum samples for cytology, and (if the diagnosis is still unknown) a CT or MRI of the chest. These patients also require thorough skin examinations and rectal examinations, and stool should be screened for occult blood. Men require careful testicular and prostate examinations, and women need careful breast examinations. If this evaluation is not productive, an abdominal CT scan (for occult renal carcinoma) should be obtained. The yield of upper and lower gastrointestinal series is too low to make them worthwhile in this setting. If the diagnosis remains obscure, stereotactic brain biopsy (or surgical resection when there is only one lesion) is necessary.

Even before the diagnosis is established, many patients require treatment for the mass effect produced by the edema surrounding the metastases. Dexamethasone usually produces dramatic reduction in brain edema and clinical symptoms. The optimal dose is not known. A common practice is to give a loading dose of 10 mg, followed by 4 mg four times a day, although one study suggested that doses as low as 1–2 mg four times a day may be equally effective and less toxic. When the mass effect is so great that there is a risk of cerebral herniation, higher initial doses are typically used, and hyperventilation and osmotic diuresis may also be necessary (see Chapter 11).

Seizures occur in approximately 25% of patients with brain metastases and are treated with anticonvulsants according to standard principles (see Chapter 5). For patients who have not yet seized, prophylactic antiepileptic drugs are usually not recommended, except for patients with metastatic melanoma, which has a high incidence of hemorrhage.

In 5–10% of patients with systemic cancer, there is clinical evidence of spread to the meninges. This spread has been given a variety of labels, including leptomeningeal metastasis, carcinomatous meningitis, or meningeal carcinomatosis. It can occur with almost any cancer but is most commonly associated with breast cancer, leukemia, lymphoma, lung cancer, and melanoma, in that order. Leptomeningeal metastasis can present in several ways. It can cause meningeal irritation, producing a syndrome resembling meningitis. Patients may present with symptoms of hydrocephalus when the cancer cells block CSF outflow. Tumor cells in the meningeal spaces may also compress nerve roots or cranial nerves as they leave the neuraxis, resulting in multiple cranial neuropathies or polyradiculopathies. The diagnosis is usually made by cytologic examination of the CSF. Individual samples may be negative, so patients may require three or more lumbar punctures before the diagnosis is established. Additional CSF tests that may be helpful include flow cytometry (looking for a monoclonal population of B cells or T cells, especially in patients with hematologic malignancies) and assays for specific tumor markers. A spinal MRI scan is probably more sensitive than a single CSF cytology analysis, showing meningeal enhancement in 76–87% of patients with leptomeningeal metastasis, but this finding is less specific than positive cytology. Meningeal enhancement on MRI scans can occur in normal subjects after a lumbar puncture, so it is best to obtain the MRI scan before performing any lumbar punctures. Intrathecal chemotherapy combined with radiation therapy helps to prolong life, but even with optimal treatment, life expectancy for patients diagnosed with leptomeningeal metastasis is 6 months.

Cancers also can metastasize to the peripheral nervous system. Tumor cells can invade the brachial plexus and the lumbosacral plexus, and this is the first symptom of cancer in some patients. Individual peripheral nerves or muscles can also be sites of metastasis, but this is less common. Focal metastases in the peripheral nervous system are usually treated with radiation therapy.

Tumors can also cause remote effects without metastasizing; these manifestations are called *paraneoplastic syndromes* and are usually diffuse rather than multifocal. Examples include cerebellar degeneration, various forms of polyneuropathy (pure sensory neuropathy is the most specific), Lambert-Eaton myasthenic syndrome, dermatomyositis, and encephalopathy. Paraneoplastic syndromes appear to be caused by autoimmune phenomena. Different syndromes are associated with specific abnormal antibodies, which have a direct pathogenic effect in some of the syndromes, but may just be an epiphenomenon in others. In about 60% of patients with paraneoplastic syndromes, neurologic symptoms precede other manifestations of cancer. Prompt diagnosis may permit the underlying cancer to be identified and treated earlier than would have been possible otherwise.

B. Central Nervous System Infections

Infectious agents can reach the CNS either by direct spread (e.g., from the sinuses or the inner ear) or via the bloodstream. When infections reach the CNS, the resulting damage can be focal (e.g., an abscess or focal myelitis), multifocal (multiple abscesses or multiple discrete sites of nervous system involvement), or diffuse (meningitis or encephalitis). This section concerns focal and multifocal infectious processes. Meningitis and encephalitis are discussed in Chapter 12, although encephalitis due to herpesviruses is also discussed later in this section.

1. Abscesses

An abscess is a localized area of suppuration and necrosis that forms when an appropriate organism reaches a relatively hypoxic region of the body where host defenses are inadequate to eradicate the infection. Initially, the region of inflammation is poorly demarcated, but over the course of two or three weeks, a well-defined fibrous capsule forms. Anaerobic bacteria, aerobic bacteria, fungi, or parasites can cause CNS abscesses.

In many ways, CNS abscesses are analogous to metastatic tumors in the CNS. Both processes produce mass lesions. The time course is characteristically subacute for abscesses and chronic for metastases, but this distinction is not always reliable. Abscesses and metastases are often indistinguishable radiographically—both characteristically appear as contrast-enhancing lesions with surrounding edema, and the area of enhancement often produces a ring around the lesion. The likely diagnosis can sometimes be established by examining spinal fluid (cytopathology for metastases, cultures for abscesses), but the yield is often low, and brain herniation sometimes occurs when a lumbar puncture is performed on a patient in whom a focal mass lesion has produced a significant elevation of intracranial pressure. For abscesses and metastases, identification of similar lesions elsewhere in the body sometimes permits a presumptive diagnosis, but definitive diagnosis usually requires direct tissue examination (i.e., biopsy or surgical resection).

The optimal treatment of a solitary CNS abscess is either total excision or aspiration under stereotactic CT or MRI guidance, in conjunction with systemic antibiotic therapy. No controlled trials have compared excision to aspiration, but aspiration is more common. Excision is usually recommended for abscesses that are multiloculated, gas containing, fungal, due to head trauma, or unresponsive to aspiration. Excision is most feasible when an abscess is solitary, superficial, and well-encapsulated. When multiple abscesses are present, systemic antibiotic therapy is the cornerstone of treatment, although the largest lesions may still be aspirated or (less often) excised. The choice of antibiotics depends on the underlying organism (or organisms), so even when neither excision nor aspiration is an option (e.g., when there are multiple small or deep abscesses), biopsy of one of the lesions may be desirable. When biopsy is not possible, patients are treated empirically, typically with penicillin or a third-generation cephalosporin (cefotaxime or ceftriaxone) in combination with metronidazole. Chloramphenicol also provides good coverage and CNS penetration but carries a greater risk of toxicity. When there are reasons to suspect a particular infectious agent, the antibiotic regimen should be tailored accordingly (e.g., antistaphylococcal agents, such as oxacillin, nafcillin, or vancomycin, should be included when abscesses occur in the setting of recent head trauma or brain surgery).

2. Infective endocarditis

Infections in the heart are ideally situated for sending colonies in all directions. Cerebral embolism occurs in 20–40% of all patients with infective endocarditis. The emboli can be either sterile or infectious. Sterile emboli result in strokes that are indistinguishable from any other cardioembolic strokes. Infectious emboli can produce strokes by occluding arteries, or they may be deposited in the meninges or parenchyma, serving as foci for the development of meningitis or abscesses. Septic emboli can also infect the walls of the cerebral arteries themselves, leading to aneurysmal dilatation (*mycotic aneurysms*). Mycotic aneurysms are rare, but dangerous, because they can rupture and cause subarachnoid, intraparenchymal, or intraventricular hemorrhage. Even unruptured mycotic aneurysms are important, because they can embolize, resulting in ischemic strokes. The mortality rate is 30% among patients with unruptured mycotic aneurysms and nearly 80% in patients with ruptured mycotic aneurysms.

The only reliable way to diagnosis a mycotic aneurysm is to visualize the intracranial arteries. Intra-arterial catheter angiography is considered the gold standard imaging modality. The traditional teaching has been that this procedure should be performed in all patients with infective endocarditis who develop strokes, because if the source of the stroke is a mycotic aneurysm, the risk of rupture is considerable. This teaching has been challenged, largely because the optimal treatment of a mycotic aneurysm—ruptured or unruptured—is unknown. Although some authorities advocate surgical resection or coiling, others favor conservative management, citing the fact that about one third of unruptured mycotic aneurysms resolve completely by the end of a standard course of antibiotic treatment for endocarditis, and about one sixth get smaller but do not resolve (one third get neither smaller nor larger, and one sixth increase in size). Thus, even in patients with stroke due to embolization from a mycotic aneurysm, it might be reasonable to defer angiography until the completion of a full course of antibiotic treatment, especially since catheter angiography has associated risks that may be considerable in patients with endocarditis, who often have multiple medical problems. Given that mycotic aneurysms occur in only 3–10% of patients with infective endocarditis, the risks of catheter angiography may outweigh the benefits. An alternative approach is to perform a magnetic resonance angiogram (MRA), but the sensitivity and specificity of MRA in this setting is unknown. Some authorities recommend catheter angiography only for patients with hemorrhagic stroke, not for those with ischemic stroke. These issues remain undecided and controversial.

My general recommendation, regardless of whether patients' strokes are ischemic or hemorrhagic, is to obtain an MRA as soon as it is safe and feasible to do so. Although identification of mycotic aneurysms and determination of their size could influence management eventually, the likelihood that this information will affect acute management is not high enough to justify the risk of catheter angiography (or even a noninvasive test like MRA, if it interferes with more pressing tests or treatment). If the MRA shows a mycotic aneurysm, then another MRA should be obtained at the conclusion of the antibiotic course. If the aneurysm is unchanged or larger, the patient will probably need surgical resection or coiling; if the aneurysm is present but smaller, a prolonged course of antibiotics would be reasonable. For patients whose initial MRA shows no mycotic aneurysm, the possibility remains that the MRA is not a sufficiently sensitive test, so those with intracerebral hemorrhage should have a catheter angiogram at the conclusion of the antibiotic course. Patients with purely ischemic stroke and a normal initial MRA may not need further testing for mycotic aneurysms unless long-term anticoagulation is being considered.

Although anticoagulation is the standard treatment for most cardioembolic causes of stroke (see Chapter 4), it is generally avoided in patients with infective endocarditis because it does not prevent the growth of vegetations and may increase the risk of hemorrhagic transformation of a stroke or rupture of a mycotic aneurysm. The one exception is endocarditis on an artificial valve, in which the risk of recurrent embolization is so high that the benefits of anticoagulation probably outweigh the risks (except in the case of S. aureus endocarditis, where the usual practice is to withhold all anticoagulation for at least the first two weeks of antibiotic therapy).

Stroke in the setting of endocarditis is not an indication for valve replacement surgery. When patients require acute valve replacement for other reasons (such as refractory congestive heart failure or perivalvular abscess), the surgery can result in further neurologic deterioration if performed within the first week or two of a stroke. For this reason, valve replacement surgery should be delayed until at least a week after the stroke, if possible.

3. Specific infectious agents

Certain infectious agents are particularly likely to produce multifocal nervous system disease. Most of these infections are relatively indolent, perhaps because more aggressive infections become symptomatic and are treated (or result in death) before they have a chance to form colonies throughout the body.

a. Human immunodeficiency virus (HIV)

Patients infected with HIV can develop dysfunction at any level of the nervous system. At least four factors predispose to neurologic involvement. First, these patients are at risk for many opportunistic infections and neoplasms that affect the nervous system. Second, HIV itself appears to have a predilection for both the CNS and the PNS and may produce symptoms directly. Third, antigenic cross-reactivity between HIV and nervous system elements may occur, so that the inflammatory reaction provoked by HIV infection results in neurologic damage. Fourth, many of the medications used to treat HIV or its complications can have neurotoxic effects.

Peripheral nervous system syndromes reported in HIV patients include polymyositis and dermatomyositis, and IBM has also been reported. These most often occur at the time of seroconversion. Some patients develop pyomyositis, a focal suppurative bacterial infection of the muscle. There also appears to be a myopathy associated with the use of zidovudine, and patients may develop a myopathy from cachexia. Four principal neuropathic syndromes are associated with HIV infection. The most common is a distal, symmetric peripheral polyneuropathy that tends to increase in incidence and severity with disease duration. This polyneuropathy is thought to be a direct effect of HIV infection, although other potential causes are often present (notably nutritional deficiencies and drug toxicity). Didanosine (ddI), zalcitabine (ddC), and stavudine (d4T) have been associated with neuropathy, and so have some of the drugs typically used to treat infectious manifestations of AIDS. The second type of neuropathic syndrome, inflammatory demyelinating polyradiculoneuropathy, is much less common than axonal polyneuropathy. Acute inflammatory demyelinating polyradiculoneuropathy (AIDP) and chronic inflammatory demyelinating polyradiculoneuropathy (CIDP) may occur in HIV-positive patients who do not have AIDS. These conditions sometimes develop at the time of seroconversion, suggesting that they are caused by the inflammatory response to HIV and not by immunosuppression or some other direct effect of HIV infection. Another, relatively rare, neuropathic syndrome is mononeuropathy multiplex, which can also occur early in the course of HIV infection. The fourth major variety of HIV-related neuropathic syndrome is progressive polyradiculopathy, typically beginning with leg weakness and bladder or bowel problems, with progression to the arms over several weeks. This generally occurs with advanced immunodeficiency. *Cytomegalovirus* (CMV) appears to be the cause in many cases. *Herpes varicella zoster* reactivation is also common in HIV-infected patients, leading to a more localized radiculopathy. Cranial nerves may also be involved in patients with zoster, mononeuropathy multiplex, AIDP, or CIDP.

In the CNS, the most common manifestation of HIV infection is HIV-associated dementia, an encephalopathy that is sometimes mistaken for depression because it usually presents with nonspecific mood changes, psychomotor slowing, and concentration problems. It rapidly progresses to generalized cognitive deterioration, often associated with pronounced apathy and social withdrawal. These patients frequently develop tremor or myoclonus. Many patients with HIV-associated dementia also develop a myelopathy, with characteristic vacuolar changes noted in the spinal cord at autopsy. Incontinence, gait disturbance, and bilateral Babinski signs are frequent late in the course of HIV-associated dementia, either as a direct result of cerebral involvement or as a consequence of myelopathy. HIV-associated dementia typically occurs in the setting of advanced immunosuppression, and it improves in response to high doses of zidovudine, suggesting that it is a direct result of HIV infection. Treatment with multiple antiretroviral medications is more effective than monotherapy.

Focal lesions in the brain and spinal cord are common manifestations of HIV-associated secondary processes, especially toxoplasmosis, cryptococcus, lymphoma, and progressive multifocal leukoencephalopathy (PML), a disease of white matter caused by the JC virus, an opportunistic papovavirus. All of these can produce mass lesions (presenting with progressive, focal symptoms, usually with a subacute time course), but they can also be asymptomatic or produce diffuse symptoms. Cryptococcus, in particular, usually manifests with meningitis that can be fairly subtle—about 85% of patients experience headaches, but fever and neck stiffness each occur in only 35% of patients. Approximately 40% of patients with cryptococcal meningitis have altered mental status. Except for cranial neuropathies, focal findings are uncommon in cryptococcal meningitis.

Because of the high incidence of mass lesions in the brain, an imaging study of the brain is usually the first test obtained in HIV-infected patients with headaches or mental status changes, even if there are no focal abnormalities on neurologic examination. When this study is normal, a lumbar puncture is usually performed to look for evidence of cryptococcal meningitis; cryptococcal antigen is present in the spinal fluid of 95% of patients with this infection, and India ink staining is positive in 70–80%. The CSF should also be evaluated for syphilis, tuberculosis, herpes simplex, and lymphoma.

When the brain imaging study is abnormal, differentiation between toxoplasmosis, lymphoma, PML, and less common conditions may be difficult. The condition that most readily responds to treatment is toxoplasmosis. Toxoplasmosis almost always represents reactivation of a latent infection, so toxoplasma IgG titers are consistently positive in patients with this manifestation, even early in the course. Thus, the standard approach in patients with HIV who have multifocal mass lesions on a brain imaging study is to check toxoplasma IgG titers, and if they are positive, to treat empirically with the antibiotics sulfadiazine and pyrimethamine, which usually produce a dramatic response in patients with toxoplasmosis. If clinical and radiographic parameters fail to improve over the next ten to fourteen days, a biopsy should be performed. A biopsy should be performed without waiting for a trial of empiric anti-toxoplasma medication when an MRI scan shows only a single lesion, because multiple lesions can be seen on brain MRI scans in most patients with toxoplasmosis. An urgent biopsy (rather than empiric toxoplasma treatment) is also indicated if the patient's clinical condition is deteriorating rapidly, or if the initial brain imaging study suggests a high risk of herniation. PML can sometimes be difficult to distinguish from toxoplasmosis and lymphoma on MRI scans, but it usually has a fairly distinctive appearance. When the scan looks typical of PML, empiric anti-toxoplasma medicine is not necessary. Polymerase chain reaction (PCR) testing of CSF for JC virus DNA can also be helpful in diagnosing PML. Highly active antiretroviral therapy (HAART) significantly prolongs survival for patients with PML, and also for patients with CNS lymphoma, who otherwise have a dismal prognosis. Cryptococcal meningitis usually responds readily to treatment with amphotericin, with or without flucytosine; the relative efficacy of amphotericin and triazole agents (fluconazole and itraconazole) for acute therapy remains unclear (although the triazoles are effective for cryptococcal suppression and prophylaxis). For both toxoplasmosis and cryptococcal meningitis, prolonged maintenance therapy is necessary to prevent relapses.

The *immune reconstitution inflammatory syndrome (IRIS)* is a rare condition characterized by a paradoxical clinical deterioration within weeks of beginning HAART. It should be suspected in patients whose CD4 count is recovering and in whom HIV RNA viral load is declining with unexpected progression of an appropriately treated infection or the new appearance of a previously undiagnosed opportunistic condition. Some patients may respond to a brief course of corticosteroids, although controlled trials are not available.

Patients with AIDS have an increased incidence of syphilis, which may be hard to diagnose because some of the traditional serologic tests are less reliable in this setting. Patients who have AIDS may require more aggressive and sustained treatment for neurosyphilis than is necessary in immunocompetent individuals. Other conditions that may affect the nervous system in patients with AIDS include Kaposi's sarcoma, atypical mycobacterial infections, nocardiosis, and fungal infections (e.g., candidiasis, aspergillosis, histoplasmosis, mucormycosis, and others). Patients with AIDS also have an increased incidence of strokes. In patients with AIDS, it is common for several different processes to affect the nervous system simultaneously.

b. Spirochetal infections

The initial clinical manifestation of syphilis (primary syphilis) is a skin lesion, or chancre, at the site of inoculation. In untreated patients, this heals spontaneously over 3–6 weeks; during this time, the spirochetes disseminate throughout the body, and in about 25–40% of infected patients, the nervous system is seeded. At this point, patients may develop the features of secondary syphilis (flu-like symptoms, rash, lymphadenopathy, and mucosal lesions). Neurologic symptoms are relatively rare; at most 5% of patients with secondary syphilis develop symptoms of aseptic meningitis (although asymptomatic lymphocytic meningitis is present in 25–40%). Some patients with disseminated organisms never manifest any symptoms of secondary syphilis. The symptoms (if any) of secondary syphilis resolve without treatment over a period of weeks to months, and patients enter a latent stage in which there are no clinical manifestations of infection for months to years. In 10–30% of untreated patients, the latent stage is followed by tertiary syphilis, which is characterized by skin, osseous, cardiovascular, or neurologic manifestations.

Neurosyphilis refers to nervous system involvement at any stage of syphilis. Most patients with neurosyphilis, regardless of the stage, are asymptomatic—only 4–6% of untreated patients with syphilis ultimately develop neurologic symptoms. These patients typically display one of several distinctive clinical syndromes. The earliest is the aseptic meningitis that can occur within the first 1 or 2 years after the initial infection, often associated with cranial nerve involvement. Meningovascular syphilis can occur 1–10 years, but typically 5–7 years, after the initial infection. It is characterized by diffuse meningeal infiltrates and inflammation and fibrosis of arteries, causing brain and spinal cord lesions that may be focal, multifocal, or diffuse. The most delayed neurologic manifestations of syphilis are general paresis and tabes dorsalis, which generally occur 10–30 years after the initial infection. General paresis is a condition of diffuse cortical dysfunction, producing dementia, upper motor neuron findings, myoclonus, seizures, dysarthria, and pupillary abnormalities. Tabes dorsalis results from involvement of the posterior nerve roots as they enter the spinal cord. Typical symptoms are loss of proprioception, ataxia, lightning-like pains, and urinary incontinence. Deep tendon reflexes are usually absent in the lower extremities, though Babinski signs may be present when there is co-existent general paresis. The pupils are abnormal in more than 90% of patients; various abnormalities can occur, but the most characteristic finding is small, irregular, and unequal pupils that do not constrict in response to light but constrict with accommodation.

Diagnosis of neurosyphilis is based on serologic studies and spinal fluid analysis. Two types of serologic tests are currently available (tests using PCR or monoclonal antibody reagents hold promise but are still experimental). Nonspecific antibodies, such as the VDRL or rapid plasma reagent (RPR), are present in the blood of almost all patients with secondary syphilis but revert to normal in about 25% of patients with late syphilis. Their presence in the CSF is diagnostic of neurosyphilis, but their absence does not exclude the diagnosis. Specific treponemal antibodies, such as fluorescent treponemal antibody (FTA) or microhemagglutination–*Treponema pallidum* (MHA-TP), are also present in the blood of nearly all patients with secondary syphilis, and persist throughout life even when the infection itself is eradicated. They are therefore a reliable indicator of previous syphilitic infection, but they do not indicate whether the infection is still active. In a patient with clinical features suggestive of neurosyphilis, the first diagnostic test should be to check the serum FTA or MHA-TP. If the result is negative, this practically excludes the possibility of neuro-syphilis (these antibodies may be undetectable in early stages of primary syphilis, but those patients do not exhibit neurologic manifestations). If the FTA or MHA-TP result is positive, this simply means that the patient had an active syphilis infection at some point in the past. To determine if the infection is currently active in the CNS, a lumbar puncture should be performed, and the presence of any of the typical abnormalities (i.e., elevated white blood cell count, increased protein concentration, or positive VDRL) warrants treatment for neurosyphilis with high doses of IV penicillin for 10–14 days.

Lyme disease, like syphilis, can result in neurologic complications months or years after the initial infection. The initial rash at the site of the tick bite is analogous to the initial chancre of syphilis—it can resolve without treatment, but meanwhile spirochetes disseminate throughout the body. The most common neurologic manifestation is subacute or chronic meningitis that typically begins a few weeks to a few months after inoculation. The usual symptoms are headache and stiff neck, often with associated mood changes and difficulty concentrating. These symptoms are frequently mild and usually resolve even without treatment, so this stage of the disease is probably unrecognized in many cases. Cranial nerve palsies (almost always including one or both facial nerves) and radicular pain sometimes accompany the meningitis. Even in untreated patients, actual parenchymal infection of the brain or spinal cord is very rare, but when it occurs it can result in focal deficits or encephalitis. Patients with Lyme disease can also develop peripheral polyneuropathy.

Borrelia burgdorferi, the agent that causes Lyme disease, can almost never be cultured from the blood or spinal fluid, and even spinal fluid PCR has a 40–50% false-negative rate (probably because of the organism's relative scarcity in body fluids), so diagnosis is based on clinical characteristics and serologic antibody studies. Most laboratories use enzyme-linked immuno-sorbent assay (ELISA) techniques, which—like the specific treponemal antibody assays for syphilis—indicate a history of exposure, but not necessarily active infection. Moreover, they are neither 100% specific nor 100% sensitive. When ELISA testing suggests Lyme disease but the diagnosis remains uncertain, Western blot assay can provide specificity by identifying the specific antigens to which the patient's antibodies react. Consensus criteria for what should be considered a positive result now exist, although they may sacrifice some sensitivity for specificity, and they do not apply to patients with negative ELISA results. Antibody testing on the spinal fluid can be helpful, but again, sensitivity and specificity are less than 100%, especially in chronic disease.

Although evidence suggests that oral antibiotic regimens can be effective for patients with neurologic manifestations of Lyme disease, most clinicians treat with IV ceftriaxone, cefotaxime, or penicillin for at least two weeks. Many experts recommend a 4-week course, although this is not based on evidence from randomized trials. Doxycycline or chloramphenicol are options for patients allergic to penicillin and cephalopsorins.

c. Tuberculosis

Mycobacterium tuberculosis can spread to the nervous system via the bloodstream either during the initial infection or with subsequent caseation at the primary site or other sites. The resulting tuberculous foci (tubercles) can then remain dormant in the CNS for months or years before producing clinical symptoms. The most common neurologic manifestation is tuberculous meningitis, which occurs when a suitably located subpial tubercle grows or ruptures into the subarachnoid or intraventricular space. This meningitis is most marked at the base of the brain, ultimately forming a thick, gelatinous mass that engulfs the cranial nerves and blood vessels passing through it. Less often, tubercles located deep in the brain parenchyma may grow large enough to present as a mass lesion (a tuberculoma).

Tuberculous meningitis usually begins with a several-week prodrome of headache, malaise, personality change, and low-grade fever. The headache eventually becomes more severe and continuous, and patients develop nausea, vomiting, neck stiffness, confusion, papilledema, and cranial nerve abnormalities. Focal deficits (such as hemiparesis, paraparesis, and ataxia) can result from local pressure, venous congestion, or strokes that occur because blood vessels passing through the region of basilar meningitis become inflamed and thrombosed. Approximately 10% of adults and a higher proportion of children develop seizures. Patients subsequently progress to stupor and coma, with death typically occurring within two months of the onset of illness in untreated patients, but occasional patients follow a more indolent course over many months or even years.

The diagnosis of tuberculous meningitis can be extremely difficult to establish, and antituberculous treatment often must be initiated even when the diagnosis is only presumptive. A positive tuberculin skin test is helpful, but a negative test is not, because false-negatives are common in all forms of tuberculosis. Similarly, evidence of active tuberculous infection elsewhere in the body is helpful when present, but not when absent, because the nervous system can be the only site of active infection. CSF is usually the most important guide to diagnosis (see Table 12.1 in Chapter 12). Typical findings are elevated opening pressure, increased protein (usually 100–500 mg/dl), reduced glucose (<45 mg/dl in 80% of patients), and moderate pleocytosis (100–300 white blood cells per mm^3 in most patients). The cellular reaction is predominantly mononuclear, but polymorphonuclear cells may predominate in a significant minority of patients, especially early in the course. Mycobacterial cultures from the CSF require weeks to months for detectable growth, and even then the false-negative rate is at least 25%. The yield is increased by sending samples from several lumbar punctures (usually repeated on a daily basis); there is no need to delay treatment for this, because the yield from cultures remains good even after several days of therapy.

The long delay and high false-negative rate for cultures have prompted a search for alternative means of diagnosis. PCR techniques provide nearly 100% specificity but a sensitivity of at most 75%. Use of ELISA methodology may enhance sensitivity, and promising results have been reported with an assay for mycobacterial ribosomal RNA. Other tests that require further evaluation include a rapid culture technique and spinal fluid assays for substances that are believed to be unique to M. tuberculosis, including tuberculostearic acid and adenosine deaminase.

The optimal treatment regimen for tuberculous meningitis has not been established. Current recommendations are to treat for two months with four drugs, isoniazid, rifampin, pyrazinamide, and ethambutol (although streptomycin can be substituted for ethambutol). After two months, the regimen can be simplified to isoniazid and rifampin, as long as the organism is fully sensitive to them. These drugs are continued for 4–7 more months. The specific agents used and the duration of therapy may be modified depending on the likelihood of drug resistance. Patients taking isoniazid should take pyridoxine (vitamin B6) concurrently to prevent neuropathy. Adjunctive corticosteroids appear to help limit or even prevent the neurologic consequences of tuberculous meningitis, though this has never been convincingly demonstrated. They are typically administered to patients with increased intracranial pressure, spinal block, focal neurologic signs, or depressed level of consciousness. Tuberculomas can usually be adequately treated with medications, although the lesions are sometimes resected when the diagnosis is uncertain. Surgical procedures are sometimes required to treat increased intracranial pressure or hydrocephalus.

d. Herpesviruses

Herpesviruses have a tendency to lie dormant in the nervous system for years at a time, periodically reactivating and causing clinical symptoms. Several distinctive syndromes can result. The most serious is herpes simplex encephalitis (HSE). This is mainly due to *Herpes simplex virus type 1*, which causes HSE in adults, whereas *Herpes simplex virus type 2* is the principal cause of neonatal HSE and adult aseptic meningitis. HSE is the most frequent cause of fatal encephalitis, and it is the most common identified cause of acute, sporadic encephalitis. About two thirds of cases are due to reactivation, and a third are due to primary infection resulting from exposure to contaminated saliva or respiratory secretions. The clinical presentation is similar to that of any other form of encephalitis, with a prodromal phase characterized by malaise, fever, headache, and sometimes behavioral changes. The distinctive feature of HSE is a tendency to involve the frontotemporal lobes predominantly, resulting in focal signs and symptoms in at least 50% of patients. These include hemiparesis, aphasia, visual field abnormalities, and cranial nerve deficits. Florid behavioral changes, amnesia, seizures, stupor, and coma are also common. The clinical course is extremely variable, with some patients progressing to coma within a few days but other patients stabilizing and demonstrating only a mild to moderate encephalopathy for several weeks.

Spinal fluid examination typically reveals a lymphocytic pleocytosis (50–500 cells per mm^3) with mild protein elevation and normal or moderately reduced glucose. In 25–40% of patients, red blood cells are present in the CSF. Regions of abnormal signal and microhemorrhage, especially in the temporal lobes, may be evident on MRI scans, and unilateral or bilateral periodic lateralized epileptiform discharges in the frontotemporal regions are characteristic EEG findings. PCR testing for viral DNA in the spinal fluid is the most reliable diagnostic test (other than brain biopsy, which is now performed only rarely, primarily in atypical cases or when PCR testing is not available). PCR testing has an estimated sensitivity of 98% and a specificity approaching 100%, although false-negative results may be more common in the first 24–48 hours of illness. Whenever HSE is a realistic possibility, it is best to initiate empiric treatment with acyclovir (30 mg/kg per day in three divided doses for at least 14 days) while awaiting CSF PCR results. The mortality rate in patients treated with acyclovir and supportive care is 20–30%, compared with 70%–80% mortality in untreated patients.

Herpes varicella-zoster virus remains latent in neurons of sensory ganglia after resolution of the primary infection (varicella, commonly called chickenpox). Zoster, or "shingles," occurs when the virus is reactivated years later. The risk of zoster increases with increasing age and decreasing immune function, but it may occur even in immunocompetent young people. The most common manifestation is sharp, burning pain in a dermatomal distribution, most often in a thoracic dermatome, followed two to five days later by a characteristic rash in the same distribution (though some patients never develop the rash). Another typical area of involvement is on the forehead in the territory of the ophthalmic division of the trigeminal nerve (*zoster ophthalmicus*). The most common neurologic complication is postherpetic neuralgia, which occurs in roughly 10% of all patients with zoster but in up to 50% of patients older than 60 years. Postherpetic neuralgia is characterized by steady, burning pain with superimposed lightning-like pains in the distribution of the preceding skin involvement, persisting for more than 4 weeks after the rash disappears. The area is often extremely sensitive to touch.

Acyclovir, famciclovir, and valacyclovir have all been shown to reduce the duration of the rash and the acute pain if they are initiated within seventy-two hours of the onset of the rash. Famciclovir and valacyclovir are generally preferred over acyclovir because they have also been shown to reduce the duration of postherpetic neuralgia. Unfortunately, none of these agents has been shown to reduce the incidence of postherpetic neuralgia. For this reason, the development of a vaccine was a major advance. Compared to patients who receive placebo, elderly patients who receive the varicella vaccine have a 61% reduction in the incidence of shingles and a 67% reduction in the incidence of postherpetic neuralgia. Other options for acute treatment of shingles include steroids (when given in conjunction with an antiviral drug, and only in patients with no contraindications), tricyclic antidepressants, anti-epileptic drugs (especially gabapentin, pregabalin, and carbamazepine), opioids, and local anesthetics (including lidocaine patch and capsaicin cream).

Other neurologic complications of zoster can occur when the virus spreads from the sensory nerve to involve other components of the nervous system. For example, spread to the anterior root can cause focal weakness, usually in the distribution of the nerve root that corresponds to the affected dermatome. Spread of the virus to the spinal cord may result in myelitis, and more diffuse spread may result in encephalitis or aseptic meningitis. About a third of patients with zoster ophthalmicus develop abnormalities of other cranial nerves, especially the third nerve. Other potential complications of zoster ophthalmicus include ocular involvement (in about 20% of patients) and, rarely, a thrombotic cerebral vasculopathy that results in delayed contralateral hemiparesis. Patients with these syndromes of more extensive nervous system involvement are usually treated with IV acyclovir, although its efficacy remains unknown. Ramsay Hunt syndrome (*zoster oticus, zoster auricularis,* or *zoster cephalicus*) is thought to represent spread of the virus from the geniculate ganglion of the facial nerve. It is characterized by vesicular eruption in the external auditory meatus accompanied by ipsilateral facial weakness, and often by hearing loss, tinnitus, or vertigo. Cranial nerves V, IX, and X are frequently involved, and there may be severe pain in the territories of these nerves.

e. Parasitic infections

Parasites are ideally adapted to colonize multiple sites in the nervous system and other organ systems without provoking overwhelming host responses. Many of these organisms are uncommon in the United States, but they account for significant worldwide morbidity and mortality. Parasitic infections that are particularly likely to involve the nervous system include malaria, toxoplasmosis, trypanosomiasis, amebic infections, strongyloidiasis, trichinosis, onchocerciasis (the fourth leading cause of blindness in the world), schistosomiasis, paragonimiasis, echinococcosis, and cysticercosis (the most common cause of adult-onset epilepsy in developing countries and increasingly common in the United States). Detailed descriptions of these parasites, their life cycles, and the diseases they cause are available in textbooks of infectious diseases.

f. Potential agents of bioterrorism

In recent years, the risk of bioterrorism has required physicians to become aware of some pathogens that would otherwise be primarily of historical interest. Some of these agents can affect the nervous system.

About 95% of cases of anthrax are of the cutaneous form, and of these, spontaneous healing occurs in 80–90% of untreated patients. The rest develop bacteremia, which can lead to a fulminant and rapidly fatal hemorrhagic meningoencephalitis. Meningoencephalitis may occur in up to 50% of cases of inhalational anthrax. This is the form of the disease most likely to be used as an agent of bioterrorism, although it accounts for only about 5% of cases of naturally acquired anthrax. Patients typically present with fever, headache, vomiting, and delirium; they may also have seizures, myoclonus, increased tone, and focal abnormalities. Patients should be treated with IV ciprofloxacin or doxycycline, together with one or two antibiotics with in vitro efficacy, such as rifampin, clindamycin, or vancomycin.

Because of the successful global eradication of smallpox in 1980, immunization was discontinued. If bioterrorism results in the re-emergence of smallpox, historical experience suggests that neurologic complications will be uncommon, but some patients may develop encephalomyelitis 5–16 days after the onset of the typical rash. This can result in headaches, seizures, varying degrees of mental status change (up to and including coma), or a flaccid paralysis resembling poliomyelitis. Encephalomyelitis can also occur after vaccination, especially in children.

Meningitis can occur with any of the forms of plague (bubonic, septicemic, and pneumonic), but it is uncommon. It is treated with intravenous chloramphenicol. Tularemia produces a variety of localized syndromes, but dissemination can also occur, associated with meningitis, encephalitis, or Guillain-Barré syndrome. Tularemia is treated with intramuscular streptomycin.

Botulism as a tool of bioterrorism would be disseminated via the toxin, not the actual infection. As discussed in Chapter 6, botulinum toxin acts at presynaptic receptors to block release of acetylcholine and thereby prevent transmission at the neuromuscular junction, resulting in severe weakness. Diplopia, blurred vision, and ptosis are often the first symptoms, followed within 72 hours by dysarthria, dysphagia, and flaccid paralysis. Patients are treated with antitoxin and meticulous supportive care.

IV. Inherently Multifocal Diseases

A. Multiple Sclerosis

Multiple sclerosis (MS) is the prototype of an inherently multifocal CNS disease. Most patients have discrete attacks of CNS dysfunction that arise over hours to days, typically last two to six weeks, and improve partially or completely over weeks or months. Early in the disease, the attacks occur at an average of once a year, but after the fifth year the frequency falls to an average of one attack every two years. The attacks can affect any pathway in the CNS, but the most common presenting symptoms involve the spinal cord (50%), optic nerve (25%), or posterior fossa structures (20%). Spinal cord lesions can produce numbness, paresthesias (e.g., tingling), dysesthesias (including Lhermitte's phenomenon), pain, weakness, stiffness, clumsiness, urinary urgency, incontinence of bladder or bowels, constipation, or impotence. Lhermitte's phenomenon is an electric sensation passing down the back and into the limbs, provoked by neck flexion. It can occur with any condition affecting the posterior columns of the cervical spinal cord, including vitamin B12 deficiency or extrinsic cord compression. Optic nerve lesions can manifest with blurred vision, loss of vision, or eye pain. Brainstem or cerebellar involvement can result in diplopia, dysarthria, dysphagia, clumsiness, vertigo, numbness, or weakness. The most common symptoms of MS are weakness in one or more limbs (40%), optic nerve symptoms (22%), paresthesias (21%), diplopia (12%), vertigo (5%), and urinary symptoms (5%). Tremor, fatigue, and cognitive impairment are common, especially in longstanding disease. Patients may also experience paroxysmal symptoms, including seizures, trigeminal neuralgia (see Chapter 12), other intermittent pains, episodic dysarthria or ataxia (usually lasting less than 20 seconds), and dystonic episodes (sometimes called "tonic seizures").

In an individual patient, it is extremely difficult to predict when the attacks will occur, what sites in the nervous system will be involved, the severity of the symptoms, and the degree of recovery. Four general categories of clinical progression have been defined:

(1) *Relapsing-remitting*: clearly defined attacks (relapses), with no disease progression during the periods between the attacks. Patients typically recover from the attacks, but not always, and the recovery may be either partial or complete. If they have attacks from which they do not fully recover, their overall condition may deteriorate over time.

(2) *Primary-progressive*: continued disease progression from onset (though there may be occasional plateaus or temporary periods of minor improvement).

(3) *Secondary-progressive*: initial relapsing-remitting course, followed by continued progression (though there may be occasional plateaus, superimposed relapses, or temporary periods of minor improvement).

(4) *Progressive-relapsing*: continued progression from onset, but with clear superimposed relapses followed by partial or full recovery. There is continuing progression during the periods between relapses.

A minimum duration of 24 hours is arbitrarily required for symptoms to be classified as relapses. At onset, 85% of patients have a relapsing-remitting course, but by ten years, 50% of the patients whose course was originally relapsing-remitting have evolved to a secondary-progressive pattern. About 10% of patients have a primary-progressive course, and about 5% have a progressive-relapsing course. MS affects women more than men (in a ratio of 2:1), and it preferentially affects young adults, with the age at onset typically between 10 and 59 years, although it can begin in early childhood or in later life. Primary-progressive MS tends to affect men and women equally, with a later age of onset.

Even in patients with relapsing-remitting disease, imaging studies show changes between relapses, suggesting that the disease is not truly "in remission." Nonetheless, patients who have less frequent clinical relapses early in the disease tend to be less disabled later in the course. Patients who have minimal disability after five years of disease (i.e., patients who have recovered nearly completely from their relapses to date) also have a better prognosis.

The pathologic hallmark of MS is the demyelinating plaque. Macroscopically, plaques are well-demarcated areas of discoloration that can occur anywhere in the white matter; microscopically, they are perivascular collections of macrophages and lymphocytes (CD4+ T-cells based on immunoreactivity), with numerous demyelinated axons demonstrated on myelin stains. Although the axons themselves are less prominently affected, they are reduced in number compared to normal brain, and axonal transection is common. Aggressive investigation has failed to identify a consistent infectious agent or other common factor responsible for inciting the inflammation, but environmental and genetic factors both play a role.

The diagnosis of MS is based on a history of "two or more CNS lesions separated in space and time," confirmed on physical examination. Many diseases can cause recurrent symptoms in a single location (e.g., seizures, TIAs, intervertebral disc herniation), and many monophasic illnesses are multifocal or diffuse (e.g., infections, metabolic disturbances), but very few conditions cause multiple, discrete episodes of transient dysfunction involving more than one area of the CNS. Of those that do, MS is by far the most common. Thus, when a patient's history and examination provide compelling evidence of two or more CNS lesions separated in space and time, it is usually reasonable to look for evidence of a systemic inflammatory disease, such as systemic lupus erythematosus, but otherwise, no diagnostic testing is required.

Several diagnostic tests can be used to supplement the history and examination, but no test is completely reliable. More than 90% of patients with a clear diagnosis of MS (based on history and examination) have typical abnormalities on MRI scans of the brain or spinal cord. Similar abnormalities can be helpful in establishing the diagnosis when the clinical evidence is strongly suggestive, but not diagnostic. For example, at the time of presentation for one symptom, patients may report a history of a different symptom in the past, but the only abnormalities on neurologic examination correspond to the current symptom. In this situation, MRI evidence of disseminated lesions (especially when they appear to be chronic, and the MRI also shows an acute lesion that corresponds to the current symptom) can establish the diagnosis. A consensus panel has published a set of criteria for diagnosing MS, including explicit discussion of situations like this in which the history and physical examination do not completely establish dissemination in space and time, but MRI scans (and sometimes additional tests) provide sufficient evidence to confirm the diagnosis. Although the MRI signal changes that occur in MS have characteristic features, they are not specific—identical findings can result from other inflammatory conditions, ischemia, trauma, metabolic abnormalities, or even neoplasms (see Figures 10.1 and 10.2). The MRI scan can only be interpreted reliably in the context of the history and examination.

The second most useful test in patients whose diagnosis can not be established from history and physical examination is CSF testing. Patients with MS produce antibodies (especially IgG) within the CNS, commonly demonstrated with two tests. One of these tests is the IgG index, defined as:

$$\text{IgG index} = [\text{IgG(CSF)}/\text{albumin(CSF)}] / [\text{IgG(serum)}/\text{albumin(serum)}]$$

The ratio of IgG to albumin is used to be sure that an elevated IgG is not simply a manifestation of a generalized increase in protein. The normalization of this ratio in CSF with respect to the same ratio in serum is necessary to be sure that an elevated CSF IgG does not simply reflect

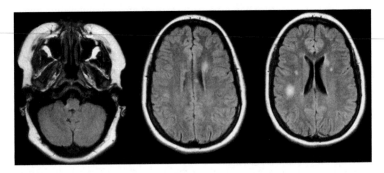

Fig. 10.1 MRI (FLAIR sequence, axial plane) images showing typical demyelinating lesions in a patient with relatively mild MS. (*Source:* Preston DC, Shapiro BE. Neuroimaging in neurology: an interactive CD. Elsevier, 2007).

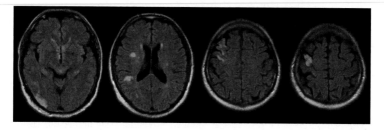

Fig. 10.2 MRI (FLAIR sequence, axial plane) images showing multiple small strokes in the distribution of multiple branches of the right middle cerebral artery (MCA). (*Source:* Preston DC, Shapiro BE. Neuroimaging in neurology: an interactive CD. Elsevier, 2007).

passive migration of serum IgG across the blood-brain barrier in a patient with systemic inflammation. The other commonly used CSF marker of IgG production within the CNS is the presence of oligoclonal bands on electrophoretic analysis of CSF. Electrophoresis of CSF from normal subjects usually produces a homogeneous blur of immunoglobulin. Patients with MS typically have a number of discrete bands distinct from the background, representing antibody produced by one or more clones of plasma cells. Bands that are present in the spinal fluid but not in the serum indicate active inflammation within the nervous system. Neither an elevated IgG index nor the presence of oligoclonal bands is specific for MS as opposed to other causes of CNS inflammation, but in certain clinical settings this information can be very helpful.

In some cases, when the physical examination does not provide compelling evidence for more than one CNS lesion, evoked potentials can be useful. These are essentially measures of the speed with which sensory information reaches the brain (which is dependent on the function of myelinated pathways). EEG activity is recorded just before and just after a sensory stimulus. Because of the large amount of random activity in a routine EEG, the specific response to the stimulus cannot be distinguished from the background noise after a single stimulus. For this reason, the same stimulus is presented repetitively, and time-locked EEG activity is recorded. When these repetitive records are averaged, activity that is unrelated to the stimulus is likely to be randomly distributed across the recordings, sometimes positive and sometimes negative, and the sum is likely to be near zero. In contrast, activity that is a response to the stimulus will occur at the same delay after the stimulus on each recording, and the signal will be reinforced by summing across recordings. The resulting waveform can then be compared to normal controls, or even better, to the analogous waveform in the same subject stimulated on the opposite side. Abnormal function of the sensory pathway results in a prolonged latency of the signal (or, less reliably, reduced amplitude or complete absence of the signal). This may provide evidence of a clinical lesion not apparent on the neurologic examination. The standard evoked potential tests are visual, auditory, and somatosensory. The ones that most often provide useful information in diagnosing MS are the visual evoked potentials. Of course, abnormal evoked potential results do not in and of themselves provide information about the underlying cause of dysfunction or when it occurred, but taken in the context of the history and examination, they can sometimes be very helpful.

Because the diagnosis of MS requires demonstration of at least two episodes, the diagnosis can NEVER be established at the very onset of the disease. Nonetheless, certain clinical presentations are very characteristic of MS – notably optic neuritis, transverse myelitis (i.e., a spinal cord lesion with CSF evidence of inflammation), and a brainstem or cerebellar lesion with inflammatory CSF. Patients who present with one of these "*clinically isolated syndromes*" and MRI scans showing multiple white matter lesions have a high probability of developing MS. Conversely, each of the clinically isolated syndromes can occur in patients who never proceed to manifest any subsequent neurologic symptoms, and this outcome is much more likely if the MRI scan is normal or nearly normal.

Another group of patients who do not have two discrete clinical episodes separated in time are patients with primary-progressive MS. In these patients, the diagnosis requires a consistent history and examination, CSF evidence of inflammation, MRI (and sometimes evoked potential) demonstration of multifocal lesions, and a progressive course (documented on physical examination or serial MRI scans). Particular caution is required before making the diagnosis in these patients, so that a focal or multifocal structural process is not overlooked.

One condition that can be particularly difficult to distinguish from MS is *acute disseminated encephalomyelitis*, or *ADEM*. This is a multifocal condition that typically begins abruptly and progresses over hours, often with associated fever, headache, neck stiffness, and depressed level of consciousness. It is more common in children than adults, and there is typically a history of an antecedent infection (or, less often, vaccination). Some patients with ADEM subsequently develop MS, but not all.

Some patients develop optic neuritis and transverse myelitis, either separately or simultaneously, but they never develop any other MS lesions. A growing body of evidence indicates that this is a distinct condition, called *neuromyelitis optica* (NMO), or *Devic's syndrome*. It is associated with a specific auto-antibody to aquaporin 4, a water channel. MRI scans of the spinal cord in patients with NMO characteristically show demyelinating lesions that extend over more spinal segments than a typical MS lesion, and MRI scans of the brain are usually normal.

Six disease-modifying agents have been approved for use in MS. Three of them are different preparations of interferon beta. Two of these (Avonex and Rebif) are different formulations of interferon beta-1a, and one (Betaseron) is a formulation of interferon beta-1b. All three of these interferon preparations have been shown in controlled trials to reduce the frequency of relapses in patients with relapsing-remitting MS, and they also (in most studies) reduce the progression of MRI abnormalities and clinical disability in these patients. There appears to be a dose effect. In particular, using the standard dosing regimens, the total dose of Avonex per week is lower than the weekly dose of either of the other two agents, and Avonex was found to be less effective than each of them in head-to-head trials. Betaseron and Rebif have not been directly compared to each other. The results with these three agents in patients with secondary-progressive MS have been inconsistent. Patients may form neutralizing antibodies after receiving any of the interferon preparations; it remains unclear how often this affects response to treatment.

The fourth approved agent is glatiramer acetate (Copaxone), a polypeptide that was initially developed as a synthetic analogue of myelin basic protein for use in experimental animal models of inflammatory demyelinating disease. It has also been found to reduce relapse frequency in patients with relapsing-remitting disease. It may also slow the progression of disability, although these results are less convincing. In head-to-head trials, the clinical efficacy of glatiramer was similar to the efficacy of each of the high-dose forms of interferon beta (Rebif and Betaseron), although MRI outcome measures were better for interferon beta in two of the studies.

The fifth approved disease-modifying agent is natalizumab (Tysabri), a monoclonal antibody against the T-cell adhesion molecule α4 integrin. Like glatiramer and the three interferon beta drugs, natalizumab reduces the frequency of relapses and the degree of clinical and MRI progression in patients with relapsing-remitting MS. When analyzed in terms of relative risk reduction, the beneficial effect of natalizumab (for each of the standard clinical and MRI outcome measures) is greater than that observed in most trials of glatiramer or interferon beta, although when analyzed in terms of absolute risk reduction, the agents are comparable (except for a smaller benefit with low-dose interferon beta than with all of the other agents). Natalizumab has not been compared to any of the other agents in a head-to-head trial. Unfortunately, a few patients receiving natalizumab have developed PML; the estimated risk is about 1 per 1000 patients treated, and the risk appears to increase with the number of treatments received. Because PML is an incurable disease that is often disabling or fatal, natalizumab is generally reserved for patients who have failed other therapies, and it is available only to patients who register with a special prescribing program restricted to healthcare providers who enroll with the manufacturer and certify that they will evaluate patients carefully before each monthly infusion. Furthermore, although some studies have found that combination therapy of natalizumab with other disease-modifying agents may provide added benefit, this practice is currently discouraged because of the concern that it might increase the risk of PML.

The sixth approved medication is mitoxantrone (Novantrone), a chemotherapeutic agent that was shown to reduce the relapse frequency and rate of disease progression both in patients with relapsing-remitting MS and in patients with a secondary-progressive course. Mitoxantrone is the only drug with an FDA-approved indication for secondary-progressive MS. Unfortunately, cardiac toxicity has been observed in patients who received high cumulative doses of mitoxantrone, so current practice is to limit the duration of MS treatment with this agent to about three years. As a result, it is generally not considered a first-line drug.

All of these drugs are very expensive, and they are all administered parenterally (Betaseron and Rebif subcutaneously 3 times a week, Avonex intramuscularly once a week, glatiramer subcutaneously once a day, natalizumab intravenously once a month, and mitoxantrone intravenously once every 3 months). The three forms of interferon frequently produce flu-like symptoms, and the two intravenous medications require intensive monitoring for adverse effects. Thus, patients who take these drugs are making a substantial commitment, and they must have realistic expectations or they are likely to get frustrated by what they perceive as a lack of effect. They must be advised that although the medications reduce the number of relapses by roughly a third, they do not prevent relapses completely. Although the medications slow disease progression, they do not halt it, and they certainly do not reverse it. Because there is no way for an individual patient to know how many relapses would have occurred or how quickly the disease would have progressed if left untreated, there is no way to gauge the benefit of treatment on an individual basis.

Despite these limitations, patients with relapsing-remitting MS should be encouraged to start glatiramer or one of the formulations of interferon beta as early in the course as possible. Patients with a clinically isolated syndrome deserve special mention. As discussed above, patients with a clinically isolated syndrome can not be considered to have MS, but their risk of eventually developing MS is very high if they have substantial white matter lesions on MRI. Controlled trials have demonstrated that treatment with glatiramer or interferon beta in this setting is beneficial. The decision regarding which specific agent to use (whether for a patient with MS or for a patient with a clinically isolated syndrome and a positive MRI) must be based on side effects, convenience of administration, cost, and recognition that higher weekly doses of interferon are more effective (but less well tolerated) than lower doses.

A variety of other treatment modalities for relapsing-remitting MS remain unproven, although some studies have shown a benefit. These modalities include IV immunoglobulin, plasma exchange, rituximab, alemtuzumab, and daclizumab. Many patients are eagerly following the promising results that have been reported with oral agents, particularly fingolimod and cladribine. An FDA advisory committee has recommended approval of fingolimod. Positive results have also been reported with the oral medications laquinimod, fumarate, and teriflunomide.

The optimal treatment for NMO is not known; for the most part, it is treated in the same way that MS is treated, but the chance of a good response may be lower than it is for MS. Based on positive results in uncontrolled trials, some authorities advocate the use of rituximab.

Glucocorticoids, such as prednisone and methylprednisolone, appear to accelerate the recovery from an acute MS relapse, but there is no consistent evidence for any long-term benefit. These agents should be considered for relapses that result in considerable discomfort or dysfunction, but they should not be used too frequently because of the high incidence of complications.

Symptomatic treatment is at least as important as disease-modifying therapy. Physical therapy, bladder and bowel regimens, drugs to reduce spasticity, and psychologic support are essential components of patient management. Certain symptoms respond to specific medications. Controlled trials have established that amantadine is effective in alleviating fatigue, but only some patients note a benefit, and the response is often incomplete. Modafinil, methylphenidate, and selective serotonin reuptake inhibitors may also be helpful. Dalfampridine, a sustained release form of 4-aminopyridine, is a potassium channel blocker that produces mild improvement in walking speed and lower extremity strength in patients with MS. Patients with trigeminal neuralgia are treated with carbamazepine, gabapentin, or the other standard agents used for this disorder. Lhermitte's phenomenon often responds to carbamazepine and gabapentin, also. The paroxysmal dystonic episodes of MS usually respond dramatically to carbamazepine, phenytoin, or gabapentin. Tremors respond to the same treatments that are effective for tremor in non-MS patients.

No medication is currently approved for patients with primary progressive MS. A variety of forms of immunosuppression or immunomodulation have been studied, including cyclophosphamide, azathioprine, cyclosporine, methotrexate, cladribine, linomide, total lymphoid irradiation, phosphodiesterase inhibitors, monoclonal antibodies, and bone marrow transplant, but the results have been mixed.

B. Connective Tissue Diseases

Connective tissue diseases characteristically involve widespread organ systems throughout the body, including the nervous system. Organ damage can be caused by immune complex deposition, vasculopathy, granuloma formation, or secondary damage due to musculoskeletal abnormalities. All levels of the nervous system can be affected. In some patients, nervous system dysfunction is the initial or the predominant symptom of the disease. Because these patients typically have multifocal neurologic deficits, they often resemble patients with MS. The main clues to the correct diagnosis are serologic tests and the eventual development of systemic symptoms.

Systemic lupus erythematosus (SLE) is the connective tissue disease most commonly associated with neurologic dysfunction. Neurologic manifestations occur at some stage of the disease in 50–75% of patients, and the initial manifestations of the disease are neurologic in as many as 3% of patients. Neuropsychiatric abnormalities—including cognitive impairment, psychosis, and alteration of consciousness—are the most common neurologic manifestations of SLE. Seizures are also common, usually in an active phase of the disease. Focal neurologic deficits in patients with SLE sometimes result from focal inflammation, but they are usually due to stroke (which, in turn, is most often related to a hypercoagulable state; see Section D). Cranial or peripheral nerve involvement is present in 12–47% of unselected patients with SLE evaluated with electrodiagnostic studies, but only about half of these patients report symptoms. The most common peripheral manifestation is a distal, symmetric polyneuropathy, but mononeuropathy multiplex also occurs.

The main CNS manifestations of *rheumatoid arthritis* result from compression of the spinal cord or brainstem due to arthritic changes in the spinal column. Rheumatoid nodules frequently form in the meninges, but they are usually asymptomatic. Symptomatic CNS vasculitis is rare in patients with rheumatoid arthritis. In contrast, peripheral nerve involvement is common, occurring in 10% of patients. It may take the form of mononeuropathy multiplex (due to either vasculitis or multiple sites of nerve entrapment) or a distal sensorimotor polyneuropathy.

CNS manifestations occur in fewer than 10% of patients with *Sjögren's syndrome*, although some have suggested that these complications may be underreported. Psychiatric symptoms, cognitive problems, meningoencephalitis, seizures, and focal cerebral and spinal cord deficits have all been described, and the clinical presentation may sometimes be confused with MS. Peripheral nervous system manifestations are more common than CNS involvement. The most distinctive is a pure sensory neuronopathy, affecting the dorsal root ganglia and often resulting in sensory ataxia ("pseudoataxia") due to profound loss of proprioception. Other neuropathies that can occur in Sjögren's syndrome include distal, symmetric, sensorimotor polyneuropathy, painful sensory neuropathy (without ataxia), autonomic neuropathy, mononeuropathy multiplex, cranial neuropathies (especially trigeminal sensory neuropathy), and entrapment neuropathies (especially carpal tunnel syndrome). Patients may develop focal myositis. Polymyositis and dermatomyositis may also accompany Sjögren's syndrome, but such cases are usually considered secondary Sjögren's (i.e., Sjögren's that is associated with another connective tissue disease).

Progressive systemic sclerosis (scleroderma) only rarely affects the CNS, but focal CNS lesions have been reported on occasion. Trigeminal neuropathy is more common, and peripheral entrapment neuropathies, particularly carpal tunnel syndrome, may occur. There have been occasional reports of a sensorimotor polyneuropathy, with pathology suggesting a microangiopathy. Most patients have diffuse muscle weakness, and some degree of abnormality is present on electrodiagnostic studies and muscle biopsy in the majority of patients; about 20% of patients have elevated creatine kinase levels.

The neurologic features of *mixed connective tissue disease* (like the systemic features) overlap with those of SLE, rheumatoid arthritis, progressive systemic sclerosis, and polymyositis. The most common neurologic feature is aseptic meningitis. Trigeminal neuralgia and trigeminal sensory neuropathy are also common. Psychiatric manifestations, movement disorders, and seizures also occur.

Between 10–40% of patients with *Behçet's disease* have neurologic signs or symptoms. The most common neurologic manifestation is aseptic meningitis. There may be focal lesions at any level of the nervous system, with the brainstem and basal ganglia being the most commonly affected sites. Lesions often occur simultaneously at multiple locations, and clinical fluctuations are common, sometimes leading to an incorrect diagnosis of MS. Misdiagnosis is particularly likely in the 5% of patients who present with neurologic symptoms. Cerebral venous thrombosis may affect up to a third of patients with neurologic manifestations of Behçet's disease. Peripheral nervous system manifestations are rare in Behçet's disease.

Polyarteritis nodosa (PAN), also called periarteritis nodosa, is the prototypical vasculitic condition. It is a necrotizing vasculitis of small- and medium-sized muscular arteries with preferential involvement of vessel branch points. Up to 80% of patients have neurologic manifestations, especially in the peripheral nervous system. PAN may produce an acute stroke syndrome with focal manifestations or a global syndrome characterized by headache and encephalopathy. The encephalopathy may present either acutely or chronically. Mononeuropathy multiplex is the classic peripheral nervous system manifestation, but distal, symmetric polyneuropathies, radiculopathies, and plexopathies also occur. Other systemic necrotizing vasculitides, including *allergic angiitis and granulomatosis (Churg-Strauss syndrome), overlap syndrome,* and *Wegener's granulomatosis,* can all produce similar neurologic manifestations. In addition, the respiratory tract granulomas of Wegener's granulomatosis can extend to involve neighboring nervous system structures, especially the optic nerve in the orbit.

Primary angiitis of the CNS is a rare vasculitis restricted to small and medium-sized arteries of the CNS. The clinical manifestations resemble the CNS manifestations of PAN without the systemic symptoms. *Primary peripheral nervous system angiitis* is an analogous condition in the peripheral nervous system.

Patients with neurologic manifestations of connective tissue diseases are treated in the same way as patients with manifestations in other organ systems, typically with immunosuppressive agents, including corticosteroids and cytotoxic agents. Wegener's granulomatosis is particularly responsive to cyclophosphamide.

C. Sarcoidosis

Sarcoidosis is a chronic, multisystem disorder of unknown cause characterized by noncaseating granulomas in several organs. It affects the nervous system in approximately 5% of patients, and the neurologic involvement is similar in many ways to what occurs in tuberculosis. As with tuberculosis, there may be either parenchymal granulomas or meningeal involvement, particularly involving the meninges at the base of the brain and producing multiple cranial neuropathies. The most common neurologic manifestation of sarcoidosis is transient unilateral or bilateral facial nerve palsy. Cranial nerves II, V, VIII, IX, and X are also commonly involved, but any cranial nerve can be affected.

The most common site of parenchymal involvement is the hypothalamus, leading to diabetes insipidus or other endocrine abnormalities. Other intracranial sites may also be involved, resulting in focal signs or obstructive hydrocephalus. Spinal cord involvement can produce a transverse myelopathy. Noncranial peripheral neuropathy occurs in 9–26% of patients with neurosarcoidosis. The most common pattern of involvement is a chronic sensorimotor polyneuropathy, but mononeuropathy multiplex, pure sensory neuropathy, and plexopathy have also been described. Sarcoidosis commonly affects muscles. Typical granulomas are found on muscle biopsy in up to 50% of patients with sarcoidosis, but these are usually asymptomatic.

When clinical and radiologic findings suggest neurosarcoidosis, the most reliable way to establish the diagnosis is to demonstrate the typical pathologic findings in a tissue specimen. Radiologic evidence alone is not specific enough to permit a definitive diagnosis, and even the pathologic findings are not entirely specific, as noncaseating granulomas can occur in a number of other diseases, including infections and malignancies. Serum levels of angiotensin-converting enzyme (ACE) are typically elevated in patients with sarcoidosis, but this test is neither specific nor sensitive. In patients with neurologic manifestations of sarcoidosis, CSF ACE levels are more likely to be abnormal than serum ACE levels, but they are still normal in approximately 40% of patients with neurosarcoidosis, and they are sometimes abnormal in patients without neurologic involvement.

Patients with neurosarcoidosis usually improve when treated with corticosteroids, but untreated patients can also experience spontaneous remissions, and no controlled trial of corticosteroids in neurosarcoidosis has ever been conducted. Because prednisone at a dose of 0.5–1.0 mg/kg per day has been shown to be effective for most pulmonary cases, this dose usually is initiated for neurologic manifestations also. Uncontrolled reports suggest that immunosuppressive medications, such as cyclosporine, methotrexate, azathioprine, cyclophosphamide, chlorambucil, mycophenolate, infliximab, etanercept, pentoxifylline, and thalidomide may be useful in patients with neurologic manifestations who fail to respond to steroids or who do not tolerate a steroid taper. Although radiation therapy is ineffective for pulmonary manifestations of sarcoidosis, uncontrolled reports indicate that it may be beneficial for neurosarcoidosis.

D. Coagulation Disorders

The physiologic pathways involved in maintaining hemostasis are complicated and can be compromised in many ways. Patients with hemophilia or other diseases predisposing to hemorrhage are usually diagnosed early in life because of uncontrolled bleeding after trivial injuries. Nervous system hemorrhages in these patients are treated as they would be in other patients. Hypercoagulability may occur because of a well-defined abnormality in the coagulation or fibrinolytic systems (primary hypercoagulable states) or in association with some other clinical condition in which the exact pathophysiology of thrombosis is unknown (secondary hypercoagulable states). The most common causes of primary hypercoagulability are resistance to activated protein C (most often due to a mutation in the gene for factor V Leiden), a mutation in the gene for prothrombin G20210, antithrombin III deficiency, protein C and protein S deficiency, and abnormalities of plasminogen or plasminogen activator. Most of these conditions are particularly associated with venous thromboembolism, and they are treated with anticoagulant medications. Causes of secondary hypercoagulable states include malignancy, pregnancy, congestive heart failure, extensive trauma, diabetes, nephrotic syndrome, vasculitis, and medications (including oral contraceptives and l-asparaginase). Many of these same conditions, but especially malignancies, can lead to nonbacterial thrombotic endocarditis, which results in an even higher incidence of nervous system involvement due to embolization. An increased risk of thrombosis and stroke is also associated with a heterogeneous family of antibodies known as antiphospholipid antibodies. Lupus anticoagulant and anticardiolipin antibody are two overlapping but not identical groups of antibodies included in this family. These antibodies occur not only in patients with SLE but also in association with other connective tissue diseases, infections, neoplasms, and drugs, and they may be found in otherwise normal individuals. The optimal treatment for most secondary hypercoagulable states remains unknown; warfarin does not confer any additional benefit over aspirin. Thrombotic thrombocytopenic purpura (TTP), an extremely rare, life-threatening microcirculatory disorder, responds to plasma exchange.

V. Discussion of Case Histories

Case 1. In a right-handed patient, aphasia is almost always due to a lesion in the left hemisphere. In this case, the patient is nonfluent with relative sparing of comprehension, suggesting a left frontal lesion. This could not possibly account for the left-sided weakness, which is most likely due to a lesion in the right frontoparietal cortex, given the involvement of face, arm, and leg and the associated sensory loss. A single lesion large enough to produce both the aphasia and the left hemiparesis would involve such an extensive region of cortex bilaterally that impaired consciousness would be expected. Thus, the patient appears to have two separate lesions. The time course is acute, suggesting multifocal vascular disease. This has developed in the setting of an acute or subacute systemic illness. In an IV drug abuser, this clinical picture is suggestive of acute bacterial endocarditis. This patient is also in a risk group for AIDS, which is also associated with an increased risk of stroke, but it would be an unusual coincidence to develop fever, malaise, and cerebrovascular complications simultaneously as a result of HIV infection.

Cerebral emboli suggest left-sided valvular involvement, which is common in endocarditis whether or not the patient abuses IV drugs (in contrast to right-sided involvement, which is much more common in drug abusers than in any other group). Almost all patients with left-sided involvement have a heart murmur at some stage of the disease, but this may be absent on initial presentation.

The most important step in diagnosis is isolation of an organism from the blood. At least three separate venous blood cultures should be drawn. Echocardiography provides useful additional information, but a negative test does not rule out endocarditis. The sedimentation rate is almost always elevated in this condition, but it is nonspecific. An imaging study of the brain should also be performed, because even though the cerebral lesions are most likely ischemic, hemorrhages and even abscesses remain possible. An MRI/MRA provides good lesion visualization, and it is also the best noninvasive technique for detecting mycotic aneurysms. Finally, HIV testing should be offered to the patient, as the results will have an obvious impact on her future medical condition even if unrelated to her current problem.

Even before culture results are available, empiric broad-spectrum antibiotic treatment should be initiated. This should cover *Staphylococcus aureus*, as well as many species of streptococci and gram-negative rods. One such regimen consists of nafcillin, ampicillin, and gentamicin. In areas where nafcillin-resistant *S. aureus* species are common, vancomycin should be substituted for nafcillin. Anticoagulation is generally not used in this setting.

Case 2. The examination corroborates this man's report of left lower extremity weakness. The hyperreflexia there indicates an upper motor neuron lesion (i.e., a left-sided lesion in the spinal cord or low medulla, or a right-sided lesion above the medulla). The left afferent pupillary defect indicates a lesion anterior to the optic chiasm on the left. A single lesion could not produce both deficits without impairing consciousness. Thus, this patient has a multifocal condition. Based on his history, the two lesions appeared eight months apart, and the left eye symptoms actually resolved in the interim. Accordingly, there is evidence of multiple CNS lesions separated in space and time, and this patient meets criteria for the diagnosis of MS. Although some connective tissue diseases can mimic MS, these would be unlikely in a patient who has had no other systemic symptoms, even after two years of neurologic symptoms.

Given the convincing examination findings, no additional diagnostic tests are necessary. Most practitioners would obtain an MRI scan of the brain in this setting, as it is the single test most likely to lend support to the diagnosis, but a normal scan would not rule out MS. It would also be reasonable to order serologic testing for SLE and other connective tissue diseases.

Because the current exacerbation began 3 weeks ago, has not progressed, and is still producing only mild dysfunction, many clinicians would elect not to treat it acutely. Others would recommend a brief course of steroids, generally IV methylprednisolone followed by a rapid prednisone taper. With three exacerbations in a 2-year period, this patient should be strongly encouraged to begin one of the forms of interferon or glatiramer.

Probably the most important aspect of management at this stage of the disease is patient education. Misconceptions about MS are widespread, and many patients assume that the disease is rapidly disabling or even fatal. Although patients need to be aware that they could eventually become severely disabled, it is equally important that they realize that there is also potential for a relatively benign course. Approximately 15% of patients with MS are able to continue working at full capacity on a long-term basis. Estimates of the percentage of patients able to walk without assistance 15 years after symptom onset vary between 30–70%. Unfortunately, there are no reliable prognostic indicators, and patients must understand that the course is unpredictable. Patients who have minimal disability after 5 years of disease (i.e., patients who have recovered nearly completely from their relapses to date) have a better prognosis than other MS patients.

Case 3. In this woman, multiple cranial nerves are impaired. A mass lesion in the pons and medulla could conceivably cause this, but with such extensive bilateral impairment in the brainstem, long-tract signs (such as limb weakness, spasticity, hyperreflexia, ataxia, and sensory loss) would be expected, and alteration of consciousness would also be likely. Involvement of the cranial nerves as they exit the brainstem is therefore more plausible. In addition, she has signs and symptoms consistent with a right S1 radiculopathy. This suggests a meningeal process producing multifocal involvement of nerve roots and cranial nerves as they leave the neuraxis. The chronic time course suggests a neoplastic process, such as leptomeningeal metastasis or lymphomatous meningitis, but chronic inflammatory conditions such as tuberculous meningitis, Lyme disease, connective tissue diseases, and neurosarcoidosis should also be considered. Diagnosis depends on CSF examination and a search for other systemic manifestations of these conditions.

In this case, CSF cytopathology revealed lymphomatous cells, and there was no evidence for any other systemic involvement. The diagnosis of primary leptomeningeal lymphoma was made. This is an extremely rare condition. The patient was treated with craniospinal radiation and intrathecal methotrexate, but symptoms continued to progress and she died six months after diagnosis.

III

Common Symptoms

Chapter 11

Acute Mental Status Changes

I. Case Histories

Case 1. You are called by a nurse at 3 p.m. to evaluate a 72-year-old diabetic woman for an acute alteration in mental status. She had been admitted to the hospital yesterday for evaluation of exertional chest pain and had undergone cardiac catheterization earlier today. When you arrive, you find the nurse struggling to restrain the patient, who is awake but agitated and unable to follow commands. The patient makes occasional attempts at speech, but everything she says is unintelligible. She seems to be able to move her limbs symmetrically and withdraws to noxious stimulation in the arms and legs. With difficulty, you examine her further but find no focal abnormality.

Case 2. A 19-year-old college student has been brought to the emergency department by friends after they found him unconscious in his dorm room. He had been to a fraternity party the night before and reportedly looked well at 1 am, just before heading to his room. His friends report that he is "not a party animal"; he rarely, if ever, drinks alcohol and never uses drugs. On examination, his pulse is 110 and his blood pressure is 120/70. Temperature is slightly elevated at 38.3°C. Respirations are 24 per minute. Neurologic examination reveals no response to voice and only brief eye opening to noxious stimulation. Pupils are equal and reactive, and the doll's eyes response is absent. Reflexes are depressed but present, and the plantar responses are mute.

Questions:

1. What initial approach should be taken with both of these patients?
2. How does each clinical setting affect your diagnostic considerations and the workup?
3. How will you manage each of these cases?

Case 3. A 38-year-old weekend softball player was brought to the emergency department after being hit on the left side of the head with a bat. When first hit he had severe pain and stumbled, but did not lose consciousness. He was able to speak to his teammates and initially refused to go to the hospital. On arrival in the emergency department, he was able to speak to the triage nurse without difficulty and signed all of his admission papers. When you first examine him twenty minutes later, he requires constant stimulation to stay alert. The left pupil is slightly larger than the right, but both react to light. The rest of his examination is normal.

Case 4. You are asked to evaluate a 20-year-old woman who was thrown from a horse and hit her head on the ground. There was no loss of consciousness at the time of the fall. She has a severe headache but otherwise feels all right. On examination, she is alert and conversant. Her mental status is normal and she has no focal abnormalities on neurologic examination. She has a large occipital laceration.

Questions:

1. What is the proper approach to these two patients?
2. What determines whether a patient who has sustained a head injury needs a head CT scan? When do you need the assistance of a neurosurgeon?
3. Which head injury patients can be sent home, and what advice do you give them?
4. What problems can follow head injury?

II. Background Information

A. Definitions

coma a state in which subjects lie with eyes closed and demonstrate no conscious responses to external stimuli, even after vigorous attempts to rouse them

consciousness awareness of self and the environment, with the ability to react to internal and external stimuli

delirium an acute, transient, fluctuating confusional state characterized by impairment in maintaining and shifting attention, often associated with agitation, disorientation, fear, irritability, illusions (misperceptions of sensory stimuli), or hallucinations (imagined perceptions with no basis in the external world) *encephalopathy* any state of altered level of consciousness or clouded sensorium

minimally conscious state a condition of severely altered consciousness in which there is minimal but definite behavioral evidence of awareness of self or environment

obtundation a condition of mild to moderate reduction of consciousness in which subjects appear to be asleep, with reduced interest in the environment; they respond sluggishly to verbal or slightly painful stimuli, but when the stimulation stops they slip back into their previous state of reduced alertness and environmental interaction

stupor a state of unresponsiveness resembling deep sleep, from which subjects can be roused only by vigorous and repeated stimulation, and even then they tend to have reduced alertness

vegetative state a condition characterized by the complete absence of behavioral evidence for awareness of self or of the environment, but with preserved capacity for spontaneous or stimulus-induced arousal, including a sleep-wake cycle

B. Focal Mental Status Changes vs. Altered Level of Consciousness

Acute mental status changes can be either focal (such as aphasia, neglect, or visual hallucinations) or diffuse (such as delirium or stupor). Acute, focal mental status changes, like other acute, focal symptoms, are usually due to TIAs, strokes, or seizures (or—less often—migraines). These conditions are covered in other chapters. This chapter focuses on acute, diffuse mental status changes, and specifically, acute changes in level of consciousness.

C. Physiology of Normal and Altered Consciousness

Consciousness can be thought of as consisting of three components: arousal, awareness, and cognition. As discussed in Chapter 9, the ascending reticular activating system (ARAS) is the major system of the brain mediating *arousal*. Unlike sleep, in which the ARAS activity is modulated in a precise, cyclical pattern, stupor and coma are characterized by nonspecific suppression of ARAS activity. *Awareness* is poorly understood, and not even well-defined, but it seems to be closely related to the ability to direct and maintain attention. Thus, this aspect of consciousness may be mediated by the prefrontal cortex and its connections, especially with the thalamus. *Cognition* is a function of widespread cortical networks.

It follows that altered consciousness can result from damage to the thalamus or ARAS, and also from widespread cortical damage. Many metabolic abnormalities, including hyponatremia, hypernatremia, hypoglycemia, hyperglycemia, hypomagnesemia, uremia, hepatic dysfunction, hypothyroidism, hypoxia, acidosis, alkalosis, and a host of toxins, can cause such damage. A structural lesion can only affect consciousness if (1) it directly involves the ARAS in the brainstem or thalamus, (2) it is located elsewhere, but it is so large that it exerts pressure on the ARAS, or (3) it is so extensive that it produces diffuse, bilateral cortical damage.

Delirium can be considered the mildest form of altered level of consciousness. It is characterized by inattentiveness and confusion. Patients may be agitated or withdrawn, combative or cooperative, but the consistent feature is that they can not engage in a sustained conversation or anything else that requires sustained, lucid thought processes. Obtundation, stupor, and coma are more severe alterations of consciousness. Individuals in these states are not only unable to maintain attention, they are unable to maintain arousal. Patients who are obtunded can be aroused by stimuli of varying intensity, such as shouting or shaking. In stupor, patients can be aroused only with extremely vigorous stimuli, and as soon as the stimulation ceases, the patients become unresponsive again. In the most extreme form of altered consciousness, coma, patients are unarousable no matter how vigorously they are stimulated.

These levels of altered consciousness form a continuum, rather than a set of discrete steps. In recent years, functional imaging techniques (such as PET and functional MRI) have suggested that some patients with minimal behavioral response nonetheless have patterns of brain activity that suggest residual cognitive function. Traditional approaches to classification may require modification in the future.

III. Approach to Acute Changes in Level of Consciousness

Whether a patient is delirious, stuporous, or comatose, the potential causes are the same. When you evaluate a patient with any of these conditions, you should address the potential causes in order from most urgent to least urgent. For the less urgent causes, you have time to be analytical and individualize the management plan, but for the most urgent conditions, diagnosis and therapy should proceed rapidly and systematically. The initial management of these patients should be almost automatic. Conceptually, the evaluation should proceed in the following order:

A. ABCs (airway, breathing, circulation)

B. Oxygen, glucose, naloxone

C. Pupils, doll's eyes, motor asymmetry

D. Other electrolytes, renal, hepatic, temperature

E. Everything else

In practice, it is often convenient to take some steps out of order. For example, the blood necessary for the tests in step D can be drawn and sent to the laboratory along with the glucose in step B. In fact, as with any other medical emergency, there are bound to be many things happening at once, producing a sense of controlled anarchy. The evaluation may simultaneously reveal several potential causes of altered mental status, which makes it even more important to have a clear idea of which problems must be addressed most urgently.

A. ABCs: Airway, Breathing, Circulation

As in most other clinical emergencies, the most important initial management goal is to ensure the adequacy of cardiopulmonary function by evaluating the patient's ABCs (Airway, Breathing, Circulation). All other evaluations should be deferred until it is clear that blood pressure and ventilation are adequate. Even if ventilation is adequate, it should be monitored closely, as patients with a depressed level of consciousness are at risk for both hypoventilation and aspiration. If there is any hint that ventilation is failing, elective intubation should be considered.

B. Oxygen, Glucose, Naloxone

Once it is clear that cardiopulmonary function is adequate, you must explicitly address the possibilities of hypoxia and hypoglycemia. Both conditions can be fatal or result in irreversible damage if left untreated for even a short period, but both can be corrected rapidly once recognized. In fact, patients should be treated empirically for hypoxia and hypoglycemia unless rapid and reliable testing is available. Empiric treatment for possible narcotic overdose should be administered at the same time.

The only reliable way to assess oxygenation is to measure it directly. A clear airway and normal breathing pattern are no guarantee that oxygenation is adequate. A pulmonary embolus, interstitial pneumonitis, or anything else that produces a significant ventilation-perfusion mismatch may cause hypoxia without significantly altering breathing. Arterial oxygen saturation must be determined either with a pulse oximeter or with an arterial blood gas measurement. The blood gas has the advantage of providing additional useful information about pCO_2 and pH, but a pulse oximeter, when it is available, is faster. As a general rule, it should be assumed that there will be a brief but significant delay in obtaining the necessary information about oxygenation status, and during that delay the patient should empirically be given 100% oxygen by face mask. Although this concentration of oxygen could theoretically lead to respiratory arrest in patients with chronic CO_2 retention who are dependent on hypoxia for respiratory drive, this situation is rare and represents a far less significant risk than the danger of giving insufficient concentrations of oxygen to correct hypoxia.

The issues involved in treating hypoglycemia are analogous to those involved in treating hypoxia. If a reliable glucose measurement is not immediately available, the patient should be treated empirically by giving a 50 ml IV bolus of a 50% dextrose solution ("one amp of D50") immediately after sending a venous sample to the laboratory. The risk that this treatment could cause hyperglycemia and thereby exacerbate brain injury is far outweighed by the risk of untreated hypoglycemia. If there is any possibility that the patient might have thiamine deficiency (because of alcoholism or malnutrition), 100 mg of IV thiamine should be given with the dextrose to avoid precipitating or inducing Wernicke's encephalopathy.

The final empiric treatment that should be administered at this stage is naloxone (Narcan), 0.4–0.8 mg IV, unless the cause of coma is obvious. This measure is not as urgent as oxygen or glucose administration because patients often recover fully from narcotic overdose even when it is prolonged. Like oxygen and glucose, however, naloxone is a generally benign treatment that can produce dramatic reversal of mental status changes in the appropriate situations. This rapid improvement may be sufficient to establish the diagnosis and save the patient from more invasive and expensive diagnostic testing. When the clinical setting makes benzodiazepine toxicity particularly likely, you should also give flumazenil.

While treating for drug overdose, you should also consider the possibility of drug withdrawal. In particular, alcohol withdrawal can produce a delirious state (*delirium tremens*) characterized by agitation, confusion, hallucinations, and autonomic overactivity, including fever, tachycardia, and profuse sweating. This condition typically occurs 3 or 4 days after the last drink; common settings are alcohol detoxification programs or several days after a patient is incarcerated or admitted to a hospital. You should always consider this diagnosis in delirious patients, even if they have no known history of alcohol abuse. The main goals of treatment are to address the autonomic overactivity, maintain hydration and electrolyte balance, and prevent self-injury. To this end, large doses of benzodiazepines may be required to control agitation. Less severe alcohol withdrawal produces tremulousness and agitation; a similar picture can occur with benzodiazepine or barbiturate withdrawal.

C. Pupils, Doll's Eyes, Motor Asymmetry

After addressing the most urgent conditions that can affect mental status—systemic derangements like hypotension and hypoglycemia—the possibility of structural brain damage must be considered. Not until this point in the evaluation does the neurologic examination become critical. The most urgent structural problem is cerebral herniation, in which a mass lesion located above the tentorium expands downward and puts pressure on the brainstem, resulting in a depressed level of consciousness. The most useful elements of the examination for assessing herniation are the pupillary light reflex and the vestibulo-ocular reflex (assessed by examining the response to the doll's eyes maneuver or ice water caloric testing; see Chapter 2).

The clinical features of herniation differ depending on whether the downward expansion originates on one side or in the midline. A mass lesion located laterally in one cerebral hemisphere typically exerts pressure on the ipsilateral temporal lobe, causing the medial aspect of the temporal lobe, the uncus, to herniate over the free tentorial edge (*uncal herniation*). This puts pressure not only on the midbrain, but also on the third nerve, which exits the midbrain at this level, so the first sign of uncal herniation is an ipsilateral third nerve palsy. Because of the impaired level of consciousness, the abnormal eye movements may be difficult for the examiner to appreciate, so the most prominent feature is usually a large, unreactive pupil on the same side as the mass lesion (although occasionally the herniating temporal lobe pushes the midbrain to the other side and compresses the contralateral third nerve, so the dilated pupil may be on the "wrong side"). In contrast, when the downward expansion occurs in the midline (*transtentorial herniation*), it exerts pressure first on the thalamus, and then on the midbrain, where it disrupts both the parasympathetic and the sympathetic circuitry mediating pupillary constriction and dilation. As a result, both pupils are unreactive to light and they are fixed at an intermediate size.

If the herniation progresses beyond the level of the midbrain and reaches the pons, it can disrupt the circuitry that mediates the vestibulo-ocular reflex, because the afferent limb of the reflex is in the vestibular nerve (cranial nerve VIII), which enters the brainstem at the pontomedullary junction, and the efferent limb depends on the pontine gaze center adjacent to the abducens (cranial nerve VI) nucleus. This can occur regardless of whether the herniation originated laterally or in the midline, but either way, by this stage the patient will already have pupillary abnormalities—a fixed, dilated pupil in uncal herniation, and mid-size, unreactive pupils in central transtentorial herniation. This leads to a useful rule: *In a comatose patient, if the pupils are normal but the doll's eyes response is not, the coma is not due to herniation.*

To rephrase, when a comatose patient has an abnormal doll's eyes response but the pupils respond normally to light, a systemic metabolic abnormality is more likely than a structural lesion. This situation is surprisingly common, primarily because the doll's eyes response is relatively fragile and can be disrupted by even mild metabolic abnormalities, especially from exogenous toxins (notably benzodiazepines and barbiturates). In contrast, the pupillary reflex is resistant to such disturbances and is often preserved when altered mental status is due to metabolic causes. This is not always true, of course – in particular, a variety of drugs can affect pupillary size (see Table 11.1)—so when the pupillary responses and doll's eyes responses are *both* abnormal, the cause of coma could be *either* structural or metabolic. Nonetheless, patients with abnormal doll's eyes responses but intact pupillary responses are common enough that the rule is well worth remembering. Also note that unless drugs are applied directly to just one eye, they affect both pupils equally. When the pupillary responses are markedly asymmetric, you should suspect a structural lesion.

Table 11.1 Drugs that Commonly Affect Pupil Size

Large Pupils	Small Pupils
Anticholinergics	Cholinergics (e.g., glaucoma eyedrops)
Sympathomimetics (e.g., bronchodilator inadvertently splashed in eye; cocaine; amphetamine)	Cholinesterase inhibitors
	Opiates

Even when there is no evidence of active herniation, it is important to determine whether the patient's altered level of consciousness is due to a structural lesion. The main feature to look for is asymmetry—of reflexes, sensory function, or motor responses. Even though many components of the standard neurologic examination must be modified or eliminated when impaired cognitive function prevents full patient cooperation (see Chapter 2), deep tendon reflexes and resistance to passive manipulation can still be assessed, and the response to painful stimulation of the limbs often provides important information. An asymmetric withdrawal response to pain can signify hemiparesis or hemisensory loss. When evaluating responses to painful stimuli, you should distinguish purposeful withdrawal from local reflex responses and also from central reflexes (decorticate or decerebrate posturing). A useful technique to avoid confusion is to pinch the inner aspect of the arm or leg. Abduction of the stimulated limb is purposeful withdrawal; adduction or extension may indicate a local reflex or decerebrate posturing. Flexion of the hip, knee, or ankle may simply be a local reflex, and flexion of the elbow may indicate decorticate posturing.

When the examination suggests an expanding structural lesion, you should immediately obtain a brain imaging study (usually a CT scan), while contacting neurosurgeons to alert them that their help might soon be necessary. Even before the CT scan is done, you may need to initiate the treatment measures described in Part IV, Section B, if the physical examination provides compelling evidence that intracranial pressure (ICP) is significantly increased.

When the physical examination suggests that the altered mental status is most likely due to a metabolic cause, you can defer a brain imaging study and proceed with the next steps in the evaluation. If the diagnosis remains obscure after that, a brain imaging study may still be necessary eventually, but it is a lower priority than in patients whose examination suggests a structural lesion.

D. Other Electrolytes, Renal, Hepatic, Temperature Abnormalities

At this point in the diagnostic process, all of the true emergencies have already been considered, and you can spare a little time for deliberation. Many of the remaining causes of altered mental status are serious conditions requiring prompt treatment, but they can only be corrected gradually. Rapid treatment is impossible for some of these conditions and potentially dangerous for others.

Hyponatremia, hypernatremia, hypocalcemia, hypomagnesemia, hepatic disease, and uremia can all produce a wide spectrum of mental status changes, from irritability to coma, and there is nothing specific about the clinical picture associated with any one of them (except that the presence of tetany suggests hypocalcemia or hypomagnesemia). Laboratory testing is required for diagnosis. As noted earlier, the necessary laboratory tests should generally be requested at the same time that blood samples are sent for glucose and blood gas determinations, so the results will be available by the time this step in the evaluation process is reached. Treatment for each of these conditions is discussed in textbooks of internal medicine.

Body temperatures below approximately 34°C or above 39–40°C can produce mental status changes ranging from agitation or lethargy to stupor or coma. They can also produce many systemic abnormalities, including many of the metabolic derangements listed in the previous paragraph. These metabolic problems are often resistant to treatment until the underlying thermal disorder has been corrected. Treatment of hyperthermia and hypothermia is discussed in textbooks of intensive care medicine and emergency medicine.

E. Everything Else

The first four steps in the evaluation process address problems that are common, and patients often have more than one of these problems. For example, a hyperglycemic patient will often be dehydrated, resulting in both hypotension and hyponatremia. Narcotic overdose may be associated with hypothermia and hypotension. Thus, it is usually appropriate to proceed through all of the first four steps even if one of the initial steps has already revealed an abnormality. For the majority of patients with acutely altered mental status, those four steps will uncover the likely cause (or causes). It is only necessary to search further when the first four steps have been unrevealing or when something specific in the patient's history or examination suggests another potential cause (e.g., a febrile patient should be evaluated for infection, even if hypotension and hypoglycemia have already been discovered).

Narcotics are not the only drugs that can produce altered mental status. Drugs with anticholinergic activity (including atropine, scopolamine, and tricyclic antidepressants), amphetamines, cocaine, LSD, and phencyclidine are other potential culprits. You should explicitly ask the patient's friends and relatives about drug use. A brief search may reveal an empty pill bottle or an unfilled prescription. A urine toxin screen should be sent whenever a possibility of a drug overdose exists.

Patients may be agitated or stuporous in the postictal period after a seizure (see Chapter 5). The diagnosis is straightforward when the seizure was witnessed or when the patient is known to have epilepsy but may not be suspected when this information is unavailable. Patients discovered in bed in the morning with altered consciousness may have had a seizure in their sleep. Make every effort to find witnesses and question them about abnormal movements or behavior preceding the alteration in mental status and about any history of similar events. Again, a search for medications or prescriptions may be helpful.

Seizures may be difficult to recognize in patients who already have a depressed level of consciousness, because the motor manifestations may be subtle or absent. In one study, 8% of comatose patients with no overt evidence of seizure activity were found to be in nonconvulsive status epilepticus on EEG. Moreover, some patients in complex partial status epilepticus are conversant and interactive, with surprisingly subtle mental status changes. Thus, clinicians should always be alert to the possibility of subclinical seizure activity, and obtain an EEG whenever the cause of an acute mental status change remains unclear. Unexplained fluctuations in mental status should also increase the clinician's suspicion of subclinical seizures. Sometimes, prolonged EEG monitoring is required in order to establish this diagnosis.

Bacterial, viral, and fungal meningitis and encephalitis can all cause alterations in mental status. Fever, stiff neck, and headache are all clues to the diagnosis. Subarachnoid hemorrhage can mimic meningitis. The approach to these disorders is discussed in Chapter 12. Mental status changes also occur with sepsis and even with apparently localized infections such as pneumonia or urinary tract infections (especially in elderly or demented patients), presumably because of clinically undetectable spread of the organism to the nervous system or because of metabolic effects of the infection. If the first four steps of the evaluation are unrevealing, patients should generally be evaluated with chest x-ray and cultures of blood, sputum, urine, and spinal fluid, even if they are afebrile and have normal white blood cell counts.

Other inflammatory conditions, such as lupus and primary angiitis of the CNS, may also produce acute mental status changes. Hyperthyroidism, hypothyroidism, addisonian crisis, and Cushing's syndrome (either iatrogenic or endogenous) are other potential causes. Unless there are specific features pointing to these diagnoses, they should only be considered when more common conditions have been excluded.

IV. Special Circumstances

A. Head Trauma

When a patient has sustained trauma to the head, there is no mystery about the cause of altered mental status. Even so, the initial evaluation should proceed through the same steps as for any other cause of altered mental status in order to assess the patient's overall condition and to exclude additional causes of encephalopathy. Indeed, these other factors may even have precipitated the head trauma (e.g., a motor vehicle accident could have resulted from depressed consciousness caused by hypoglycemia).

Management should be aimed at determining whether the head trauma caused any structural damage to the nervous system and whether that damage will require neurosurgical intervention. Neurosurgical consultation should be obtained whenever an operative procedure may be necessary, such as with an intracranial hematoma (especially epidural or subdural); cerebrospinal fluid leak; compound, comminuted, or depressed skull fracture; or cervical spine injury.

Clues to the nature and severity of the injury can be gleaned from the history and general physical examination. For example, a patient who hit his head on a rafter while installing insulation is less likely to have sustained a serious injury than a patient who was violently struck in the head with a club. You should carefully inspect and palpate the head and scalp for evidence of laceration, fracture, or hematoma. If you detect any scalp lacerations, probe them with a sterilely gloved finger to exclude the presence of a fracture or foreign body. You should inspect the periorbital and temporal regions for evidence of ecchymoses, which could indicate basilar skull fracture, and examine the nares and external auditory canals for evidence of a cerebrospinal fluid leak or hemotympanum.

Progressive focal abnormalities on neurologic examination increase the likelihood that the patient has suffered an intracranial hemorrhage (see Chapter 3). It is also crucial to monitor changes in the patient's level of alertness that could indicate progressive brain damage. Every effort should be made to speak to someone who observed the patient's behavior at the scene of the injury and since. The level of alertness should be assessed at regular intervals.

One quick, reproducible method for assessing level of alertness is provided by the Glasgow Coma Scale (GCS—see Table 11.2). Possible scores

Table 11.2 Glasgow Coma Scale*

I. Best motor response	
Obeys	6
Localizes to pain	5
Withdraws to pain	4
Abnormal flexion (decorticate)	3
Extension (decerebrate)	2
No response	1
II. Verbal response	
Oriented	5
Confused but converses	4
Inappropriate words	3
Incomprehensible sounds	2
No response	1
III. Eye opening	
Spontaneous	4
To speech	3
To pain	2
None	1

*Coma score = score I + II + III

range from 3 to 15. Patients with a score of 8 or less are classified as severe head injury, those with scores of 9–12 are classified as moderate, and those with scores of 13–15 are classified as mild. In patients who are intubated, in whom assessment of best verbal response is impossible, the score is annotated by adding a "t" and the potential scores range from 3t–11t. The GCS score is useful for making a rough estimate of prognosis, and it is often used as a basis for deciding which patients need a head CT scan, which patients need intracranial pressure monitoring, and so forth. For example, indications for obtaining a head CT scan (after addressing ABCs) in a patient who has sustained head trauma include: (1) GCS < 15, (2) focal abnormalities on neurologic examination even if GCS = 15, (3) level of alertness declining or fluctuating,(4) cerebrospinal fluid leak, (5) suspected basilar skull fracture, (6) vomiting, (7) age > 65 years, (8) persistent retrograde amnesia, and (9) seizure.

Head injuries are often accompanied by injury to the cervical spine. Never remove a cervical collar or manipulate the neck of a head-injured patient without first excluding the possibility of an unstable cervical fracture by x-ray. Traumatic events that result in head injury can also cause intra-abdominal or intrathoracic injury, and these possibilities should not be ignored.

When thorough evaluation reveals no evidence of a process that might require surgical intervention, many patients with uncomplicated head injuries can be allowed to return home under close supervision by friends or family members. Patients' families should be instructed to awaken the patient every two hours during the first twelve hours after the injury and to return to the emergency department if the patient has reduced responsiveness, severe headache, or nausea and vomiting. Epidural hematomas, in particular, can be associated with a lucid interval in which the patient's mental status temporarily normalizes, followed by an abrupt decline in mental status. Many emergency departments provide a "head sheet" with instructions that a patient can take home; be sure that these instructions are clearly understood before allowing the patient to leave the emergency department.

In the days and weeks after a head injury, patients can develop a condition known as postconcussion syndrome, or post-traumatic syndrome, characterized by any combination of a diverse set of symptoms that include headaches, diffuse pain, abnormal sensation, weakness, vertigo, difficulty with thinking and memory, depression, hypersomnolence, behavioral changes, and seizures. The mechanism underlying this syndrome is not understood, and there is an ongoing debate about the role played by secondary gain and compensation issues. Treatment is symptomatic. Fortunately, the symptoms usually resolve spontaneously over a period of months, although they may last several years in some patients.

B. Increased Intracranial Pressure

The only definitive treatment for increased ICP is elimination of the underlying cause. In many cases, this requires a neurosurgical procedure. Several measures can reduce ICP transiently, limiting neurologic deterioration while awaiting definitive treatment. Unfortunately, every available strategy has potential risks. Perhaps the safest intervention, once you have established that the patient has a stable cervical spine, is to remove the cervical collar and anything else that might interfere with venous drainage from the head. For similar reasons, many clinicians elevate the head of the bed to 30°, although this is more controversial because it can also reduce arterial blood flow to the head. Ventilator pressures should be minimized, to improve the pressure gradient for venous return from the head.

Hyperventilation results in decreased arterial pCO_2, which induces cerebral vasoconstriction and hence a reduction in intracranial blood volume. This technique lowers ICP within two to thirty minutes, but the effect is transient. Furthermore, this treatment requires intubation and mechanical ventilation, and carries the risk of ischemia if the vasoconstriction is excessive. For this reason, levels of pCO_2 below 25 mm Hg should be avoided; some authors recommend a target of 35 mm Hg.

Hyperosmolar agents that do not readily cross the blood-brain barrier produce an osmotic gradient that pulls fluid out of the brain parenchyma and into the blood vessels. An osmotic diuresis also occurs because these agents are not reabsorbed from the renal tubule. It is not clear which of these effects is most significant in lowering ICP. Some maintain that the main effect of hyperosmolar agents is improved perfusion due to the decreased viscosity of blood that results from the increased intravascular water content. In any event, the effect is transient, presumably because the agents eventually do permeate tissue barriers, eliminating (and eventually reversing) the osmotic gradient. The most commonly used osmotic agents are hypertonic saline or mannitol, 0.25–1.5 g/kg over 10–20 minutes, administered in a 20% solution (100 g of mannitol in 500 ml of D5W). The same dose can be repeated every 4–6 hours. Serum osmolality is sometimes used as a treatment end point.

Paralytic agents and sedatives, such as pentobarbital, can reduce the toxic by-products of brain metabolism that occur with brain injury. Unfortunately, they can also cause hypotension, leading to reduced cerebral perfusion, and they can make it difficult to evaluate the neurologic examination. Consequently, this approach is generally considered a second-line therapy. Induced hypothermia can also slow the metabolic processes that lead to permanent cell damage or death after brain injury. In the setting of a hypoxic-ischemic event, such as a cardiac arrest, this treatment improves outcomes. This treatment has not been shown to be beneficial in patients with head trauma, however.

For tumors and abscesses, increased ICP is usually a result of edema formation around the lesion. In this setting, glucocorticoids often produce dramatic improvement. In fact, improvement may be so dramatic that the underlying lesion is no longer evident on imaging studies, complicating subsequent attempts to establish a specific diagnosis and management plan. Thus, when a brain biopsy of a mass lesion may be necessary, glucocorticoids should generally be deferred until immediately before the procedure as long as the patient's medical condition and neurologic status are stable. A typical glucocorticoid regimen is 10 mg of IV dexamethasone (Decadron), followed by 4 mg every six hours, but the optimal dosing regimen is unknown. There is no evidence that steroids are effective in treating edema related to ischemic or hemorrhagic stroke or in treating edema related to metabolic or hypoxic injury.

These measures do not in any way constitute definitive treatment of increased ICP. They are at best temporizing maneuvers to minimize deterioration while awaiting definitive treatment. Neurosurgical consultation should be requested as soon as possible whenever operative intervention is a consideration. The neurosurgeon may also elect to monitor ICP directly by means of an epidural, subdural, or intraventricular catheter, using these measurements to guide therapy.

C. Brain Death

With the development of mechanical ventilators and other means of artificial support, it has become possible to maintain some bodily functions indefinitely. As a result, philosophical questions regarding the definition of death have immediate practical relevance, especially with the advent of organ transplantation. Is it ethical to remove organs from a donor whose heart is still beating?

The concept of brain death was formulated primarily because of the issues raised by these new technologies. The United States and almost every industrialized nation in the world formally recognize the principle that conscious and unconscious brain functions are fundamental to human life, so a person who has permanent loss of all brain function is dead. Explicit rules governing the determination of brain death have been developed. In essence, they require that there be no evidence of cortical or brainstem function. Other than reflexes mediated at the level of the spinal cord, there should be no response to noxious stimuli. There must be no response to visual or auditory stimuli. All brainstem reflexes must be absent, including the pupillary reflex, vestibulo-ocular reflex—assessed with both the oculocephalic (doll's eyes) maneuver and the ice water caloric procedure, corneal reflex, gag reflex, and the respiratory reflex in response to hypercarbia. Finally, the cause of coma must be known and it must be irreversible.

Determination of brain death is necessary only in specific circumstances. The most common reason to assess for brain death is to decide if a patient is eligible to be an organ donor. Much less commonly, disagreements among family members and caregivers require formal determination that a patient is actually dead, rendering further medical treatment pointless. Most decisions about withdrawal of medical support do not involve brain death, however. Many comatose patients who still have some brainstem function have a poor prognosis. In such cases, even though the patient is clearly not brain dead, it is appropriate to withdraw support if family members agree that this is what the patient would have wanted. Published guidelines are available to help determine the prognosis in patients with coma due to a hypoxic-ischemic event.

V. Discussion of Case Histories

Case 1. The initial approach to this patient should be the evaluation discussed in the body of this chapter: (1) ABCs; (2) oxygen, glucose, naloxone; (3) pupils, doll's eyes, motor asymmetry; and (4) other electrolytes, renal, hepatic, temperature. Particular concerns in this setting would be the possibilities of hypoglycemia (if she was given her usual doses of insulin or oral hypoglycemic agents despite being NPO for the procedure), drug toxicity (from opiates or sedatives given for the catheterization), or multiple cerebral emboli dislodged from the heart or aorta because of the catheterization (less likely given the nonfocal examination).

Comment: In this case, none of the initial steps provided an explanation for the patient's altered mental status. Careful review of her medication chart revealed that she had received several sedative-hypnotic drugs before and after the catheterization. After she was successfully controlled with soft restraints, her physicians ordered a sitter to stay by her bedside and she gradually returned to normal. She had little recall of her agitated state. Follow-up examinations were normal.

Case 2. The initial management of this patient is the same as that in Case 1. Starting to get the picture? This is the initial approach that should be followed in *all* cases of diffuse altered mental status. The normal pupillary response in a patient with no doll's eyes response is strong evidence that the cause of this patient's coma is toxic/metabolic.

Comment: Despite the history given by his friends, this patient had opiates and benzodiazepines on a urine toxin screen, and drug ingestion was the ultimate diagnosis. A lumbar puncture was performed because of the patient's fever, and the results were normal. His remaining blood tests, including complete blood cell count and electrolytes, were normal. He awoke quickly after receiving naloxone and went home a day later.

Case 3. This patient has progressively worsening mental status, and his asymmetric pupils suggest a structural lesion of the brain. A neurosurgeon must be consulted urgently because of these findings.

Comment: He had suffered a fractured skull with laceration of the middle meningeal artery and epidural hemorrhage (consistent with his lucid interval). Prompt evacuation of the hematoma saved his life, and he went home after a 2-week hospital stay.

Case 4. Because the patient has a normal mental status and normal neurologic examination, she can be allowed to go home (after the laceration is stitched) if friends and family members agree to observe her closely.

Comment: Aside from mild residual headache, she felt well at a follow-up visit 4 weeks later.

Chapter 12

Headache

I. Case Histories

Case 1. A 28-year-old man came to the emergency department complaining of the worst headache of his life, starting 12 hours ago. He first started having headaches when he was 16 years old, but they used to occur only 2 or 3 times a year. In the last two years they have been more frequent, up to twice a week. They always start on one side of the head—usually the right, but sometimes the left—and progress to involve the entire head. They are associated with photophobia and nausea. They usually go away if he takes two aspirin and lies down in a dark room. His current headache is qualitatively similar to his previous headaches, but more severe. The pain is continuing to get worse, even though he has taken eight aspirin.

Questions:

1. What diagnoses should be considered?
2. What tests are necessary?
3. What treatment would you give?

Case 2. A 54-year-old man with a history of chronic obstructive pulmonary disease and hypertension has come to your office for his routine quarterly check-up. He mentions in passing that he has been having daily headaches for the past 3 or 4 months. They are always on the right side of his head. The pain is not severe, just a nagging ache that usually gets better when he takes two aspirin and goes away completely when he takes two more aspirin 4 hours later. He can live with the pain at this level, but he thought he should mention it because he never used to have headaches at all. On examination, he has his baseline level of wheezing, and a chronic cough. You note a mild left hemiparesis, and when you point it out he says he never noticed it before, but it's probably just because he is strongly right-handed and hardly uses his left side. You also find mild but definite hyperreflexia on the left, and he tends to extinguish left-sided stimuli on double simultaneous stimulation.

Questions:

1. What diagnoses should be considered?
2. What tests are necessary?
3. What treatment would you give?

II. Approach to Headache

Four questions must be addressed in evaluating and managing a patient with headaches:

1. Is the situation an emergency?
2. Are the headaches primary or secondary?
3. If the headaches are secondary, what is the underlying cause?
4. If the headaches are primary, which of the established headache syndromes do they most resemble?

Question 1 is addressed in Part IV. Question 2 is addressed in Parts V and VI. Question 3 is addressed in Parts IV and V, and Question 4 in Part VI. Part III presents some background information.

III. Background Information

A. Primary vs. Secondary Headaches

Headaches can occur independently of any other disease processes (*primary headache disorders*) or they can be associated with a wide variety of underlying neurologic and systemic conditions (*secondary headache disorders*). The pathophysiologic mechanisms are incompletely understood. Most research has focused on migraine headaches, with the tacit assumption that other headache syndromes, both primary and secondary, have similar mechanisms.

B. Pathophysiology of Migraine

One fundamental concept is the phenomenon of neurogenic inflammation. The trigeminal nerve—like any sensory nerve—is analogous to a riverbed, with numerous tiny tributaries joining to form the main channel. When a peripheral branch of the trigeminal nerve is stimulated, an electric impulse travels up the axon toward the cell body. Along the way, the impulse passes numerous branch points marking the sites where other peripheral "tributaries" join the main stream. At each branch point, the electrical impulse splits into two signals that propagate in opposite directions. One impulse proceeds "downstream" along the main channel toward the nerve cell body, while the other travels "upstream" along the tributary, away from the cell body to the peripheral terminal, where it stimulates release of neuropeptides that provoke an inflammatory response. This, in turn, activates other nearby branches of the trigeminal nerve, sending additional electrical impulses toward the cell body, and establishing a positive feedback loop that results in an ever-growing pain signal.

A second fundamental concept is that ascending pain pathways in the nervous system are modulated by descending, inhibitory pathways. These modulatory pathways ordinarily prevent the process of neurogenic inflammation from surpassing a certain level of activity. In migraine, this modulatory process appears to be impaired.

The third fundamental concept is cortical spreading depression. This is a phenomenon characterized by dramatic ionic shifts and changes in electrical excitability and blood flow that march across large regions of the cortex unrelated to arterial territories. In experimental animals, a variety of stimuli can trigger this phenomenon. Several lines of evidence suggest that cortical spreading depression in humans is responsible for the neurologic symptoms that are often prominent in migraine.

The factors that trigger neurogenic inflammation and cortical spreading depression in migraine are not known, and the sequence and interrelationships of these processes remain unclear. Perhaps patients with migraine have a hyperexcitable cortex, predisposing them to experience episodes of cortical spreading depression in response to relatively trivial stimuli. The spreading depression might result in reduced activity in the descending pain modulatory pathways, allowing the process of neurogenic inflammation to get out of control. It is conceivable that neurogenic inflammation is itself one of the stimuli that can trigger cortical spreading depression. Although much remains unknown, it is clear that several different neurotransmitter systems are involved. Serotonergic pathways play a particularly prominent role.

Just as it is not clear what initiates neurogenic inflammation and cortical spreading depression in migraine, it is not clear what terminates these processes—but something does. Migraine is a self-limited process. As such, although the clinical manifestations of migraine can be extremely unpleasant and disabling, migraine does not represent a medical emergency.

Other primary headache syndromes do not constitute emergencies, either. In contrast, secondary headaches reflect the urgency of the underlying cause.

IV. Headache Emergencies: Subarachnoid Hemorrhage and Bacterial Meningitis

The two causes of headache that require urgent management are subarachnoid hemorrhage (SAH) and bacterial meningitis. For both of these conditions, early intervention has the potential to be life-saving and to reduce the likelihood of residual deficits. Patients with SAH must be evaluated for an aneurysm so that it can be repaired before it bleeds again and causes further damage. Bacterial meningitis is an extremely aggressive condition that has a high mortality rate; antibiotics must be started as early as possible in the course. The principal situations in which to consider the diagnoses of bacterial meningitis and SAH are:

1. a severe headache that is *qualitatively* different from any headache the patient has ever experienced before, and/or

2. a headache that is accompanied by fever, stiff neck, or a focal neurologic abnormality not documented with the patient's previous headaches.

Either of these situations represents an emergency—the patient must be assumed to have either a subarachnoid hemorrhage (SAH) or bacterial meningitis until proven otherwise. Note that this approach is a little different from (and, in my opinion, more reasonable than) the common practice of assuming that all patients complaining of the "worst headache of my life" have a life-threatening illness until proven otherwise. Any patient with chronic headaches who happens to develop a particularly severe headache can legitimately complain of "the worst headache of my life." In fact, any patient who goes to the trouble of coming to an emergency department will probably use this or a similar phrase to make the staff appreciate the severity of the pain. The important thing to determine is whether this headache is *qualitatively* different from other headaches the patient has experienced in the past. If the difference is only quantitative—that is, if the patient has a long history (>1–2 years) of similar headaches, and the current one is simply lasting longer or hurting more than usual—no diagnostic studies are required, and the patient can be treated with medications appropriate for his or her chronic headache syndrome. On the other hand, if the current headache is different in character from anything the patient has ever experienced before, *this is an emergency!*

There is no completely reliable method to distinguish SAH from meningitis based on clinical characteristics. The onset of pain is typically more abrupt in SAH, and fever is more common (and usually more pronounced) in meningitis, but there are exceptions to these generalizations. Patients should be evaluated for both conditions simultaneously, and empiric intravenous antibiotics for bacterial meningitis should be administered immediately (2 g of either cefotaxime or ceftriaxone, plus 1 g of vancomycin for resistant pneumococcal strains; in immunocompromised patients, ampicillin should be added to cover *Listeria monocytogenes*, and in patients with impaired cellular immunity or in patients with likely nosocomial infection, ceftazidime should be substituted for the cefotaxime or ceftriaxone for better coverage of resistant gram-negative bacilli). Antibiotics should only be deferred if the clinical suspicion of meningitis is low and the patient is afebrile with completely normal cardiovascular, respiratory, and mental status. Conversely, if bacterial meningitis seems likely, dexamethasone should be given with or just before the first dose of antibiotics (although the benefits of this practice have been demonstrated most clearly for children with meningitis resulting from *Haemophilus influenzae* and adults with meningitis resulting from *Streptococcus pneumoniae*).

The diagnostic test for meningitis is a lumbar puncture (spinal tap). Once antibiotics have been given, CSF must be obtained promptly, or cultures may be falsely negative. Because SAH can also be diagnosed by examining the CSF, one reasonable approach would be to perform a lumbar puncture immediately in any patient with a severe, unprecedented headache. This is an invasive test, however, with the potential to provoke herniation in patients who have a cerebral mass lesion. SAH can be visualized on a noncontrast CT scan in 95% of patients scanned in the first 48 hours, so if a CT scan can be obtained immediately, it should be done before doing a lumbar puncture. If the CT scan clearly establishes the cause of the headache (either SAH or a mass lesion), a lumbar puncture is not necessary. If there is any possibility that the CT scan will introduce a delay of an hour or more, however, the CT scan should be omitted and a lumbar puncture performed immediately, unless the examination strongly suggests that the patient has a mass lesion.

Even when a CT scan can be obtained immediately, it will fail to detect at least 5% of cases of SAH. Thus, if the CT scan is normal, the next step is to perform a lumbar puncture – both to evaluate further for subarachnoid hemorrhage and to diagnose meningitis. If there are no white blood cells in the CSF, no further antibiotics are necessary. If there are more than five white blood cells per mm^3, however, the patient should receive additional antibiotics for presumed bacterial meningitis. A CSF white blood cell count less than 100 per mm^3, a lymphocytic predominance, and a normal CSF glucose increase the likelihood that the meningitis is viral rather than bacterial (see Table 12.1), but there are exceptions to all of these rules, so IV antibiotics should be continued until cultures have been negative for 48 hours.

The hallmark of SAH is the presence of red blood cells in the CSF. This must be distinguished from a traumatic tap, in which local blood vessels are punctured during the procedure and blood enters the CSF at the puncture site. For this reason, whenever SAH is a consideration, it is imperative to use a centrifuge to spin down the CSF immediately. Blood cells that have been present for twelve hours or more will already have started to break down, producing xanthochromia (a yellow tinge to the supernatant). If all the blood present in the CSF was introduced at the time of the lumbar puncture, the cells will not yet have started to break down. They will aggregate at the bottom of the tube and the supernatant will be completely colorless.

If the CT or lumbar puncture suggests SAH, neurosurgical consultation should be obtained immediately. The patient will need an angiogram to search for the source of hemorrhage. If an aneurysm is present, the patient should be admitted to a closely monitored bed in a dark, quiet room. The goal is to avoid clinical deterioration and to occlude the aneurysm by clipping or coiling within three days of the initial hemorrhage (see Chapter 4), before the period when vasospasm is most likely. Severe hypertension should be treated, but hypotension should be avoided–it is usually best to use short-acting agents that can be stopped quickly if necessary. Oral nimodipine should be started, because a regimen of 60 mg every 4 hours has been shown to improve outcomes, although the mechanism of benefit is not clear.

V. Other Secondary Headaches

In patients who do not have subarachnoid hemorrhage or bacterial meningitis, the next step is to consider other systemic or neurologic causes of secondary headache. Although these are not emergencies in the same sense as SAH or bacterial meningitis, many of them require fairly urgent treatment. These conditions are often apparent from the patient's medical history or examination. You should be sure to ask whether the patient

Table 12.1 Typical CSF Patterns in Meningitis

	Normal adult	Bacterial meningitis	Viral meningitis	Fungal meningitis	TB meningitis
CSF pressure	< 200 mm H_2O	200-500 mm H_2O	Normal	Mildly elevated	Elevated
White blood cells	0-5 cells/mm^3	> 1000 cells/mm^3	10-200 cells/mm^3	50-800 cells/mm^3	100–300 cells/mm^3
Predominant cell type	Lymphocytes	Neutrophils	Lymphocytes	Lymphocytes	Lymphocytes
Protein	15-45 mg/dL	> 100 mg/dL	15-100 mg/dL	40-500 mg/dL	100–500 mg/dL
Glucose	> 50% of serum glucose	< 40% of serum glucose	Normal	10-40 mg/dL	< 45 mg/dL
Gram stain	Negative	Positive	Negative	Positive	Negative
Cultures	Negative	Positive	Negative	Positive	Positive (eventually)

developed any other symptoms at about the same time the headaches began, and whether they started or stopped any medications at about that time.

A. Viral Meningitis or Encephalitis

Viral meningitis is not really an emergency, because there is no specific treatment, so delayed diagnosis does not affect outcome. The clinical presentation is essentially indistinguishable from that of bacterial meningitis, however, so these patients need a lumbar puncture urgently. As explained in Part IV, a CT scan should be done first if it can be done expeditiously, because SAH is also in the differential diagnosis, and antibiotics should be administered empirically unless bacterial meningitis seems truly implausible. Both the clinical features and the spinal fluid findings tend to be less dramatic in viral meningitis than in bacterial meningitis (see Table 12.1), but there is sufficient overlap that it is usually safest to continue treating empirically with antibiotics until bacterial cultures have been negative for 48 hours. A reverse-transcription PCR assay for enteroviral RNA in the CSF is commercially available, and if clinical experience confirms the high specificity reported in initial studies, it will be useful for identifying patients who do not require empiric antibiotics.

The clinical features of viral meningitis and viral encephalitis overlap considerably, but as a rule, fever, headache, and stiff neck are more prominent than mental status changes in patients with meningitis, and the converse is true in patients with encephalitis. Seizures may occur with either, but they are more common in encephalitis. About 10% of patients with encephalitis due to West Nile virus develop flaccid paralysis because of involvement of motor neurons in the anterior horns of the spinal cord. Most cases of viral meningitis are due to enteroviruses and enter the bloodstream from the intestines. This is also the source of some cases of viral encephalitis, but most cases of viral encephalitis are caused by arboviruses injected directly into the bloodstream by an insect vector, usually a mosquito or a tick. Diagnosis is usually based on serologic testing of the blood or spinal fluid. As is the case with viral meningitis, there is no specific treatment available for most types of viral encephalitis. Patients with viral encephalitis often develop associated problems that require hospitalization, and the prognosis is generally much worse for encephalitis than for meningitis. The one type of viral encephalitis for most types of which treatment is available is Herpes simplex encephalitis (HSE). As discussed in Chapter 10, clinicians should remain mindful of this diagnosis, and they should start acyclovir empirically whenever HSE is a realistic possibility.

B. Fungal or Tuberculous Meningitis

The clinical presentation of tuberculous meningitis was discussed in Chapter 10; the clinical features of fungal meningitis are similar. In general, both tend to be more indolent than viral meningitis, and they can occasionally smolder for months or even years. The spinal fluid findings for both fungal and tuberculous meningitis are generally intermediate between those of viral meningitis and those of bacterial meningitis (see Table 12.1). The treatment of tuberculous meningitis was discussed in Chapter 10. Fungal meningitis is treated with amphotericin or other anti-fungal agents.

C. Mass Lesions

The vast majority of patients with headaches have primary headaches, not secondary headaches, and even among the secondary causes of headache, mass lesions are rare. Patients whose headaches are due to structural abnormalities in the brain, such as tumor, abscess, stroke, parenchymal hemorrhage, subdural or epidural hematoma, or hydrocephalus, typically have papilledema or focal neurologic abnormalities. The main exception to this rule is when the lesion is of recent onset, because it might not have produced any focal findings or papilledema yet. My general rule is that if the patient has a history dating back a year or longer of headaches that are qualitatively similar to the current headaches (even if they have recently become more frequent or more severe), and if there are no focal findings or papilledema on examination, I reassure the patient and do not order an imaging study. When those conditions are not met—i.e., when the headaches began less than a year ago or the examination reveals papilledema or a focal abnormality—obtain a brain MRI. If it shows a mass lesion, subsequent evaluation and management depend on the appearance of the lesion and the patient's risk factors.

D. Giant Cell (Temporal) Arteritis

Temporal arteritis, also known as giant cell arteritis, is a generalized disorder of medium and large arteries that occurs almost exclusively in patients over 50 years of age. It can result in a variety of focal neurologic deficits, or it may present with generalized mental status changes, but it usually presents with head pain that is dull and superficial, with superimposed lancinating pains. It may be unilateral or bilateral, and although it is often temporal, it may occur in any location. Patients frequently report temporal artery tenderness and jaw claudication. About 40–50% of patients also have polymyalgia rheumatica, manifested by pain and stiffness of the limbs. Permanent bilateral blindness occurs in up to 50% of untreated patients, so even though the clinical course is self-limited and lasts only one to three years, prompt treatment is essential.

A sedimentation rate should be checked in all patients older than age 50 with headaches of recent onset. The sedimentation rate is a useful screening test because it is elevated in 95% of patients (and >100 mm/hour in 60%), but it is not specific. Sensitivity can be improved by simultaneously checking the C-reactive protein, but even combining these tests, an abnormal result is not specific for temporal arteritis. The diagnosis should be confirmed with a temporal artery biopsy. When the clinical suspicion is high enough, a temporal artery biopsy should be performed even if the sedimentation rate and C-reactive protein are normal. As it happens, false-negative biopsies are fairly common, because the pathologic process is often patchy, so if the biopsy result is negative and the clinical suspicion is high, a repeat biopsy should be performed on the contralateral temporal artery. Patients should be treated with either high-dose (1.5–2 mg/kg per day) prednisone or high-dose IV methylprednisolone (125–250 mg loading dose, followed by 1 g/day or 0.5–1 mg/kg every 6 hours) for up to 3 days, followed by oral prednisone at a dose of 1 mg/kg/day. The temporal artery biopsy should be obtained as soon as possible, to minimize the duration of this high-dose steroid treatment if it is not necessary. If the diagnosis is confirmed, patients should remain on this dose of prednisone for at least 4–6 weeks, with a subsequent slow taper guided by clinical symptoms and sedimentation rate.

E. Idiopathic Intracranial Hypertension (IIH; Pseudotumor Cerebri)

Idiopathic intracranial hypertension (IIH) is, as the name implies, a condition in which intracranial pressure is elevated for no known reason. It is most common in obese women of childbearing age. The headache is typically diffuse, with no distinctive characteristics. Most patients also report transient or persistent visual symptoms. Some patients report that moving from sitting to standing or from lying to sitting can precipitate or exacerbate the headache or visual symptoms. Almost all patients with IIH have papilledema, which is the main clue to the diagnosis. Some patients have unilateral or bilateral sixth nerve palsies. Patients with presumed IIH need a brain imaging study to exclude a mass lesion, followed by a lumbar puncture to document elevated intracranial pressure (and to exclude inflammatory disease as the cause). IIH is generally a self-limited condition, but it may lead to permanent visual loss. It is usually treated with acetazolamide (Diamox), a carbonic anhydrase inhibitor. Topiramate (Topamax) also inhibits carbonic anhydrase, and its potential side effect of weight loss is often desirable in patients with this condition. Patients who do not respond to medication are sometimes treated with lumboperitoneal shunting or fenestration of the optic nerve sheath.

F. Spontaneous Intracranial Hypotension

Spontaneous intracranial hypotension is characterized by a postural headache, precipitated or aggravated by sitting up or standing, and relieved by lying down. It is similar to the headache that can occur after a lumbar puncture, but it has no apparent precipitant. Patients may also experience blurred vision, visual field defects, diplopia (especially from sixth nerve palsy), dizziness, nausea, vomiting, hyperacusis, tinnitus, or mental status changes. MRI scans typically show diffuse dural enhancement and features suggesting a "sagging brain." In some of these patients, but not all, evaluation reveals a spinal fluid leak. The condition often resolves spontaneously after several weeks, but when it doesn't, it may respond to treatment with hydration, caffeine, corticosteroids, intrathecal or epidural saline infusion, or epidural blood patch. When these measures fail, an aggressive search for a CSF leak should be conducted, and if one is found, it should be repaired surgically.

G. Cerebral Venous Thrombosis

Cerebral venous thrombosis typically causes headaches and focal neurologic symptoms. Seizures are also common. The widespread use of MRI has led to increasing recognition of this condition in patients whose only symptom is headache. Cerebral venous thrombosis primarily occurs in patients who have a coagulation disorder or who are severely dehydrated, so such patients probably should have an MRI/MRV (magnetic resonance imaging with magnetic resonance venography) even if their headaches appear to be innocuous. This condition is typically treated with intravenous heparin, and sometimes with direct installation of a thrombolytic agent into the thrombus.

H. Arterial Dissection

Arterial dissection is another condition that is being recognized more often with the advent of MRI scans. The diagnosis is usually suspected when patients present with TIAs or strokes, especially in the setting of recent head trauma or cervical manipulation, but these patients often say that they have had a fairly non-specific headache or neck pain dating from around the time of the trauma. This suggests that arterial dissection may occur much more often than appreciated. The optimal management strategy is not known, but these patients are usually anticoagulated for at least three months.

I. Systemic Conditions

Headaches can occur with a wide variety of systemic infections, autoimmune diseases, neoplasms, endocrine disorders, and metabolic disturbances. Almost every class of medication can provoke headaches in some patients. A thorough discussion of all of the substances and conditions that can cause secondary headaches would, in effect, be a textbook of medicine (and pharmacology). In most cases, the characteristics of the headache are nonspecific, and the underlying condition is diagnosed based on other features of the illness (or, in the case of medications, based on a focused history and sometimes a trial off medication).

J. Secondary Headache Syndromes with Diagnostic Ambiguity

1. Sinus disease

Patients with acute sinusitis often experience headaches that are typically exacerbated by changes in head position. The diagnosis is usually apparent because these patients also have nasal discharge, congestion, conjunctival injection, cough, and sinus tenderness. Sphenoid sinusitis may be difficult to detect because the sphenoid sinus does not communicate directly with the nasal passages, so patients may experience headaches without any of the other associated symptoms that are typical of sinusitis. Patients with sphenoid sinusitis are at substantial risk for developing meningitis and require a prolonged course of antibiotic therapy, often intravenously.

The role of *chronic* sinusitis in producing headaches is less clear. Many patients with chronic headaches have some opacification in one or more sinuses on imaging studies, but many patients without headaches have similar findings. There is no compelling evidence that these patients respond to antihistamines, antibiotics, or sinus surgery, so they should be treated with the same medications used for tension and migraine headaches.

2. Temporomandibular joint disease

Structural malalignment of the temporomandibular joint can produce both local and referred pain. There is wide variation in the way this diagnosis is made, and the condition is probably overdiagnosed. Still, if a patient reports a correlation between chewing and headaches, and if the temporomandibular joint is easily dislocated on examination, the diagnosis should be considered. Initial treatment is usually a soft diet; jaw bracing and surgery are used for more severe cases.

3. Postconcussion (or posttraumatic) syndrome

It is common for patients who have had head trauma to develop headaches. The pain is often continuous, but waxes and wanes in severity. These patients often report memory difficulties, sleep disturbance, mood swings, depression, neck and back pain, dizziness, and diffuse sensory symptoms. Imaging studies are usually normal (but should be obtained once, to exclude chronic subdural hematomas and to exclude structural problems in the spine if the patient has symptoms there). Superimposed legal and disability issues often complicate this syndrome, and because all features are subjective, there is no way to rate the severity of this condition or even to be sure it is present. In most cases, the symptoms resolve spontaneously—usually within a year—but they sometimes last as long as 3 years. In approximately 10% of patients, symptoms persist beyond that point. While waiting for resolution, only symptomatic treatment is available. The headaches should be treated in the same way as migraine and tension headaches; antidepressants are often used because the patients also have symptoms of depression.

VI. Primary Headaches

As explained in Parts IV and V, certain characteristics should prompt you to evaluate patients for secondary headaches that might require prompt or even urgent treatment: (1) headache onset (or clear change in character, not just severity or frequency) within the past year, (2) fever and stiff neck, (3) focal abnormalities on neurologic examination, (4) papilledema, (5) acute or subacute mental status changes, (6) strong correlation between headache and body position, and (7) prominent systemic symptoms. Most patients have none of these characteristics—they have a long history of similar episodes, a normal neurologic examination, no fever or neck stiffness, and no other features to suggest a secondary headache disorder.

These patients have a primary headache disorder, and the next step is to classify their headaches as carefully as possible so that the appropriate treatment can be given. This classification is based purely on the history.

A. Migraine and Tension Headaches

Most patients with headaches have symptoms that fall somewhere on a spectrum that includes the symptoms of migraine and tension headaches. These have traditionally been viewed as two completely separate conditions with distinct etiologies, but many investigators believe that they may simply be varying manifestations of a single underlying pathophysiologic process. Certainly, many patients report that they have some headaches that are typical of migraine and other headaches with features characteristic of tension headaches. It is also common for individual headaches to have some attributes of migraine and other characteristics that suggest tension headache. The same medications are effective for treating both classes of headache. Despite this overlap, it is useful to characterize patients' headaches as precisely as possible in order to monitor them over time and assess their response to therapy. A detailed characterization may also be useful if the distinction between migraine and tension headache is ultimately shown to have therapeutic implications. At present, management is the same whether patients have migraines, tension headaches, or some combination.

Migraine headaches are typically unilateral (although the side of the headache may vary from one episode to the next). The pain is usually throbbing or pulsing. Nausea, vomiting, photophobia, and phonophobia are common accompaniments. Some patients develop focal neurologic symptoms or signs. The most common are visual (scintillations and scotomata), but focal numbness, weakness, aphasia, dysarthria, dizziness, and even syncope may occur. Patients who experience focal neurologic symptoms during, after, or immediately before a migraine are said to have migraine with aura, and patients with no neurologic symptoms are classified as having migraine without aura.

Migraines may last from hours to days. Many patients note that specific triggers can precipitate their headaches. These can include alcohol (especially red wine), chocolate, cheese, pickled items, processed meats, monosodium glutamate, menstrual periods, weather conditions, irregular eating or sleep habits, and stress. Many patients also have a history of motion sickness, and 50–60% have other family members with headaches (compared to 10–20% of headache-free individuals).

Tension headaches are typically bilateral, often involving either the forehead or the back of the head and neck, and sometimes the entire head. The pain is described as pressure, tightness, or a squeezing sensation. Nausea may occur, but most of the other features that can accompany migraine are absent. The only common precipitating factor is stress.

Some patients with migraine or tension headaches can achieve adequate control simply by identifying and eliminating triggers. In particular, many women only develop severe headaches after starting oral contraceptives, and they may want to consider alternative forms of birth control. Even when there does not seem to be a clear correlation between the headaches and initiation of contraceptive pill use, an empiric trial off the pills sometimes produces significant improvement in headaches. A separate concern for patients on birth control pills is the risk of thromboembolic events, including stroke. Migraines, birth control pills, and smoking are all independent risk factors. The incidence of thromboembolism in young women is ordinarily so low that the increased risk with one of these three factors is still negligible. Even with two factors present, the risk is usually acceptable (although the patient should be informed of the issue). With all three factors present, however, the risk becomes more of a concern: in general, a patient with headaches should either stop smoking or stop taking birth control pills.

For most patients, elimination of trigger factors does not produce adequate headache control, and medications are necessary. Nonpharmacologic treatments such as neck stretching exercises, relaxation techniques, physical therapy, acupuncture, and biofeedback may be helpful, but they are usually not adequate to control headaches by themselves. Pharmacologic treatment is centered on two kinds of medications: abortive agents and prophylactic agents. An abortive agent is taken as soon as possible when a headache begins, with the goal of stopping the headache. A prophylactic agent is taken on a regular basis, even when the patient does not have a headache, in an attempt to prevent headaches or reduce their frequency. The most commonly used abortive and prophylactic agents are listed in Tables 12.2 and 12.3, respectively. Medications currently in development include serotonin receptor agonists, glutamate receptor antagonists, and telcagepant and olcegepant, which are antagonists of the calcitonin-gene related peptide (CGRP).

Patients with infrequent migraine or tension headaches do not require prophylactic medications if they can find an abortive agent that consistently and rapidly relieves their symptoms. The key factor in deciding whether to start a prophylactic agent is the degree to which patients' headaches disrupt

Table 12.2 Abortive Agents for Headache

Generic (Trade) Name	Dosing Regimen
Oral and Sublingual Agents	
Aspirin	325-650 mg q 4 hrs prn (some patients respond best to larger dose all at onset, up to 1950 mg)
Acetaminophen (Tylenol)	325-650 mg q 4 hrs prn
Aspirin/acetaminophen/caffeine (Excedrin, Excedrin Migraine)	1–2 pills at onset, then 1–2 pills q 4 hrs prn
Naproxen (Naprosyn, Anaprox, Aleve)	500–750 mg at onset, then 250–375 mg q 4 hrs prn
Ibuprofen (Advil, Motrin, Nuprin)	400–800 mg at onset, then 200–800 mg q 4 hrs prn
Indomethacin (Indocin)	25–50 mg at onset, then 25–50 mg q 4 hrs prn
Isometheptene/acetaminophen/ dichloralphenazone (Midrin, Duradrin, Epidrin, Isocom, Migratine, Migrazone)	1–2 pills at onset, then 1 pill q half hour prn; maximum 5 pills/day, 12 pills/week
Almotriptan (Axert)	6.25–12.5 mg at onset, may repeat once after 2 hrs prn; maximum 2 pills/day, 2 days/week
Eletriptan (Relpax)	20–40 mg at onset, may repeat once after 2 hrs prn; maximum 80 mg/day, 2 days/week
Frovatriptan (Frova)	2.5 mg at onset, may repeat once after 2 hrs prn; maximum 7.5 mg/day, 2 days/week
Naratriptan (Amerge)	1–2.5 mg at onset, may repeat once after 2 hrs prn; maximum 7.5 mg/day, 2 days/week
Rizatriptan (Maxalt); pills or orally disintegrating tablets	5–10 mg at onset, may repeat after 2 hrs prn; maximum 30 mg/day, 2 days/week [**NOTE:** intial dose 5 mg and daily maximum 15 mg if taking propranolol]

Table 12.2 (contiuned)

Generic (Trade) Name	Dosing Regimen
Sumatriptan (Imitrex)	25–100 mg at onset, then q 2 hrs prn; maximum 300 mg/day, 2 days/week
Zolmitriptan (Zomig); pills or orally disintegrating tablets	1.25–2.5 mg at onset, then q 2 hrs prn; maximum 10 mg/day, 2 days/week
Sumatriptan/naproxen (Treximet)	1 pill at onset, may repeat after 2 hrs prn; maximum 2 days/week
Aspirin/butalbital/caffeine (Fiorinal)	1–2 pills q 4 hrs prn; maximum 6 pills/day [**AVOID if possible— addictive**]
Acetaminophen/butalbital/caffeine (Fioricet, Esgic)	1–2 pills q 4 hrs prn; maximum 6 pills/day [**AVOID if possible— addictive**]
Prochlorperazine (Compazine)	10 mg at onset, may repeat q 6 hrs prn; maximum 3 days/week
Promethazine (Phenergan)	12.5–25 mg at onset, may repeat q 6 hrs prn; maximum 3 days/week
Nasal sprays	
Dihydroergotamine (Migranal)	0.5 mg (one spray) in each nostril at onset, may repeat once after 15 minutes prn; maximum 2 mg/day, 2 days/week
Sumatriptan (Imitrex)	5–20 mg (in one nostril or split between the two nostrils) at onset, may repeat after 2 hrs prn; maximum 40 mg/day, 2 days/week
Zolmitriptan (Zomig)	5 mg (one spray) at onset, may repeat after 2 hrs prn; maximum 10 mg/day, 2 days/week
Butorphanol (Stadol)	1 mg (one spray) in one nostril q hour prn; maximum 4 mg/day, 2 days/week [**AVOID if possible— addictive**]

(*continued*)

Table 12.2 Abortive Agents for Headache (continued)

Generic (Trade) Name	Dosing Regimen
Subcutaneous injections	
Sumatriptan (Imitrex)	6 mg at onset, may repeat once after 1 hr; maximum 12 mg/day, 2 days/week
Dihyroergotamine (DHE-45)	1 mg at onset, may repeat q hour up to 3 mg/day; maximum 2 days/week
Emergency room options (in addition to all of the above)	
Dihydroergotamine (DHE-45)	0.5–1 mg IV; premedicate with 10 mg metoclopramide or prochlorperazine; repeat q 8 hrs prn
Chlorpromazine (Thorazine)	25 mg IV (slowly) or 25-50 mg IM
Prochlorperazine (Compazine)	10 mg IV
Promethazine (Phenergan)	25 mg IV
Metoclopramide (Reglan)	10 mg IV
Hydroxyzine (Vistaril)	25-100 mg IM
Droperidol (Inapsine)	2.5 mg IM or IV
Ketorolac (Toradol)	30–60 mg IM, repeat q 6 hrs prn
Valproic acid (Depacon)	5–10 mg/kg IV; no faster than 20 mg/minute
Oxygen	100% by non-rebreather mask at 12 L/minute for 30 minutes
Hydrocortisone	100–250 mg IV over 10 minutes; may repeat in 8-12 hours
Dexamethasone (Decadron)	12–20 mg IV or IM; may repeat in 8–12 hours
Magnesium	1 gm IV
Narcotics	USE CAUTIOUSLY

their lives. Even patients who have found an effective abortive regimen often experience a substantial period of discomfort before the drug takes effect, and this can be severe enough to interfere with normal activities. If this happens frequently, work productivity and quality of life can be affected. Furthermore, most abortive agents seem to be less effective if used

Table 12.3 Prophylactic Agents for Headache

Generic (Trade) Name	Dosing Regimen
Nonsteroidal anti-inflammatory drugs (NSAIDs)	
Naproxen (Naprosyn, Anaprox, Aleve)	250 mg bid up to 375 mg tid
Indomethacin (Indocin)	25 mg tid up to 50 mg tid
Aspirin	81 mg qday or 325 mg q day
Beta blockers	
Propranolol (Inderal, Inderal LA)	20 mg bid up to 80 mg qid*
Nadolol (Corgard)	40 mg bid up to 80 mg qid*
Metoprolol (Lopressor, Toprol XL)	50 mg bid up to 100 mg qid*
Atenolol (Tenormin)	25 mg q day up to 50 mg bid
Calcium channel blockers	
Verapamil (Calan, Isoptin, Verelan, Covera)	40 mg tid up to 160 mg tid*
Flunarizine	5 mg qhs up to 10 mg qhs
Tricyclic antidepressants	
Amitriptyline	25 mg qhs up to 200 mg qhs (increase SLOWLY; may need to start at 10 mg qhs)
Nortriptyline	25 mg qhs up to 150 mg qhs (increase SLOWLY; may need to start at 10 mg qhs)
Serotonin/norepinephrine reuptake inhibitors	
Venlafaxine (Effexor)	37.5 mg bid up to 75 mg tid*
Monoamine oxidase inhibitors	
Phenelzine (Nardil)	15 mg tid up to 30 mg tid [Note dietary restrictions!]
Ergots	
Methylergonovine maleate (Methergine)	0.2 mg tid up to 0.4 mg tid

(continued)

Table 12.3 Prophylactic Agents for Headache (continued)

Generic (Trade) Name	Dosing Regimen
Anti-epileptic drugs	
Valproic acid (Depakote)	250 mg tid up to 500 mg qid*
Topiramate (Topamax)	25 mg bid up to 200 mg bid
Gabapentin (Neurontin)	100 mg tid up to 900 mg qid
Levetiracetam (Keppra)	500 mg bid up to 1500 mg bid
Antihistamines	
Cyproheptadine (Periactin)	4 mg tid up to 8 mg qid
Miscellaneous	
Riboflavin	400 mg q Day up to 400 mg bid
Magnesium oxide or trimagnesium dicitrate	300 mg bid
Feverfew (*Tanacetum parthenium*)	50–82 mg/day
Butterbur (*petasites hybridus*)	50 mg bid up to 75 mg bid
Coenzyme Q	100 mg/day up to 300 mg/day
Botulinum toxin (BOTOX)	Up to 100 Units IM distributed among muscles of neck and forehead q 3 months

* Long-acting preparations can be given less frequently

too frequently. In fact, patients who take abortive agents on a daily basis often have particularly intractable headaches, leading to the concept of "medication overuse headache" or "rebound headache" (although the evidence supporting this concept is primarily anecdotal). For these reasons, patients with frequent headaches often need a prophylactic medication. No absolute criterion exists to determine when such treatment is necessary, but as a general guideline, a patient with more than one severe headache a week should probably be on a prophylactic medication. Some patients with only one headache a month may require a prophylactic agent if the headaches last several days and are disabling despite abortive treatment. Other patients may choose to experience several headaches a week rather than take a medication regularly, especially if their headaches are mild or they get prompt relief from an abortive agent.

The choice of which abortive or prophylactic agent to use is generally based on the side-effect profiles and dosing characteristics. For example, a patient with asthma should generally not be given a beta-blocker, but this might be the first choice in a patient with borderline hypertension. A patient with a predisposition to gastrointestinal bleeding should not be given a nonsteroidal anti-inflammatory drug, but most other patients tolerate these agents quite well (although concurrent use of aspirin and another NSAID should be avoided). A patient who can't manage to take medications regularly throughout the day should be given a medication with a long half-life. Intramuscular botulinum toxin injections are an attractive alternative for patients who are routinely unable to tolerate the side effects of oral medications; the mechanism of action is unknown.

Side-effect profiles are a particular concern in pregnant patients. No medication is considered absolutely safe during pregnancy (and similar considerations apply to women who are breast-feeding). Fortunately, headaches often subside during pregnancy. If a patient requires medication, it is best to try to control the headaches with abortive agents alone. Ergots and triptans are absolutely contraindicated. Acetaminophen is generally thought to be the safest abortive agent. Codeine may be added if necessary, but indiscriminate use has been associated with various congenital malformations. Opiates and anti-emetic agents are considered relatively safe, and isometheptene (Midrin) probably is also. If a prophylactic agent is necessary, cyproheptadine may be the safest choice, but it is not always effective. Nonsteroidals can cause premature ductus closure and consequent pulmonary hypertension; they may also increase bilirubin and impair renal function. They are generally considered relatively safe in the first two trimesters. Metoprolol (Lopressor) is also considered fairly safe. Propranolol (Inderal) has an oxytocic effect and may cause growth retardation, respiratory depression, and hypoglycemia. It carries more risk than metoprolol but may be more effective for some patients. Calcium channel blockers may be relatively safe in pregnancy, but there is a theoretical risk of reduced uterine blood flow due to hypotension. Limb reduction abnormalities, other bone deformities, and hand swelling have been reported with amitriptyline (Elavil) and nortriptyline (Pamelor). Anti-epileptic drugs should be avoided in the first trimester because of teratogenic potential.

B. Cluster Headaches

The most distinctive feature of cluster headache is the time course: the patient may go for months or years without headaches but then experiences a cluster of daily headaches. Clusters usually last 4–8 weeks and occur once or twice a year, but this is quite variable. The headaches themselves typically last 30 minutes to 2 hours (an average of 45 minutes), and the onset is explosive. Patients prefer to be upright. They often cannot sit or stand still, and many will even hit their head against a wall. Within a cluster there may be one or more headaches a day, but at least one of the headaches typically occurs at the same hour every day (patients say they "could set the clock" by them). Most of the headaches occur at night, frequently awakening the patient from REM sleep.

Like typical migraine, cluster headaches are unilateral, but unlike migraine, every headache is on the same side. Cluster headaches are frequently associated with ipsilateral lacrimation, redness of the eye, nasal congestion, and rhinorrhea. An ipsilateral partial Horner's syndrome is sometimes present during the attack, and it may persist between attacks. Whereas migraine headaches are twice as common in women as in men, cluster headaches are six times more common in men than women.

Any abortive agent used for migraine can also be used to abort a cluster headache, but certain agents are particularly effective:

1. Oxygen, 100% by mask at 8-10 L/minute for 10–15 minutes

2. Intranasal (aerosol) ergotamine, 0.36-1.08 mg (one to three puffs)

3. Intranasal lidocaine, 4% (1 ml) in the ipsilateral nostril

4. IV dihydroergotamine (DHE); see Table 12.2 for dose recommendations

5. Subcutaneous sumatriptan, 6 mg

In some cases, the cluster can be managed purely with abortive treatments (e.g., by providing a home oxygen tank). In many cases, this is not practical, however, and medication must be given to try to stop the cluster. One commonly used medication is prednisone, 80 mg per day for 1–2 weeks, followed by a rapid taper. Alternatives include verapamil (360–480 mg per day in divided doses), valproic acid (500–2000 mg per day in divided doses), lithium carbonate (600–900 mg per day in divided doses, adjusted to keep the serum level in the therapeutic range), or topiramate (50–200 mg b.i.d.). Whichever medication is used, the dose should be gradually tapered after the patient has been free of headaches for 2 weeks. For patients who have very frequent clusters (or who have entered a chronic phase, which may last 4–5 years), prophylactic medication may be necessary even between clusters. All of the same prophylactic agents may be useful, but lithium and verapamil are the ones prescribed most commonly. Surgical intervention is an option for the 10% or fewer of patients who are refractory to medications. Good results have been reported with radiofrequency thermocoagulation of the trigeminal (gasserian) ganglion, sensory root section of the trigeminal nerve, stereotactic radiosurgery, and stereotactic implantation of a stimulating electrode into the periventricular hypothalamus.

C. Trigeminal Neuralgia

Trigeminal neuralgia (tic douloureux) is characterized by a paroxysmal, "electric shock-like" pain, usually beginning at the maxilla or mandible and lasting about a second. It tends to occur in trains lasting 5–30 seconds. The pain can sometimes be triggered by lightly touching a particular spot on the face, called a trigger zone. The location of the trigger zone differs among patients. Cold wind, brushing the teeth, or chewing may also trigger the pain. It usually does not wake patients from sleep. There is often a superimposed dull, continuous ache, especially when the condition has been present a long time.

Trigeminal neuralgia is usually a benign condition, either idiopathic or associated with compression of the trigeminal sensory root by blood vessels, but it can also be associated with other structural lesions of the fifth nerve, and it occurs fairly frequently in patients with multiple sclerosis. Symptoms usually begin after age 50 but may occur as early as the teen years. The younger the patient, the greater the likelihood that the trigeminal neuralgia is secondary to some other condition, especially multiple sclerosis. An MRI scan of the brain, with special attention to the posterior fossa, should be done if the patient is younger than age 50, if there are focal abnormalities on examination, or if symptoms began or changed in character within the past two years. A substantial number of patients develop trigeminal neuralgia as a result of dental problems, including microabscesses, so all patients should be carefully evaluated for dental disease.

Initial treatment is usually with carbamazepine (Tegretol), starting at a dose of 100 mg b.i.d. or t.i.d., but increasing if necessary to doses as high as 1500 mg per day. If this is ineffective (or if its effect is only temporary), the following drugs are often effective also:

1. Baclofen (Lioresal), 10 mg b.i.d.; up to 20 mg q.i.d., if necessary

2. Gabapentin (Neurontin), 300 mg t.i.d.; up to 900 mg q.i.d., if necessary

3. Lamotrigine (Lamictal), 25 mg b.i.d.; up to 200 mg b.i.d., if necessary

4. Oxcarbazepine (Trileptal), 150 mg b.i.d.; up to 900 mg b.i.d., if necessary

5. Topiramate (Topamax), 25 mg b.i.d.; up to 200 mg b.i.d., if necessary

6. Phenytoin (Dilantin), 100 mg b.i.d.; up to 100 mg q.i.d., if necessary

7. Amitriptyline (Elavil), 25 mg q.h.s.; up to 150 mg q.h.s., if necessary

8. Valproic acid (Depakote), 250 mg b.i.d.; up to 500 mg q.i.d., if necessary

9. Clonazepam (Klonopin), 0.5 mg b.i.d.; up to 2.0 mg q.i.d., if necessary

10. For patients in the midst of a severe attack, intravenous fosphenytoin (250 mg phenytoin equivalents at 50 mg PE/minute) or anesthesia of the ipsilateral conjunctival sac with proparacaine (a local ophthalmic anesthetic) may provide acute relief

At least several of these agents should be tried before considering surgical treatment. There are two principal surgical options. The most reliable method, but also the most invasive, is microvascular decompression of the trigeminal sensory root. The less invasive method is a percutaneous lesion of the trigeminal ganglion or sensory root, either with radiofrequency pulses or with glycerol injection. Unfortunately, a few patients develop "anesthesia dolorosa" after the percutaneous procedures. This is a condition of numbness and extremely painful paresthesias over part of the face, notoriously refractory to treatment. As a general rule, microvascular decompression is probably preferable to percutaneous ganglion lesions, except in older patients or others who might be poor surgical candidates. A third option is to destroy the branch of the trigeminal nerve that is painful, usually with glycerol injection, but results are often inadequate. Other options include percutaneous balloon compression of the trigeminal ganglion and stereotactic radiosurgery.

D. Glossopharyngeal Neuralgia

The pain characteristics and clinical features of glossopharyngeal neuralgia are similar to those of trigeminal neuralgia, except that the pain typically starts in the oropharynx and extends upward and backward toward the ear (sometimes in the reverse direction). Swallowing (especially sour or spicy foods), yawning, sneezing, coughing, cold liquids in the mouth, or touching the ear can be triggers. Unlike trigeminal neuralgia, the pain frequently awakens patients from sleep. The pain sometimes is associated with syncope. Medical treatment is the same as for trigeminal neuralgia, and surgical treatment is analogous. Glossopharyngeal neuralgia is rare (trigeminal neuralgia is seventy-five times more common).

E. Chronic Paroxysmal Hemicrania and Related Conditions

Chronic paroxysmal hemicrania is also a rare condition. The clinical features of the pain and accompanying symptoms are the same as for cluster headache, but the temporal profile is different: The headaches are short (3–46 minutes, an average of 13 minutes) and recur frequently throughout the day (4–38 attacks a day, an average of 14). No nocturnal predominance is apparent, and the headaches usually occur daily throughout the year, rather than in clusters. Chronic paroxysmal hemicrania is five times more common in women than in men and is responsive to indomethacin (Indocin), though dose requirements may vary.

A similar syndrome known as SUNCT ("short-lasting unilateral neuralgiform headache with conjunctival injection and tearing") is characterized by paroxysms of pain that last 5–120 seconds, but typically 15–30 seconds, averaging 28 attacks per day (with a range of 1–77). The ipsilateral conjunctival injection and lacrimation are extremely prominent. Except for the temporal profile of the attacks, the clinical features of SUNCT are very similar to those of chronic paroxysmal hemicrania. It might seem as if the two conditions simply represent two ends of a spectrum, but unlike chronic paroxysmal hemicrania, SUNCT does not respond to indomethacin. In fact, it is resistant to most medications, but topiramate, lamotrigine, gabapentin, and carbamazepine have each been reported to be effective in some cases. Another feature that differentiates SUNCT and chronic paroxysmal hemicrania is that SUNCT is more common in men than in women.

Even briefer paroxysms of stabbing pain, lasting less than a second, are common in patients who are subject to migraine, but they can also occur in patients with no prior headache history. They have been called "ice-pick headaches" or, more generally, "primary stabbing headache." These headaches typically respond to indomethacin. At the other end of the spectrum, patients with "hemicrania continua" have a continuous, unilateral headache with superimposed attacks of more intense pain accompanied by the same ipsilateral autonomic symptoms that occur in cluster headaches and the other hemicranias. This syndrome is also responsive to indomethacin.

F. Atypical Facial Pain

Patients who do not fit cleanly into any well-defined category are classified as having atypical facial pain. They often have some features of migraine, but others of neuralgia, and other features that are not typical of either.

This diagnosis obviously has no consistent pathophysiologic correlate, and treatment is usually a matter of trial and error with medications used for one of the more well-defined conditions. As with other headache syndromes, diagnostic testing is only necessary if the neurologic examination shows focal abnormalities or if there has been recent onset or change in the character of the patient's symptoms.

VII. Discussion of Case Histories

Case 1. Even though this patient complains of the worst headache of his life, it is not qualitatively different from headaches he has been having for twelve years. If his examination is normal—in particular, if he is afebrile, with a supple neck, and no focal neurologic abnormalities—no imaging study is necessary. The patient is too young to have giant cell arteritis, so a sedimentation rate is not necessary. The features are in the migraine/tension spectrum (mostly migraine, although the progression to the entire head is atypical). He should be given an abortive agent. Nonsteroidal medications should be avoided because he has already taken eight aspirin; subcutaneous sumatriptan (Imitrex) or intravenous DHE would provide the most rapid relief. Since he is now having up to two headaches per week, he should be sent out of the emergency department with a prescription for a prophylactic agent; either naproxen (Naprosyn) or propranolol (Inderal) would be a reasonable first choice. If naproxen is prescribed, he should also be given a prescription for some abortive agent other than aspirin.

Case 2. Although this patient's headache is not severe, it has two features that increase the likelihood of an underlying systemic or neurologic process: It has only been present three months, and there are focal abnormalities on examination (localizing to the right frontal and parietal lobes). The patient seems to have some anosognosia (unawareness of his own deficits), a common accompaniment of nondominant parietal lobe lesions. Given a focal lesion and a chronic time course, a neoplasm is a prime concern (see Chapter 3). This patient needs an imaging study of the brain as soon as possible, and treatment will depend on what it shows. At the same time, he could be given symptomatic treatment for his headaches, using the same approach that would be followed in a patient with migraine or tension headaches.

Comment: A CT scan revealed a ring-enhancing lesion in the right frontal and parietal lobes, with substantial edema surrounding it. A chest x-ray showed an apical lesion in the right lung that had not been present on previous studies, the most recent of which had been obtained nine months earlier. A non-small cell lung cancer was found at bronchoscopy. The cerebral mass was presumed to be a metastasis, and the patient was started on dexamethasone to treat the cerebral edema. This eliminated the headaches, also. He was referred to an oncologist for management of his primary cancer. The patient refused resection and radiation of the cerebral metastasis.

Chapter 13

Visual Symptoms

I. Case Histories

Case 1. A 22-year-old woman has been experiencing discomfort and blurring of vision in her left eye for several days. She has never had similar symptoms before and has otherwise been healthy. She has 20/20 vision in her right eye, measured with a near vision card while her left eye is covered. With the right eye covered, she is unable to read newsprint and her acuity is 20/300. Her pupils are equal, but she has a left afferent pupillary defect. The left optic disc appears slightly pale; the right appears normal. She complains of discomfort in the left eye during testing of visual pursuit. The remainder of her examination is normal.

Case 2. A 75-year-old man complains of blurred vision in his left eye. The symptoms began several days ago and have progressed slowly. There is no eye pain. He also complains that he has been unable to chew meat because of pain in his jaw. Even with his glasses, he is barely able to count fingers with the left eye, but right eye visual acuity is normal. He has a left afferent pupillary defect and a swollen left optic disc. The remainder of his examination is normal.

Case 3. A 60-year-old woman reports episodes of loss of vision in the left eye. Each spell begins suddenly and gradually worsens over 15–30 seconds. She can not provide any details, except that at the height of the episode "everything is dark in that eye." The visual loss lasts for several minutes before resolving completely. She has no pain or other symptoms with these spells. The first episode occurred two months ago, and she has had four more episodes since. Her examination is normal.

Questions:

1. How is the approach to these patients the same?
2. How does their evaluation differ?
3. What steps must be taken urgently?

II. Background Information

A. Definitions

diplopia double vision

homonymous affecting the same side of the visual field in both eyes

heteronymous affecting different sides of the visual field in each eye

B. Overview of the Visual System

Information from each eye travels separately to the optic chiasm, where fiber pathways cross and sort themselves so that fibers carrying information from analogous portions of the visual fields of the two eyes travel together to the primary visual cortex in the occipital lobe. The visual information is subsequently forwarded to many other specialized regions of cortex where features such as form, color, depth, and motion are analyzed. Most of the individual cells in these different regions of visual cortex receive input from both eyes. For these cells to function properly, the two eyes must be exquisitely aligned. This is accomplished by the ocular motor system, which directs the output of cranial nerves III, IV, and VI in such a way that both eyes are always fixated on the same point.

When the ocular motor system malfunctions so that the two eyes fixate on slightly different points, the brain receives two visual images of the world that are a little displaced from each other. The result is diplopia. In contrast, lesions of the visual pathways produce a degraded image in the affected visual field regions, but the visual fields of the two eyes remain aligned, so patients experience loss of vision, rather than diplopia.

III. Approach to Visual Symptoms

An accurate description of visual symptoms is the key to diagnosis. Does the patient have diplopia or loss of vision? If the problem is vision loss, does it involve one eye or both, and does it involve the entire visual field of the affected eyes or only a portion of the field? Are the symptoms transient, static, or progressive? If the symptoms are transient, are there any precipitating factors? Are the episodes stereotyped, and, if so, what is the temporal progression of the symptoms?

Patients with static or progressive deficits can be examined while symptoms are present. When the symptoms are transient, however, the patient is often completely free of symptoms during the examination and may have trouble providing a detailed description of the episodes. In these cases, it is helpful to instruct patients that if they have more episodes in the future they should cover each eye in turn during the episodes and pay careful attention to how this affects their symptoms.

IV. Monocular Vision Loss

Symptoms confined to a single eye imply a lesion anterior to the optic chiasm because this is the only portion of the visual pathway that does not receive input from both eyes. The cause of monocular vision loss can usually be deduced from the age of the patient and the time course of symptoms.

Examination findings are helpful in distinguishing diseases of the optic nerve from other ocular causes of loss of vision. Unless the vision loss is mild, the "swinging flashlight test" (see Chapter 2) almost always reveals an afferent pupillary defect when the problem is in the optic nerve. A careful ocular examination (including measurement of intraocular pressure) will usually reveal disease situated in the nonneural tissue of the eye. Regardless of the cause of monocular vision loss, the most straightforward way to determine severity and follow the clinical course is to measure visual acuity in each eye separately. In a few conditions, especially glaucoma and increased intracranial pressure, visual acuity is relatively spared, so disease progression must be assessed in other ways.

A. Acute or Subacute Monocular Vision Loss in Young Patients

In young patients, the acute onset of monocular vision loss usually signifies *optic neuritis* (much less common causes include sinus mucocele, vasculitis, and optic nerve infiltration by carcinomatous or granulomatous processes). The vision loss of optic neuritis may progress over 7–10 days. Eye pain, which is usually exacerbated by eye movement, may precede or accompany the loss of vision. Optic neuritis may occur in isolation or as a manifestation of multiple sclerosis (MS). Patients should be asked explicitly about any previous neurologic symptoms that might suggest the latter diagnosis. Those with no prior history of neurologic symptoms have a 30–40% risk of developing MS within 5 years. Patients with multiple white matter lesions on MRI scan of the brain have a higher (50% or more) likelihood of developing MS, whereas only 10% of patients with completely normal MRI scans subsequently develop MS. Patients with optic neuritis who receive a 3-day course of high-dose IV methylprednisolone (followed by oral prednisone for 11 days) recover slightly more quickly than those who receive placebo, but there is no difference in visual function between the two groups six months later.

Acute vision loss can also result from traumatic injury to the eye, but this is usually obvious from the history and examination. In young diabetic patients, vitreous hemorrhage should be considered. Acute iritis typically presents with blurred vision, pain, and redness, sometimes in one eye only. Iritis can be a symptom of systemic autoimmune disease, so these patients should be asked about problems of the skin, joints, or visceral organs.

B. Acute or Subacute Monocular Vision Loss in Older Patients

In older patients, monocular loss of vision may be due to acute glaucoma, retinal detachment, macular degeneration, cataracts, or acute ischemic optic neuropathy. Glaucoma (increased intraocular pressure) is usually a chronic condition causing gradually progressive field loss, but acute obstruction of aqueous outflow results in sudden vision loss accompanied by severe eye and face pain, nausea, vomiting, and dilation of the pupil. Retinal detachment is commonly associated with myopia, diabetes, intraocular inflammation, or cataract surgery; it can also occur after trauma (even minor trauma, such as jogging). Cataracts and macular degeneration (and most cases of glaucoma) produce gradual vision loss progressing over years and are usually evident on examination.

Acute ischemic optic neuropathy is particularly important because it is sometimes caused by *giant cell arteritis (temporal arteritis),* which can usually be successfully treated but may progress to complete blindness in both eyes if left untreated. Historical clues to the presence of giant cell arteritis include headache, jaw or tongue claudication, and aches or discomfort in the shoulder and pelvic girdles (polymyalgia rheumatica). On examination, temporal pulses may be absent. Biopsy of the temporal artery is the "gold standard" for diagnosis and should be obtained whenever the clinical setting suggests giant cell arteritis, even if the sedimentation rate and C-reactive protein are not elevated (see Chapter 12). Whenever the diagnosis of giant cell arteritis is seriously considered, treatment with high-dose corticosteroids should begin immediately even if temporal artery biopsy must be delayed. Histopathologic changes will still be seen if a biopsy can be performed within two weeks of starting steroids, but the goal should be to obtain the biopsy within a few days, to avoid the risk of adverse effects from steroids if they are not necessary. A common approach is to treat with intravenous methylprednisolone (125–250 mg loading dose, followed by 1 g/day or 0.5–1 mg/kg every six hours for up to three days), but oral prednisone (1.5–2 mg/kg day) is an acceptable alternative. After the initial treatment, patients should be treated with oral prednisone (1 mg/kg/day for at least 4–6 weeks), tapering the dose very slowly thereafter (usually by no more than 10 mg every month, more slowly if clinical or laboratory evidence suggests relapse).

V. Transient Vision Loss (Monocular or Binocular)

Transient visual obscuration in one or both eyes may be caused by ischemia, migraine, or increased intracranial pressure. The visual phenomena associated with migraine are typically distinctive. Patients describe flashing lights or jagged lines on the edge of a scotoma in which vision is obscured or totally absent. The abnormal region often expands gradually or moves off toward one side of the visual field. When patients have a typical headache before, during, or after experiencing characteristic visual symptoms, the diagnosis is usually straightforward. Diagnosis can be more difficult when patients have the visual symptoms without any headache, or symptoms that are atypical in some way; it is usually prudent to evaluate these patients for vascular disease or structural abnormalities before concluding that their symptoms are due to migraine.

Transient vision loss in one eye can represent a transient ischemic attack (TIA) due to atherosclerotic disease in the ipsilateral carotid artery (or, less likely, caused by cardioembolism). The vision loss typically progresses over a matter of minutes and resolves completely within an hour—usually within minutes. Patients' descriptions of the symptoms and the time course vary greatly, and many patients just can't remember the details of how the symptoms evolved. Contrary to traditional teaching, most patients do not describe "a shade being pulled down from the top or up from the bottom," although some do. The possibility of TIAs should always be considered when patients at risk for atherosclerotic disease experience transient monocular vision loss.

Patients can also experience transient vision loss as a result of cortical TIAs, but in this case the symptoms involve only one half of the visual field, and both eyes are affected. Some patients do not report hemi-field loss, either because they did not notice it or because both sides became ischemic simultaneously (so-called "lone bilateral blindness"). Also, patients sometimes mistakenly report that they were unable to see out of one eye during the episode, so you should be sure to ask them explicitly whether they checked their vision in each eye separately. In addition to the homonymous nature of the visual symptoms, the time course and the presence of risk factors are clues to the diagnosis.

Patients with increased intracranial pressure sometimes experience transient visual symptoms triggered by even minor changes in intracranial pressure. For example, they may note visual disturbance in one or both eyes whenever they sit up from a lying position, or when they stand from a lying or sitting position. The characteristic physical finding is bilateral optic disc edema in the presence of normal optic nerve function. Increased pressure can result from obstruction of cerebrospinal fluid outflow. An appropriately placed mass lesion can cause this (see Chapter 11), or it may occur without any obvious structural cause; this is called *idiopathic intracranial hypertension,* or *pseudotumor cerebri* (see Chapter 12).

VI. Binocular Vision Loss

Soon after the visual pathways leave the optic chiasm, the input from the two eyes is aligned so closely that any lesion posterior to the chiasm produces a homonymous visual field defect. Lesions in the chiasm itself typically affect the fibers that are in the process of crossing from right to left or vice versa; these are the fibers from the nasal half of each retina, corresponding to the temporal half of each eye's visual field. The result is a *heteronymous (bitemporal) hemianopia.* As noted in Chapter 2, this lesion may go undetected by the patient, because the "bad" field in each eye corresponds to the "good" field in the other eye. The deficit is only evident when each eye is tested separately. The differential diagnosis of lesions affecting the chiasm includes pituitary adenomas, suprasellar meningiomas, craniopharyngiomas, gliomas, and internal carotid artery aneurysms.

For lesions affecting the visual pathway posterior to the optic chiasm, the differential diagnosis is based on demographic considerations and the time course of symptoms, as described in Chapter 3, and management is predicated on the underlying disease process.

VII. Diplopia

A. Localization

Diplopia can result from lesions anywhere in the ocular motor system starting in the brainstem nuclei of cranial nerves III, IV, and VI and proceeding along the pathways of those nerves to the individual extraocular muscles. Generalized diseases of muscle or the neuromuscular junction can also interfere with the ability to keep the eyes aligned, and so can anything affecting the mechanical properties of the eyeballs themselves (e.g., a soft tissue mass in the orbit restricting movement of the eyeball).

The first issue to address in a patient with diplopia is whether all of the patient's findings could be caused by dysfunction of a single cranial nerve. There are three specific patterns to recognize:

1. *Sixth nerve lesion:* limitation of abduction (lateral movement) of one eye only; all other movements intact.

2. *Fourth nerve lesion:* impaired ability of one eye to look down and in (i.e., toward the nostril); patients often compensate by tilting the entire head in the direction the affected eye cannot move (i.e., away from the affected eye).

3. *Third nerve lesion:* limitation of adduction (medial movement), supraduction (upward movement), and infraduction (downward movement) of one eye only, sometimes associated with ipsilateral ptosis and dilated pupil.

If one of these patterns is found, then the correct localization is almost always at the level of the cranial nerve or its nucleus. The same is true even if some components of the pattern are missing (e.g., a patient with a third nerve lesion may have all the eye movement abnormalities without a dilated pupil or ptosis).

If the patient's eye movement problems do not all fit into the syndrome expected with a lesion of a single cranial nerve, the next question is whether the findings could all be explained by combined lesions of two cranial nerves, especially two that are neighbors at some point in their course (such as both sixth nerves, or the left third and left fourth nerves). If so, this is the likely localization.

Whenever the cause of the eye movement abnormality appears to be malfunction of one or more cranial nerves, the next issue to address is whether the lesion is intra-axial (within the substance of the brainstem itself) or extra-axial (affecting cranial nerves after they have exited the brainstem). This requires a search for involvement of fiber tracts passing through the brainstem but not entering or exiting at that level, so that a purely extra-axial process could not possibly affect them. Thus, patients should be examined closely for limb weakness, sensory changes, ataxia, and hyperreflexia.

When a lesion of one or two cranial nerves cannot explain the pattern of eye muscle abnormality, and there is no suggestion of an intra-axial brainstem lesion, a primary muscle or neuromuscular junction problem should be considered, especially when muscles of both eyes are involved. A disease of muscle or neuromuscular junction can sometimes produce a pattern that resembles an isolated lesion of the third, fourth, or sixth cranial nerve, but this is uncommon because there is no particular reason for a generalized disease process to affect only the muscles innervated by a single cranial nerve. Meningeal inflammation or cancer can also affect multiple cranial nerves (see Chapter 10), and mechanical limitation of eye movement from structural problems in the orbit (including soft tissue swelling) should not be ignored.

B. Differential Diagnosis and Management

Diseases primarily affecting the neuromuscular junction or muscle are discussed in Chapter 6. Initial symptoms are often restricted to extraocular muscles, and sometimes these are the only muscles involved throughout the entire course of the illness. The principles of diagnosis and management are the same as for patients with these diseases who have more widespread muscle involvement.

When the localization of disease appears to be affecting one or more cranial nerves, the differential diagnosis depends on whether the process is intra-axial or extra-axial and on how many cranial nerves are affected. An intra-axial lesion can be analyzed according to the approach presented in Chapter 3, using the time course and epidemiologic factors to guide diagnosis and management. An extra-axial process affecting multiple cranial nerves is almost always caused by meningeal infiltration, either from inflammatory disease (including infection) or from neoplastic disease. Evaluation should include cerebrospinal fluid examination and a search for systemic evidence of a neoplasm or inflammatory disease. On rare occasions, meningeal biopsy may be diagnostic when less invasive studies are not.

Extra-axial involvement of a single cranial nerve is usually caused by either compression or focal ischemia. Diabetic patients are particularly likely to develop isolated third, fourth, or sixth nerve palsies, and these are generally attributed to small-vessel ischemia. As with small vessel disease elsewhere in the nervous system, no specific treatment is available; fortunately, spontaneous recovery gradually occurs in approximately 50% of cases. Compressive lesions, in contrast, often signal the need for urgent treatment, because an expanding mass at this level may go on to produce brainstem compression and death. Because treatment of a compressive lesion can potentially prevent devastating consequences, patients with extra-axial involvement of a single cranial nerve should be considered to have a compressive lesion until proved otherwise. An MRI of the brain with attention to the brainstem should be obtained as soon as possible.

The best known example of a life-threatening situation presenting with a lesion of a single cranial nerve is the "blown pupil" that occurs when a mass lesion situated laterally in one cerebral hemisphere puts medially-directed pressure on the ipsilateral temporal lobe, compressing the third nerve (*uncal herniation*—see Chapter 11). Third nerve compression may also result from an expanding arterial aneurysm, which is almost as urgent a problem as herniation, because of the high morbidity and mortality associated with aneurysmal rupture (see Chapters 4 and 12). If the aneurysm can be found and repaired before it ruptures, the patient may be spared these dire outcomes. Thus, it is important to distinguish a compressive third nerve lesion from an ischemic lesion.

Examination of the pupil can be helpful in making this distinction. In compression, the pupil is almost always abnormal. Ischemic lesions usually affect the extraocular muscles innervated by the third nerve but "spare" the pupil. When a patient has complete loss of all eye movements controlled by the third nerve, but the pupil remains normal, an ischemic lesion is likely. Exceptions occur, however, and with the widespread availability of MRI and noninvasive techniques for imaging the cerebral blood vessels (MRA and CTA), it is often simplest just to order an imaging study to resolve the question.

Treatment of a compressive lesion usually requires surgical intervention and the techniques of treating increased intracranial pressure discussed in Chapter 11.

VIII. Discussion of Case Histories

Case 1. The monocular visual symptoms indicate a lesion in the visual pathway anterior to the optic chiasm, and the left afferent pupillary defect implies that the lesion is in the left optic nerve. The relatively acute onset suggests optic neuritis in this age group, and her examination is typical of that condition.

Comment: An MRI scan of the brain showed eight white matter lesions that were 5–10 mm in diameter, and one of them enhanced with contrast. Her physician explained to her that this MRI finding in the setting of optic neuritis indicates a high likelihood of developing MS, and that disease-modifying therapies have been proven to improve outcomes in this situation (see Chapter 10). She was given a brief course of IV methyl-prednisolone to shorten the duration of her acute relapse, and after learning about the available treatment options, she decided to begin treatment with glatiramer.

Case 2. This patient also has monocular visual symptoms and a left afferent pupillary defect, again suggesting a lesion in the left optic nerve. Of the various potential causes of monocular vision loss in this age group, the time course is most consistent with acute ischemic optic neuropathy. The jaw pain when chewing (jaw claudication) suggests that this patient's acute ischemic optic neuropathy is due to giant cell (temporal) arteritis.

Comment: His sedimentation rate was greater than 100 mm/hour, and temporal artery biopsy showed arteritis. He was treated with prednisone for just over six months, and all of his symptoms resolved. The prednisone was very gradually tapered off over the subsequent six months.

Case 3. This patient had a TIA involving the retinal artery. Evaluation and management of TIAs are discussed in Chapter 4.

Both Case 2 and Case 3 represent urgent problems, because the symptoms described by each of the two patients may be associated with underlying conditions (temporal arteritis and TIAs) for which prompt treatment can prevent serious and irreversible consequences (blindness in Case 2 and stroke in Case 3).

Chapter 14

Dizziness and Disequilibrium

I. Case Histories

Case 1. A 40-year-old school bus driver is terrified that she is going to lose her job. For the past six weeks, she has been experiencing severe nausea and a spinning sensation every time she turns her head to the far right. She has stopped driving, because even though the symptoms always resolve within 30 seconds, she reasons that this is plenty of time for an accident to happen. A routine physical examination is entirely normal.

Questions:

1. Does this patient have vertigo? If so, is it central or peripheral?
2. What additional examination techniques would be useful in this case?
3. What is the likely diagnosis?
4. What additional diagnostic and treatment measures should be taken?
5. What is the prognosis?

Case 2. A 45-year-old right-handed man is "having problems walking straight." For the past 6 months, he has needed to hold on to walls or furniture for support when he walks, because it feels as if the ground slants to the left. He thinks the problem is getting worse, because three days ago he actually fell down for the first time. He has also noticed that the right side of his face "feels funny," but he thinks he may be imagining it. His handwriting is getting sloppier, but it has always been poor. He also mentions that he has had tinnitus and hearing loss in the right ear for the past 2 or 3 years, but attributes it to "all those rock concerts in college."

His examination is notable for reduced sensation on the entire right side of his face, with an absent corneal reflex on the right. He has left-beating nystagmus with a slight rotatory component, most prominent when looking to the left. His hearing is reduced in the right ear, and his right arm and leg movements are ataxic.

Questions:

1. Does this patient have vertigo? If so, is it central or peripheral?
2. What is the likely diagnosis?
3. What additional diagnostic and treatment measures should be taken?
4. What is the prognosis?

Case 3. A 60-year-old man has an unsteady gait that has been getting progressively worse over the past 6 months. He sometimes stumbles so much that others worry for his safety. He has had increasing trouble climbing ladders because of stiffness in his legs. He has a long history of mild neck discomfort. He is embarrassed to admit that he has had several episodes of urinary incontinence. On examination, his mental status and cranial nerves are normal. His gait is stiff and unsteady, and he tends to fall if not supported. The intrinsic muscles of his hands are atrophic, and he has spasticity and weakness in his lower extremities. His reflexes are brisk at the knees and ankles, normal in the arms, and symmetric throughout. He has bilateral extensor plantar responses.

Questions:

1. Does this patient have vertigo? If so, is it central or peripheral?
2. Where's the lesion?
3. What is the likely diagnosis?
4. What additional diagnostic and treatment measures should be taken?

Case 4. A 65-year-old man has finally been persuaded by his family to see a doctor for his trouble walking. He has difficulty relating a coherent history, especially regarding the time course of his symptoms, but his family is certain that his walking is getting worse. He seems afraid to walk and will only do so when he can hold on to somebody's hand. He denies incontinence but smells like urine. His examination is notable for global cognitive deficits, but they are mild. His gait is wide-based. He is very hesitant when he walks and needs significant support. His lower extremity strength and coordination are normal, however. In fact, the remainder of his examination is notable only for diffuse hyperreflexia.

Questions:

1. Does this patient have vertigo? If so, is it central or peripheral?
2. Where's the lesion?
3. What is the likely diagnosis?
4. What additional diagnostic and treatment measures should be taken?

II. Approach to Dizziness

Patients use the word "dizzy" in many different ways. It can refer to light-headedness, a sense of spinning or other movement, balance difficulty, clumsiness, confusion, or a vague sense of malaise. Thus, the first step in evaluating a dizzy patient is to clarify the nature of the symptoms the patient is experiencing. Unfortunately, many patients have trouble characterizing their symptoms. It is usually easier for them to say whether the dizziness is constant or intermittent, whether there are consistent triggers, whether anything makes the dizziness better or worse, and whether there are any associated symptoms. All of these features are helpful in classifying the dizziness and formulating a differential diagnosis.

III. Light-Headedness (Presyncope)

Light-headedness and disequilibrium are probably the most commonly experienced types of dizziness. Patients who are light-headed often say they feel as if they are about to faint, and at times they do lose consciousness. This symptom usually results from global cerebral hypoperfusion. The potential causes are discussed in Chapter 5.

IV. Vertigo

Many people (including many physicians) think that vertigo refers specifically to a sense of spinning, and this is probably the most common manifestation, but in fact, it means any false sensation of movement. Vertigo results from dysfunction of the vestibular system, either in the periphery (the labyrinth and the vestibular nerve) or centrally (the vestibular nuclei, the cerebellum, and their connections).

A. Localization

The processes that affect the peripheral vestibular system are distinct from those that affect it centrally. Several features help to distinguish central from peripheral lesions. Because the vestibular end-organ (the labyrinth) is adjacent to the auditory end-organ (the cochlea), and the vestibular and cochlear nerves remain next to each other all the way to the brainstem, hearing loss and tinnitus frequently accompany peripheral vertigo. In contrast, because the auditory pathways proceed bilaterally as soon as they enter the brainstem, a unilateral central lesion generally does not produce significant hearing loss, so it is unusual for central vertigo to be associated with prominent auditory symptoms. Instead, the typical abnormalities accompanying central vertigo include dysarthria, dysphagia, diplopia, and limb numbness, weakness, or ataxia, reflecting the fact that this portion of the vestibular pathway is located in the brainstem and cerebellum.

Both central and peripheral vertigo are commonly associated with nystagmus. The specific characteristics of the nystagmus help to distinguish between central and peripheral lesions, but there are no absolutely reliable rules. The most dependable rule is that nystagmus that changes direction depending on the direction of gaze ("multidirectional nystagmus") is usually due to a central lesion. Peripheral lesions almost always cause unidirectional nystagmus; the direction can be remembered by recalling that in testing caloric responses, cold water in one ear (which mimics a destructive lesion) results in slow deviation of the eyes toward that ear, and (in a conscious patient) the fast beat of nystagmus is away from that ear (see Chapter 2).

Peripheral nystagmus usually has both a rotational component and a translational (horizontal or vertical) component; pure horizontal, pure rotatory, or pure vertical nystagmus usually indicates a central lesion. The intensity of the subjective sensation of vertigo is often greater with peripheral lesions. There are exceptions to all of these rules, but they are usually reliable.

In summary, the nystagmus that accompanies peripheral vertigo is almost always unidirectional (with the direction of the fast beat away from the side of the lesion) and it usually has both translational and rotatory components; the nystagmus accompanying central vertigo may be either unidirectional or multidirectional, and it may be purely horizontal, purely vertical, purely rotatory, or any combination. Symptoms or signs of brainstem dysfunction suggest a central lesion; unilateral hearing loss or tinnitus suggest a peripheral lesion. Vertiginous symptoms are often more severe with peripheral lesions.

When these clinical features are not sufficient to determine whether the lesion is central or peripheral, specialized testing in a vestibular laboratory may be helpful. An audiogram can also be useful in demonstrating unilateral hearing loss that would make a peripheral disorder more likely. In theory, brainstem auditory evoked potentials (see Chapter 10) could help localize defects in the auditory pathway, but they are generally not reliable enough to be very useful. When localization remains uncertain, imaging studies of the brain (especially the posterior fossa) and skull (especially the auditory canal) may be necessary.

B. Differential Diagnosis

The differential diagnosis of vertigo depends primarily on two factors: whether the lesion is central or peripheral, and the time course of symptoms.

1. Central vertigo

Central vertigo that is getting progressively worse is usually due to a neoplasm or abscess (see Chapter 3). Central vertigo of acute onset usually signifies a vascular process (or trauma, in the appropriate setting). Recurrent, transient spells can represent transient ischemic attacks, migraines, seizures, or paroxysmal manifestations of multiple sclerosis; the time course and associated symptoms usually distinguish these possibilities (see Chapters 4, 5, 10, and 12). In particular, many patients with recurrent episodes of vertigo have a personal or family history of migraine, and anecdotal reports (but no controlled trials) suggest that their episodes of vertigo become less frequent or less severe (or both) when they take prophylactic migraine medications. Some of these patients have headaches accompanying their vertigo, but many do not. Similarly, some have other migraine features (such as visual distortion, nausea, or photophobia) at the time of their vertigo, but many do not. This condition ("migraine dizziness") remains poorly characterized and poorly understood, in part because it is not associated with specific abnormalities on examination or diagnostic tests. No diagnostic criteria have been established. Nonetheless, it is diagnosed increasingly frequently. Some people consider it to be the most common cause of dizziness in patients who report dizziness dating back several months or more, without key characteristics of a common peripheral disorder or examination findings suggestive of a structural lesion.

2. Peripheral vertigo

Peripheral vertigo that is getting progressively worse suggests inflammatory or neoplastic disease. The most common tumors in the cerebellopontine angle are meningiomas and vestibular nerve schwannomas; the latter have traditionally been referred to as acoustic neuromas, but this term is misleading, because these tumors usually arise from the vestibular division of the eighth nerve. Even so, the initial symptoms are usually auditory. Disequilibrium, ipsilateral facial numbness and weakness, and ipsilateral ataxia often develop later in the course. A few specific toxins cause progressive, bilateral eighth nerve dysfunction, notably aminoglycosides and cisplatin.

Most often, peripheral vertigo begins acutely and does not progress (though it may persist for days, weeks, or even months). In this situation, the diagnoses to consider depend on whether similar episodes of vertigo have occurred in the past.

a. Recurrent episodes

The distinction between peripheral and central vertigo may be especially difficult when the symptoms are episodic, and the patient is only available for examination during asymptomatic periods. Thus, in a patient with recurrent episodes of vertigo, even when the symptoms sound peripheral, central disorders such as migraines, vertebrobasilar TIAs, seizures, and multiple sclerosis must be considered. Most often, though, a peripheral condition is the cause.

Benign paroxysmal positional vertigo (BPPV) is the most common cause of recurrent vertigo. Patients with BPPV experience brief episodes of vertigo whenever the head is in certain positions, and they have no vertigo in other head positions. They typically report that the symptoms occur when they extend their head to look up, or when they turn over in bed. The vertigo usually begins about 5–10 seconds after the head assumes the symptomatic position. It typically lasts less than 30 seconds and almost always less than a minute. The vertigo usually becomes less severe if the head is placed in the symptomatic position several times in a row. These features can often be demonstrated by performing the *Hallpike maneuver* (Figure 14.1): Start by having the patient sit near one end of the examination table, with the body facing the far end of the table and the head turned 45° to one side. Next, help the patient recline to a supine position with the head hanging over the edge of the table and the neck extended 30–45°, still turned to the same side. Keep the patient in this position for at least 20 seconds and ask him/her to report any symptoms of vertigo, while at the same time, you are observing the patient's eyes for nystagmus. Then return the patient to the seated position, and repeat the maneuver with the head rotated 45° to the other side. To establish the diagnosis of BPPV, one of these positions should trigger a burst of upbeat and torsional nystagmus that lasts about ten to thirty seconds.

BPPV is usually due to calcium carbonate particles (otoliths) that have become dislodged from the otolith membrane and migrated to one of the semicircular canals, where they typically float free in the endolymph though occasionally they can adhere to the cupula. The condition may follow head trauma or labyrinthitis, but usually no obvious precipitant is apparent. The most common form of BPPV is posterior canal BPPV,

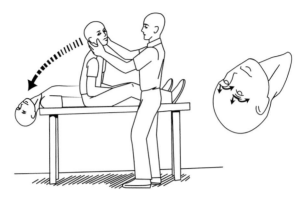

Fig. 14.1 Hallpike maneuver for diagnosing benign paroxysmal positional vertigo (BPPV); details explained in text.

which is readily treatable with particle repositioning maneuvers (typically the *Epley maneuver;* see Figure 14.2) designed to move the particles from the canal back into the central chamber of the inner ear, the vestibule.

Less common forms of BPPV involve the horizontal or anterior canals. In horizontal canal BPPV, the nystagmus is in the horizontal plane and is best triggered by having the patient lie supine and then roll over to either side. This condition does not generally respond to the Epley maneuver. In anterior canal BPPV, the Hallpike maneuver triggers a burst of downbeat, torsional nystagmus. This condition usually responds to the Epley maneuver (thereby providing evidence that the patient does not have positional downbeat nystagmus due to a central lesion, which would require neuroimaging).

Ménière's disease is characterized by episodic vertigo and tinnitus superimposed on a condition of hearing loss. The hearing loss is fluctuating and completely reversible early in the disease, but it eventually becomes progressive. The episodes of vertigo typically begin with a sensation of fullness and pressure in one ear, accompanied by tinnitus and reduced hearing in that ear. The vertigo reaches maximum intensity within minutes and slowly subsides over the next few hours, but the patient usually continues to feel vaguely unsteady and dizzy for the next few days. Nausea, vomiting, and ataxia may accompany the episodes. These attacks occur irregularly, at intervals of weeks, months, or years.

Ménière's disease is associated with increased endolymph volume throughout the labyrinth. It can occur after labyrinthitis but is usually idiopathic. It is typically treated with salt restriction and diuretics, although

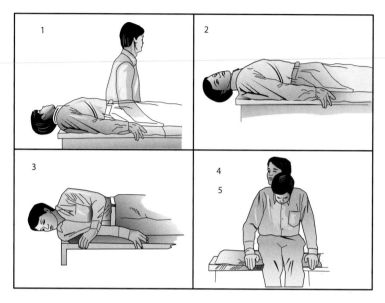

Fig. 14.2 Epley maneuver for treating posterior semicircular canal BPPV. The first steps (1) are the same as the Hallpike maneuver (note that this patient's displaced particles are in the left ear, whereas Figure 14.1 shows a patient whose problem is in the right ear). Keep the patient in the initial position (in this case, head extended 45° over the end of the table and turned all the way to the left) for at least a minute, then (2) rapidly turn the head all the way to the other side (still keeping the head extended 45° over the end of the table). Keep the head in this position for at least a minute, then (3) roll the patient's body in the direction the head is already turned, maintaining the rotated position of the head relative to the body so that the patient's face is now pointed toward the floor. Keep the patient in this position for at least a minute, then (4) have the patient sit up, maintaining the rotated position of the head relative to the body.

the evidence supporting their efficacy is anecdotal. Endolymphatic shunts have been attempted, without consistent benefit. When all else fails, ablative therapy may be attempted, because the brain can eventually habituate to the complete loss of vestibular function on one side better than it can adjust to fluctuating vestibular function. The least complicated ablative procedure is intratympanic gentamicin injection, although this does not always control the vertigo and there is a 25% risk of hearing loss in that ear.

Labyrinthectomy is more consistently effective, but also results in hearing loss. These procedures are most appropriate when patients have already lost functional hearing on the affected side. A vestibular nerve section is the procedure most likely to preserve hearing, but it is more complicated and less reliable.

Perilymph fistula is characterized by episodes of vertigo that are often precipitated by sneezing, coughing, loud noises (*Tullio's phenomenon*, which may also occur in Ménière's disease), exertion, or airplane flights. The fistula consists of a small tear in the oval window or the round window, but the mechanism by which this produces symptoms is unclear. Most patients recover spontaneously, so treatment is usually conservative: bed rest, head elevation, and measures to reduce straining. Surgical correction is possible when conservative measures are ineffective.

Dehiscence of the superior semicircular canal is a rare condition in which the part of the temporal bone that overlies the superior semi-circular canal is thin or absent. The symptoms are similar to those of perilymph fistula (including Tullio's phenomenon), together with mild low-frequency hearing loss and hypersensitivity to bone-conducted sounds (sometimes including the movement of the eyeballs in their sockets). Surgical repair can be attempted if the symptoms are debilitating, but many patients do well with conservative management.

Vestibular paroxysmia is a rare condition that is thought to result from vascular compression or another irritant of cranial nerve VIII, analogous to some cases of trigeminal neuralgia (see Chapter 12). Patients experience very brief episodes (lasting seconds or at most a few minutes) of vertigo accompanied by hearing loss, hyperacusis, or tinnitus. Like trigeminal neuralgia, this syndrome can respond to carbamazepine.

b. Single episode

Acute labyrinthitis is characterized by the sudden or subacute onset of severe vertigo, nausea, vomiting, and imbalance, sometimes associated with hearing loss and tinnitus. Symptoms are usually severe for hours to days, with residual symptoms gradually resolving over days to months. This condition may occur with a documented bacterial infection of the middle ear or in association with a systemic viral illness. When a clear bacterial cause can be found, appropriate antibiotics should be given.

Acute idiopathic unilateral peripheral vestibulopathy (also called *acute peripheral vestibulopathy* or *acute vestibular syndrome*) is an analogous and much more common condition. The symptoms usually develop over several hours, but sometimes in a matter of seconds or minutes. Patients experience intense vertigo that is worst when they move their head, but present even at rest, and most patients have nausea and vomiting. Unlike patients with acute labyrinthitis, patients with acute vestibular syndrome have normal hearing. This condition is widely presumed to be viral or postviral (specifically, reactivation of herpes simplex virus type 1) based on some epidemiologic and pathologic evidence, but the etiology has not been convincingly demonstrated. This condition is often referred to as vestibular neuritis. These patients have unidirectional horizontal and rotatory nystagmus with the fast component away from the affected ear. With the head impulse test, or head thrust maneuver (see Chapter 2), patients maintain fixation on the target when you turn their head away from the affected ear, but when you turn the head toward the affected ear, their eyes move off the target (in the direction of the head movement), so that at the conclusion of the head movement they have to make one or more corrective saccades (in the direction opposite to the way in which the head was just moving). When the head thrust maneuver does not show this abnormality, a lesion in the cerebellum or brainstem becomes a serious consideration.

In patients with acute peripheral vestibulopathy, treatment with oral methylprednisolone (100 mg a day, reducing the dose by 20 mg every 3 days) significantly enhances the recovery of vestibular function measured a year later, although no improvement in clinical outcome has been demonstrated. The only other available treatments are symptomatic and may include bed rest, antiemetics, antihistamines, and vestibular rehabilitation programs.

All of the conditions in the differential diagnosis of recurrent peripheral vertigo must also be considered in a patient with a single episode—after all, there must be a first episode even for recurrent symptoms. The specific characteristics of the patient's symptoms will determine which (if any) of these recurrent conditions are realistic possibilities. Ischemic disease merits special mention. According to traditional dogma, the blood vessels that supply the CNS portions of the vestibular system also supply brain regions that mediate other functions, so it is impossible for an ischemic lesion to produce isolated vertigo without ataxia or brainstem signs. This rule is false. With improved imaging modalities, it is now clear that some patients with small cerebellar strokes have a syndrome virtually indistinguishable from vestibular neuritis. Such patients are uncommon, however. The main situations in which a patient presenting with the acute vestibular syndrome should have an MRI scan to look for ischemia are when (1) the symptoms or examination are not typical of vestibular neuritis (for example, the patient does not have the typical pattern of nystagmus, or has a normal response to head thrust maneuver in both directions); (2) the patient has signs suggesting a lesion in the cerebellum or brainstem (such as limb ataxia, dysarthria, or asymmetric deep tendon reflexes); or (3) the patient has strong risk factors for stroke (such as a recent neck injury that might have caused a vertebral artery dissection, or multiple atherosclerotic risk factors).

V. Disequilibrium

To maintain balance, the brain must receive detailed, accurate information about the position of the body relative to the environment and generate an appropriate, coordinated motor response. Any condition that disturbs either the sensory input or the motor output can produce disequilibrium. The visual, proprioceptive, and vestibular pathways are the most important sensory systems for determining body position. The auditory pathway also contributes, but to a lesser degree. The history and examination should be directed at detecting dysfunction in any of these pathways. The Romberg test is a useful screen. Normal individuals can maintain balance with their eyes closed, because even after visual information has been removed the remaining sensory modalities are sufficient to provide a sense of body position. In contrast, patients with dysfunction of the proprioceptive or vestibular system rely heavily on visual input, and although they may be able to maintain equilibrium with their eyes open, they lose their balance when they close their eyes.

Patients with disequilibrium because of an inadequate motor response usually have difficulty maintaining their balance even with their eyes open, so the Romberg test does not apply. An inadequate motor response can result from a purely mechanical problem (such as a hip fracture), weakness, stiffness (either because of spasticity or due to extrapyramidal disease), ataxia, or cognitive deficits. All of these possibilities should be evaluated in the course of the history and the physical examination.

If any sensory or motor abnormalities that could contribute to disequilibrium are found, they should be evaluated and treated according to principles presented elsewhere in this book. For example, vestibular diseases are discussed in Part IV of this chapter, neuromuscular causes of proprioceptive disturbance are discussed in Chapter 6, normal pressure hydrocephalus (NPH) is discussed in Chapter 7, and so forth. Disequilibrium is often multifactorial; patients may have several minor abnormalities combining to produce significant impairment of balance even though each of the abnormalities in isolation would be unlikely to cause serious problems.

Treatment of gait difficulty should include an assessment of the patient's home environment. Patients with gait disturbances who have difficulty climbing stairs can be helped by a stair-lift or by moving to a ground-floor apartment or bedroom. Loose rugs are a hazard and should be removed whenever possible. Strategically placed handrails can help to make the home safer. Wall-to-wall carpeting is more easily negotiated in smooth-soled shoes than sneakers, whereas sneakers are better for walking on the sidewalk or street.

VI. Discussion of Case Histories

Case 1. This patient clearly has recurrent episodes of vertigo based on her description. The consistent relationship to a specific head position, the brevity of the symptoms, and the intensity of the vertigo all suggest a peripheral lesion, and specifically, BPPV. Positional vertigo can occasionally occur with central lesions, however, so the Hallpike maneuver should be performed. If this demonstrates the characteristic burst of upbeat and torsional nystagmus with the head to one side, it will establish the diagnosis of posterior canal BPPV. The patient can then be reassured and treated with a particle repositioning procedure, followed by a repeat Hallpike maneuver to confirm the response.

Case 2. This patient also has vertigo, because he feels as if he is falling in one direction. The association with tinnitus and hearing loss makes a peripheral lesion almost certain. The unidirectional nystagmus with both horizontal and rotatory components also suggests a peripheral lesion. The fast component of the nystagmus is toward the left, suggesting a right-sided lesion (the fact that the nystagmus is most prominent when looking to the left adds no localizing information, because nystagmus is always most prominent when the patient is looking in the direction of the fast component). With a right-sided vestibular lesion, the left vestibular apparatus is relatively unopposed, accounting for the patient's subjective impression of the ground slanting to the left. All of the examination findings are also consistent with a focal lesion located at the right cerebellopontine angle. In this case, the symptoms were progressive, with a time course of several years, suggesting neoplastic disease.

The history is typical of a vestibular nerve schwannoma, but other inflammatory and neoplastic diseases are certainly possible. This patient needs an MRI scan. If it is consistent with a vestibular nerve schwannoma, and it is relatively large, the treatment of choice is surgical excision using microsurgical techniques, with intraoperative electrophysiologic monitoring of the facial nerve. For small vestibular schwannomas, conservative management with serial imaging to monitor tumor growth may be the preferred approach; radiosurgery is also an option. The prognosis is good.

Case 3. This patient has disequilibrium, not vertigo. He has upper motor neuron signs in the lower extremities and lower motor neuron signs in the intrinsic hand muscles. Although a combination of upper and lower motor neuron signs can indicate motor neuron disease, this patient's lower motor neuron findings are confined to the distribution of the C8 and T1 nerve roots. A lesion compressing the nerve roots and spinal cord at this level would produce lower motor neuron findings locally and upper motor neuron signs in the lower extremities, while sparing structures higher up, explaining the normal arm reflexes (mediated by roots C5–C7), cranial nerves, and mental status. The symptoms have been progressive, with a chronic time course. A chronic, focal lesion is generally a neoplasm. He needs an imaging study of the cervical spine.

Comment: In this case, an MRI scan of the cervical spine showed degenerative spine changes and compression of the spinal cord. A multilevel decompressive laminectomy was performed with slight benefit.

Case 4. This patient also has disequilibrium rather than vertigo. Like the patient in Case 3, he has a gait disorder and urinary incontinence. The diffuse hyperreflexia suggests upper motor neuron involvement. Cervical spine disease is once again an important consideration, and this could be an urgent problem. In addition, however, this patient has dementia, indicating diffuse involvement of the cerebral hemispheres. It is possible that this is unrelated, as dementia and cervical spine disease are both relatively common in 65-year-old people, and some patients have both conditions just on the basis of chance. On the other hand, the triad of gait disturbance, dementia, and incontinence suggests the diagnosis of normal pressure hydrocephalus (see Chapter 7). One reasonable approach to evaluating this patient would be to obtain an imaging study of the head, and if it did not show prominent hydrocephalus, to proceed with an imaging study of the cervical spine.

Comment: In this case, a head CT scan confirmed markedly enlarged ventricles with only mild sulcal enlargement. The patient's gait disorder and incontinence resolved with shunting, and his dementia stopped progressing but did not resolve.

Chapter 15

Back Pain and Neck Pain

I. Case Histories

Case 1. A 55-year-old woman with a history of heavy tobacco use and right lung resection for cancer one year ago has come to your office because, while lifting a heavy box yesterday, she suddenly developed a sharp pain that started in her low back and shot into her right buttock, posterior thigh, and posterior leg. On examination, you note a positive straight leg raising sign on the right, slight weakness of right ankle plantar flexion, and a reduced right ankle jerk.

Case 2. A 50-year-old hypertensive, diabetic man has come to the emergency department "to get some relief." Over the years, his back would "go out" on him now and then, but he would stay in bed for a day, apply heat, and wear a corset for the next two weeks and he would be "as good as new." Six weeks ago his back went out on him again, but it did not resolve as it had previously. If anything, it seems to be getting worse. It keeps him awake at night, and he is having trouble concentrating at work. He has no pain in his legs, and no difficulty with bladder or bowel function. His examination is notable only for obesity, tight muscles throughout the lower back, and mild tenderness in that region. He has no tenderness along the spine. His motor examination, reflexes, and sensory examination are all normal.

Questions:

1. What diagnoses should be considered?
2. What tests should be ordered?
3. What treatment should be prescribed?

II. Approach to Back or Neck Pain

There are two principal questions to address in evaluating a patient with back or neck pain:

A. Does the patient have a condition that might require urgent treatment?

B. Even if it isn't urgent, will the patient require surgery?

A. Emergency Situations

Patients with symptoms or signs suggesting rapidly progressive damage to the spinal cord or multiple nerve roots need an urgent MRI scan (or, occasionally, a myelogram) of the involved area of the spinal canal. If a soft tissue mass is compressing the spinal cord or multiple nerve roots, it could be a metastasis, an epidural abscess, a primary tumor, a hematoma, or an acute disc herniation. If the patient is already known to have cancer somewhere else in the body, and the imaging characteristics of the spinal lesion are consistent with metastasis, the patient can be treated accordingly. If the imaging characteristics are ambiguous, especially in a patient with no known cancer, the patient will generally need a surgical procedure to establish a diagnosis and at the same time to decompress the lesion (and sometimes to stabilize the spine).

Even without evidence of neurologic deterioration, any patient with known cancer who develops back or neck pain requires an MRI scan (or in rare circumstances, a myelogram) of the painful region to look for a spinal metastasis. Only when the likelihood of metastatic disease is extremely low (i.e., the pain is characterized as a dull ache confined to the paraspinal area, the patient has had no recent constitutional symptoms such as fever or weight loss, the neurologic examination is completely normal, and plain x-rays of the symptomatic region of the spine are benign) is it safe to treat the patient symptomatically without further testing.

If a patient is found to have spinal cord compression due to a metastatic lesion, high-dose dexamethasone (Decadron) should be started immediately and arrangements made for direct decompressive surgery, followed by radiation therapy (based on the results of one randomized trial and a number of uncontrolled series). If a patient is found to have a vertebral metastasis without evidence of spinal cord compression, or if there are multiple vertebral metastases, the patient should receive radiation therapy without surgical decompression.

If imaging studies do not reveal a compressive lesion, patients with focal signs or symptoms should be evaluated for noncompressive causes of the neurologic abnormalities. For example, patients with myelopathy should be evaluated for transverse myelitis, vitamin B12 deficiency, and other inflammatory and metabolic conditions.

B. Non-urgent Indications for Surgery

Even when patients do not require urgent decompression, their back or neck pain could still be caused by a structural lesion that might eventually require surgical intervention. The main indications for surgery are the following:

1. Spinal cord compression,
2. Compression of one or more nerve roots causing persistent motor deficits or abnormal control of bladder or bowels,
3. Lumbar spinal stenosis, or
4. A mass lesion of unknown etiology.

Surgery is also performed on occasion when patients have pain that is refractory to all nonsurgical treatment, if the pain is in a distribution that clearly corresponds to the structural lesion.

Thus, patients who have symptoms or signs that suggest lumbar spinal stenosis or damage to the spinal cord or to one or more nerve roots should have an MRI scan (or myelogram) of the appropriate region of the spinal canal. The imaging study can be scheduled electively to be done within the next few weeks as long as the patient has no known cancer, no erosive bone lesions on plain films of the spine, and no clinical evidence of rapid progression.

III. Specific Conditions Causing Back or Neck Pain

A. Musculoskeletal Pain

In the vast majority of patients with back or neck pain, the pain is diffuse, with no specific signs or symptoms to suggest damage to individual nerve roots. This is a very common problem, but it is not well understood. It is generally thought to be a musculoskeletal problem related to frequent excessive stress on the bones, muscles, and connective tissue elements that support the back. The pain generally improves over time even in untreated patients. If the neurologic examination is normal, further diagnostic testing is unnecessary. In the past, patients with low back pain were routinely instructed to stay at strict bed rest for two weeks or more, but the evidence indicates that patients who are instructed to continue with their ordinary activities have better outcomes than patients assigned to bed rest.

Treatment approaches include physical therapy, heat, ultrasound, analgesics, nonsteroidal anti-inflammatory drugs, tricyclic antidepressants, some anti-epileptic drugs (notably gabapentin), acupuncture, yoga, chiropractic manipulation (for the low back, *not the neck*, because of the risk of arterial dissection with neck manipulation), and soft tissue injections (with anesthetic agents, steroids, or botulinum toxin). The evidence that any of these treatments can change the long-term course of the condition is weak, although most provide at least temporary relief. A reasonable approach is to prescribe a nonsteroidal anti-inflammatory drug and to instruct the patient to continue a moderate level of activity, but to focus on correct postures and avoid major back strain or lifting. Recovery occurs within four weeks in 90% of patients. Physical therapy should be considered in those who fail to improve. Patients may require trials of several medications or physical therapy regimens.

B. Disc Herniation

A herniated intervertebral disc can exert pressure on a nerve root and produce pain. This is far less common than musculoskeletal pain. The classic history for a lumbosacral disc herniation is a sudden pain in the low back during heavy lifting, later radiating into one lower extremity in a band conforming to the distribution of the L5 or S1 nerve root. Pain in this distribution is often referred to as *sciatica*, but this term should be avoided because it has been used in so many different ways that it is ambiguous. The pain of a herniated disc is worst when sitting and is exacerbated by coughing, sneezing, or straining at bowel movements. These classic features are not always present, however. For example, many patients have no precipitating event, some patients have only lower extremity pain with no back pain, and others have the opposite.

A straight leg raising sign is usually present: patients experience extreme pain when the hip is passively flexed while holding the knee extended. This pain is exacerbated by dorsiflexion of the ankle and relieved by flexion of the knee. This sign is sensitive but not specific. Some patients with a herniated disc will have weakness in the distribution of the involved nerve root, and some may have reduction of the relevant tendon reflex. When the nerve root irritation is severe, abnormalities may be detected on EMG and motor nerve conduction studies.

For cervical disc herniation, the antecedent injury—when there is one— often involves rapid head turning. Pain or numbness extends from the neck into one arm or the medial scapula, conforming to the territory of a single cervical nerve root (or two adjacent nerve roots). Patients may also have weakness, atrophy, and hyporeflexia in the distribution of the affected nerve root.

For both cervical and lumbar discs, the risk of neurologic impairment is greatest when the herniation is in the midline, rather than laterally. In the case of a cervical disc, this can put pressure on the spinal cord, which can affect function of the lower extremities, bladder, or bowels. Patients with cervical disc herniation may have little or no neck pain, presenting instead with gradually progressive gait disturbance. Many of these patients are found to have completely normal strength in the lower extremities; their gait problems are primarily a result of spasticity. When a lumbar disc herniates centrally, it can compress the cauda equina, resulting in diffuse lower extremity weakness and numbness, as well as loss of bladder and bowel control.

Disc herniation, like musculoskeletal pain, is incompletely understood. Although the symptoms suggest nerve root irritation, and imaging studies show impingement on the nerve root by the disc, many patients' symptoms resolve without resolution of the imaging abnormalities. Other patients with no history of any pain or neurologic symptoms have disc herniation as an incidental finding on imaging studies. The degree of inflammatory reaction around the nerve root may be an important factor in determining whether a herniated disc produces symptoms.

The symptoms of disc herniation, like those of musculoskeletal pain, often resolve even without specific therapy. The same treatment modalities are used, with the same lack of clear evidence that they improve the already favorable natural course of the disease. Controlled trials of bed rest excluded patients with evidence of radiculopathy or myelopathy, so it is not known whether bed rest is helpful for patients with disc herniation, but it is often prescribed. Epidural steroid injections are commonly administered, also, although their benefit has not been clearly established. Decompressive surgery is another option. Randomized trials have shown no significant difference in long-term outcome between patients treated surgically and patients treated conservatively, although the rate of perceived recovery is faster for patients in the surgical group. The efficacy and indications for minimally invasive procedures (such as microdiscectomy or percutaneous discectomy) relative to traditional open discectomy have not been established. Surgery is usually reserved for patients who have failed to respond to conservative treatments (especially bed rest, analgesics, and physical therapy), patients with substantial motor deficits (especially when they are progressive), or patients with involvement of bladder or bowels. Patients who do not fall into one of these categories should be treated in the same way as patients with musculoskeletal pain, and imaging studies may not even be necessary.

C. Spinal Stenosis

Over time, there may be growth of bony elements in the spinal canal, resulting in significant narrowing of the canal (especially when superimposed on a congenitally narrow canal). In the cervical spine, this produces the same symptoms as a disc herniation, and the management is analogous. In the lumbar canal, spinal stenosis often produces a syndrome known as neurogenic claudication—pain in the low back or legs provoked by standing and relieved by bending over or sitting down. Unlike vascular claudication, the pain is related to position and not to exertion (walking is no worse than standing, and riding a bike may produce no pain at all). This condition is less likely than disc herniation to respond to conservative measures and generally requires surgical decompression.

IV. Discussion of Case Histories

Case 1. This patient has characteristic features of an acute S1 radiculopathy and most likely has a disc herniation at L5–S1. Even so, with the history of recent cancer, you must be sure she does not have a metastatic lesion at this level. You should order an urgent MRI (or if it is not possible, a myelogram) of the lumbosacral spine. If metastatic disease is present, start dexamethasone (Decadron) and arrange radiation therapy; if it is not, prescribe a nonsteroidal anti-inflammatory drug, activity modification, and a gentle stretching program.

Case 2. This is an example of musculoskeletal pain. There is no radiation of the pain along a nerve root, and there are no focal findings on examination. The long history of similar problems makes it very unlikely that the patient has a new structural lesion, and no imaging studies are necessary. This kind of pain may be just as severe as the pain from a herniated disc or metastatic cancer. The patient has already discovered for himself several of the conservative measures that are often used to treat this problem. Because his symptoms persist despite these measures, he should be given a prescription for a nonsteroidal anti-inflammatory drug and possibly a tricyclic antidepressant (which may be synergistic), while undergoing a physical therapy program designed to teach him gentle stretching exercises and educate him about correct posture. Ultimately, weight loss would help to relieve the mechanical stress on his spine and might prevent future exacerbations.

Chapter 16

Incontinence

I. Case Histories

Case 1. A 55-year-old multiparous woman complains of "accidents" with her bladder whenever she sneezes or coughs. Otherwise, she is able to void normally and has no bowel or sexual dysfunction. She has no other symptoms and her neurologic examination is normal.

Case 2. A 40-year-old man with limb-girdle muscular dystrophy has had episodes of bowel and bladder incontinence for the past several months. He has no difficulty sensing when he "needs to go." He has started using a bedside commode, and this has solved his problem with nocturnal incontinence, but he still has difficulty when he is away from his home. He has started scouting out the restrooms whenever he goes to a new place, because he can avoid accidents as long as he can make it to the restroom quickly enough. He has also noticed progressive difficulty with walking over the past year. He has no sensory symptoms. His sexual function has been normal. His examination is notable for profound proximal weakness of the legs and arms, and a slow, waddling gait. Perianal sensation and anal wink reflex are normal. Deep tendon reflexes are normal and plantar responses are flexor.

Case 3. A 60-year-old woman with chronic back pain due to degenerative lumbar spine disease has developed urinary incontinence characterized by frequent dribbling of small amounts of urine without any sensation of a need to void. She has also noted mild lower extremity weakness and an increase in her baseline lower extremity numbness. Examination is notable for weakness of ankle dorsiflexion, absent ankle jerks, and numbness on the lateral borders of the feet and in the perianal region. Rectal tone is decreased.

Questions:

1. What is the likely explanation for each patient's incontinence?
2. Which of these is an urgent problem?

II. Background Information

The normal bladder stores a large volume of urine at low pressure. Continence is maintained (generally unconsciously) by contraction of muscle fibers in the bladder neck (internal sphincter) and urethra (external sphincter). A micturition reflex is triggered when a sufficient volume of urine collects in the bladder. Except at extremely high bladder volumes, a normal individual is able to inhibit this reflex until a socially convenient time. The reflex produces a coordinated event in which the internal and external sphincters open and the detrusor muscle in the bladder wall contracts, while the junctions between the bladder and the ureters are compressed to prevent reflux toward the kidney. The coordination between bladder and sphincter contraction is largely mediated by a micturition center in the pons.

The majority of detrusor motor innervation is cholinergic from the pelvic parasympathetic plexus, which derives from the S2–S4 nerve roots. Sympathetic adrenergic fibers originating at the T10–L2 levels provide the major motor innervation of the distal ureters, trigone, and bladder neck. Voluntary sphincter control is mediated by the pudendal nerve, which is derived from the S2–S4 nerve roots.

III. Approach to Incontinence

Incontinence is a particularly distressing symptom for patients and their families, and this would be reason enough to evaluate it promptly. In addition, although incontinence is not an emergency in and of itself, it sometimes indicates the presence of an underlying neurologic condition that must be addressed urgently. This chapter focuses on urinary incontinence, but the same principles apply when evaluating neurologic causes of fecal incontinence. Neurologic conditions more often produce urinary incontinence than fecal incontinence, and when both occur, urinary incontinence generally appears first.

Two questions must be addressed in evaluating a patient with urinary incontinence:

A. Is the problem related to nervous system control of bladder function?

B. If so, what level of the nervous system is involved?

A. Neurologic vs. Urologic Causes of Incontinence

The most common cause of incontinence is weakness of the mechanical structures supporting the urethral sphincters. This produces *stress incontinence*, characterized by leakage of small amounts of urine during any activity that results in increased intra-abdominal pressure, such as coughing or sneezing. In normal individuals, increased abdominal pressure is transmitted equally to the bladder and proximal urethra, so that the pressure across the sphincter remains constant. Stress incontinence occurs when there is relaxation of pelvic floor musculature and partial herniation of the proximal urethra through the pelvic floor, so that increases in abdominal pressure result in an increased pressure gradient across the sphincter. This problem is common in elderly women, especially those who have had several vaginal deliveries. It is unusual in men unless their urinary sphincters have been damaged during past surgery. There are generally no associated abnormalities on neurologic examination. Treatment consists of pelvic floor exercises, pessaries (instruments placed in the vagina to support the uterus), and various surgical procedures designed to augment the mechanics of the external sphincter.

The term functional incontinence applies to any condition that results in difficulty reaching a toilet quickly in a patient whose bladder, its associated sphincters, and their nerve supply all function normally. The most self-evident example is a patient in mechanical restraints. Limb pain or weakness may be less obvious, but no less an obstacle to patient mobility. Confused patients may manifest functional incontinence simply because they can't find the bathroom. Making the diagnosis of functional incontinence can sometimes be tricky, especially when the condition limiting mobility is a neurologic problem that could also be affecting bladder function directly. The main question is whether the problem would persist even if the patient could get to the bathroom quickly. It sometimes suffices to ask this directly. If patients have trouble answering this question, they should be asked whether they can recognize when the bladder is full and whether they can inhibit urination for a brief time. Functional incontinence is managed by maximizing mobility, providing adult diapers, and placing commodes in strategic locations in the home.

A damaged urinary sphincter may be inadequate to maintain a tight seal, resulting in leakage of urine from the bladder. This can be caused by neurologic injury or may be the result of prior surgery or trauma. The standard surgical procedures for stress incontinence are not helpful in this condition, but use of a pubovaginal sling is effective. In males, an artificial urinary sphincter can be inserted. Other non-neurologic causes of incontinence include medication side effects (e.g., diuretics and alpha-adrenergic antagonists), volume overload, diabetes mellitus, diabetes insipidus, urinary tract infection, and reduced bladder compliance.

B. Central vs. Peripheral Nervous System Causes of Incontinence

Lesions at any level of the nervous system can cause incontinence. The main localizing distinction is between a *spastic bladder* and a *flaccid bladder*. Patients with a spastic bladder experience *urge incontinence*— a sudden, uncontrollable urge to void, with complete emptying of the bladder contents. In patients with a flaccid bladder, the muscle in the bladder wall does not contract either voluntarily or reflexively; these patients tend to retain urine, and the bladder expands passively until its capacity has been surpassed, at which point urine may leak out in small volumes. This is called *overflow incontinence*. Unlike stress incontinence, this can occur even without any elevation of intra-abdominal pressure.

A spastic bladder indicates an upper motor neuron problem and can result from lesions in the brain or spinal cord. Associated symptoms and examination findings may permit a more precise localization. For example, limb hyperreflexia and a sensory level suggest myelopathy. The coexistence of dementia and gait disorder suggests normal pressure hydrocephalus (see Chapter 7). Other dementing illnesses may also result in incontinence because of disinhibition.

A flaccid bladder corresponds to a lower motor neuron lesion. It can result from any condition that disturbs the nerves that supply the bladder after they have exited the spinal cord. For example, overflow incontinence is the typical pattern that occurs in patients with diabetic polyneuropathy. Associated symptoms and signs again provide clues to the site of pathology; a patient with sacral numbness, leg weakness, and hyporeflexia at the ankles and knees, for example, may have a lesion of the cauda equina. Overflow incontinence can also occur in patients who have an upper motor neuron lesion that is below the level of the pontine micturition center. Such lesions produce not only a spastic bladder but also *detrusor-external sphincter dyssynergia*, in which the timing of bladder and sphincter contraction is poorly coordinated so that the bladder contracts against a closed sphincter. This condition often leads to ureteral reflux.

When historical information and examination findings are insufficient to discriminate between a flaccid bladder and a spastic bladder, useful information may be obtained from urodynamic studies, in which the bladder pressure is measured at different volumes. The point at which the subject feels an urge to void and the point at which the urge to void cannot be overcome are recorded, as is any residual volume in the bladder after voiding. This study is called a cystometrogram. Even if a complete urodynamic study is not feasible, the post-void residual can be measured by catheterizing the bladder immediately after the patient voids spontaneously.

Neurogenic incontinence is treated by addressing the underlying neurologic problem to the extent possible. When there is a structural lesion affecting the spinal cord or the cauda equina, urgent decompressive surgery may be necessary. In addition, symptomatic improvement can often be achieved using anticholinergic medications to inhibit bladder wall contraction. Commonly used drugs include oxybutynin (Ditropan), tolterodine (Detrol), solifenacin (Vesicare), darifenacin (Enablex), trospium (Sanctura), and fesoterodine (Toviaz). In principle, alpha-adrenergic agonists can be used to enhance sphincter tone, but side-effects limit the use of this class of medication. Timed voiding may help prevent the bladder from filling to the point where reflex emptying occurs. Patients are often counseled to limit their evening fluid intake to minimize nocturia, but the effectiveness of this approach has not been proven. Electrical stimulation of the S3 nerve root or the pudendal nerve has been advocated for selected patients. In some patients, catheterization is necessary, especially when detrusor-external sphincter dyssynergia is present.

IV. Discussion of Case Histories

Case 1. This patient is describing typical stress incontinence. In the absence of other symptoms or examination abnormalities, no tests are indicated. This is not an urgent problem. Treatment is described in Part III, Section A.

Case 2. This patient has functional incontinence that is the result of deteriorating ability to walk because of his progressive muscle disease. The diagnosis is based on the history and examination; no tests are indicated. This is a serious but not urgent problem. Treatment of the incontinence is described in Part III, Section A. Unfortunately, no treatment is available for his underlying muscular dystrophy.

Case 3. This patient's incontinence is an important clue to an urgent neurologic problem. The lower extremity weakness and decreased reflexes suggest a lower motor neuron problem, and this is consistent with the flaccid character of her urinary symptoms. The distribution of her weakness and sensory abnormalities (including abnormal sacral sensation) suggests involvement of several different nerve roots bilaterally, and the most likely lesion localization would be the cauda equina. The time course is difficult to determine. Her urinary symptoms are subacute, but she has had chronic back pain and lower extremity numbness. This suggests a chronic process that has recently accelerated. A chronic, focal lesion is most likely a tumor. This patient needs an imaging study urgently, and she may need emergency surgery for diagnosis and decompression.

Comment: An MRI scan of the lumbosacral spine showed a prominent disc herniation with compression of multiple sacral nerve roots. This is yet another example of how the rules of Chapter 3 are approximations, lumping many different "new growths" into the category of neoplasm. Even so, cancer was a realistic possibility, and use of the rules resulted in the appropriate diagnostic test with the correct level of urgency. This patient was taken for decompressive surgery immediately, because a delay could have resulted in permanent loss of bladder and bowel function.

IV

Bookends

Chapter 17

Pediatric Neurology

I. Case Histories

The five questions below apply to all of the case histories that follow:

1. What additional historical information would be most useful?
2. Which parts of the neurologic examination would most likely provide helpful data?
3. What diagnoses should be considered?
4. How should the patient be evaluated?
5. How should the patient be managed?

Cases 1 and 2: Spells

Case 1. A 5-year-old boy was well until about a month ago, when he started having spells characterized by speech arrest and subtle, unilateral facial twitching. The episodes last one to five minutes. During the spells, he appears to understand what people say to him, and he sometimes says a few words. He has had at least twenty such episodes so far.

Case 2. An 8-year-old boy has been exhibiting unusual repetitive movements for the past three months. For the first two months, he repeatedly blinked his eyes and jerked his head. These symptoms resolved spontaneously, but they were followed two weeks later by intermittent episodes of repetitive hand clapping and throat clearing.

Cases 3 and 4: Ataxia

Case 3. Seven days after a 7-year-old girl developed chickenpox, her parents noted that she was very unsteady. She was able to sit up, but she was unable to walk. She was mentally alert, and when she was lying down she had normal strength in all four limbs.

Case 4. A 4-year-old boy has been experiencing occasional headaches for the past several months. He has also had some vague stomach problems and vomiting over the same period. For the past week, his gait has been increasingly unsteady, and he has fallen a few times.

Cases 5 and 6: Toe Walking

Case 5. A 3-year-old girl has always walked on her toes. Her parents were initially told that this would probably resolve, and they are concerned because it hasn't. The patient and her twin sister were born at gestational age 32 weeks. The patient has made regular developmental gains, but all motor milestones have been delayed relative to her twin.

Case 6. A 3-year-old boy has recently developed a tendency to walk on his toes. He was born at term, and his initial development was considered normal, although he lagged a little behind his twin sister in all aspects of development. He walked at age 18 months. He has always had trouble running or climbing stairs, but recently he has been stumbling and falling more frequently.

Cases 7, 8, and 9: School Problems

Case 7. A 7-year-old girl has been referred for unusual behavior and problems at school for the past three months. She had been a model student last year, but lately her school performance has been inconsistent. The girl's teacher has observed that she often appears to be daydreaming, and she sometimes fails to complete tasks. The family had noted similar behavior at home but had not considered it abnormal.

Case 8. A 9-year-old boy has just transferred to a new school, and an initial evaluation indicates that he is 18 months behind in his reading skills. He has previously been diagnosed as dyslexic and hyperactive, and he is being treated with methylphenidate (Ritalin). The boy's parents and pediatrician all think that his attention and behavior have improved markedly with this treatment. The boy's family is also concerned because he has not learned how to ride a bicycle, and he is awkward and uncoordinated.

Case 9. A 10-year-old boy is being evaluated for a decline in school performance over the past six to nine months. He had always been an "A" student before but is now failing in all subjects. He is apathetic and insolent to his teacher, who says that he "seems like a different boy." His parents divorced about a year ago, and the boy's difficulties were initially attributed to psychosocial stress. He has had no headaches, seizures, or loss of motor skills.

II. Developmental Considerations

Children are immature. This is hardly a revelation, yet it expresses a fundamental principle of human biology. Although the human brain has an enormous capacity for complex processing, most of its potential is unrealized at birth. In other species, a newborn is able to walk, swim, or fly almost immediately, with full adult function acquired within a few years at most. In humans, the process takes more than a decade (and, of course, "some kids never grow up"). This confers great flexibility, allowing children to develop functions that are directly adapted to their particular environment. In essence, the process results in "custom-made" brains, rather than assembly line products. The most obvious example is language. Different cultures, different regions, and above all, different eras have vastly different vocabulary needs, and the rate at which evolution proceeds is far too slow to accommodate them. Instead, heredity provides a general program for linguistic processing, but environmental exposure determines the specific language elements that an individual acquires. The same principle of developmental plasticity applies to most aspects of perception, motor function, and cognition. Without plasticity, there would be no learning.

Developmental plasticity is the main feature distinguishing pediatric neurology from adult neurology. The diagnostic principles presented in the first three chapters of this book still apply, but many of the nervous system functions typically assessed in adults are not fully operational until months or years after birth. Obvious examples are walking, talking, and control of bladder and bowel function. Incontinence in an adult patient is clearly abnormal and suggests a set of specific lesion sites (see Chapter 16). Incontinence in a pediatric patient may be significant or not, depending on the patient's age. The same is true of the inability to walk or talk. Conversely, some reflexes normally present in infancy disappear as children age. Thus, a child's developmental stage determines how the examination is interpreted and how it is performed.

The effects of disease also vary depending on an individual's developmental stage. The developing nervous system is extremely vulnerable to some injuries that have little effect on the mature nervous system, whereas developmental plasticity permits more complete recovery from some injuries in children than in adults.

This chapter is not meant to be a comprehensive survey of the vast array of diseases that affect the developing nervous system. Rather, the goal is to present a general approach to some of the more common clinical situations that occur primarily in the pediatric population.

III. Hypotonic Infants

Newborn infants have very limited behavioral repertoires. The most common manifestation of neurologic disease at this age is abnormal motor activity. In particular, parents report a "floppy baby," and physicians observe hypotonia. There are several ways to assess an infant's tone. One way is to pull the baby by the hands from a supine to a seated position. A normal, full-term baby will flex the neck to lift the head from the surface along with the body. Another way to assess tone is to suspend the baby with the abdomen lying on your outstretched hand—normal infants will straighten their back, flex their limbs, and hold their head straight or extended. A hypotonic infant held in this way will be limp, with head and limbs drooping down over your hand. A normal infant can be held vertically by supporting the axillae, whereas a hypotonic infant tends to "slip through" the examiner's hands. The assessment of tone requires a fair amount of experience with the expected range of variation among normal infants.

Unlike adults, who manifest reduced tone with LMN lesions but increased tone with UMN lesions, infants manifest hypotonia with lesions anywhere in the motor pathway. Consequently, other features must be used to distinguish between central and peripheral lesions. Infants with peripheral hypotonia (caused by lesions at the level of anterior horn cell, nerve root, peripheral nerve, neuromuscular junction, or muscle) typically have severe weakness, with reduced or absent tendon reflexes. When hypotonia is due to lesions at the level of the spinal cord or higher, the hypotonia is usually more profound than the weakness, and tendon reflexes are normal or brisk. When the lesion is in the cerebral hemispheres, there are often additional manifestations of cerebral malfunction (such as seizures or reduced alertness).

Central hypotonia may be idiopathic, or it may result from intrauterine or perinatal hypoxic-ischemic events, chromosomal abnormalities (such as Down syndrome, Prader-Willi syndrome, or Turner's syndrome), congenital malformations, infections, and a variety of metabolic derangements including hypoglycemia, hyperbilirubinemia, hypothyroidism, leukodystrophy, and drug intoxication. Many of these conditions can be evaluated by obtaining an imaging study of the brain, checking serum electrolytes and glucose, and taking a careful history of intrauterine and postnatal drug exposure.

Some of the peripheral causes of hypotonia are hereditary (especially myotonic dystrophy, some metabolic myopathies, and some neuropathies), so the diagnosis can sometimes be made by taking a careful family history or examining family members. Approximately 15% of infants born to mothers with myasthenia gravis have hypotonia and weakness, traditionally attributed to passive transfer of maternal antibodies, although this explanation has been challenged. The average duration of symptoms is 18 days. Spinal muscular atrophies (SMAs) are hereditary forms of lower motor neuron disease. Type 1 SMA is an acute, fulminating form that begins at birth or within the first six months of life. Mothers often report marked reduction or disappearance of fetal movements during the final months of pregnancy. Type 2 SMA usually becomes symptomatic between the ages of 6 and 18 months, and type 3 after the age of 18 months (usually between 5 and 15 years of age). Types 2 and 3 are milder and more slowly progressive than type 1. Postural or kinetic tremor of the hands is common in types 2 and 3, but rare in type 1. Areflexia is typical of all three types. All three forms are caused by mutations in a gene that is known as the survival motor neuron 1 (SMN1) gene, but the specific phenotype is a function of nearby genes, including a nearly identical gene known as SMN2. The function of the protein coded by these genes is not completely understood. Infantile botulism is caused by ingestion of food (most often honey) or soil containing the bacterium, which colonizes the gut and produces toxin (in contrast to adults, who have defenses against the bacterium, and only acquire the disease by ingesting already-manufactured toxin). Detailed questions about what the child has recently eaten may be key to the diagnosis. A history of constipation is typical. Other historical information may provide clues to other metabolic or toxic conditions. Specific biochemical or genetic assays, nerve conduction studies, EMG, and muscle biopsy may help clarify the diagnosis.

IV. Developmental Delay and Developmental Regression

The process of development varies considerably from one child to the next, but it proceeds in the same general sequence and in a similar time frame in all children. When children reach developmental milestones at a slow rate that is clearly outside the normal range, it is called *developmental delay*.

This determination requires comparison to expectations for "normal" children. Because the range of normal is so broad, and the stigma associated with developmental delay is so great, this label should only be applied when a child is unequivocally outside the normal range.

When children who develop at a normal rate begin to lose some of the skills they have already acquired, it is called *developmental regression*. This diagnosis can be assigned even without reference to "normal" ranges, because it is based purely on a child's own previous development. Nonetheless, caution must be exercised in diagnosing developmental regression, because even normal children intermittently regress slightly.

An isolated, time-limited insult to the nervous system, such as an infection or head trauma, can result in developmental delay. Although the event itself may be transient, the damage it produces may severely limit or even abolish the nervous system's capacity to develop further. On the other hand, regression usually implies an ongoing disease process. Although a one-time event may retard or halt forward progress, it does not usually result in backward movement.

Developmental delay can affect various components of development—motor, language, cognitive, and social—either in isolation or in combination, and the differential diagnosis depends on the pattern of impairment. *Cerebral palsy* is defined as a nonprogressive (static) abnormality of control of movement or posture due to CNS dysfunction that is prenatal or perinatal in onset and not degenerative. The differential diagnosis includes most of the conditions (except for chromosomal abnormalities) that can cause central hypotonia in infants—note that as children mature and their nervous systems myelinate, the hypotonia is replaced by spasticity, so most patients with cerebral palsy eventually manifest spasticity rather than hypotonia. By definition, patients with cerebral palsy have delayed motor development; they may or may not have abnormal language or overall cognition.

The most common cause of an isolated delay in language development is hearing impairment. Children with language delay should have formal audiologic testing, because the language disorder may resolve once the hearing impairment is addressed. Other causes of developmental language disorders include hereditary factors and perinatal injury. In older children who have difficulty with reading and writing despite normal initial language development, dyslexia is an important consideration.

Children who have widespread cognitive delay, affecting other intellectual functions in addition to language, should still have their hearing tested, but hearing impairment is unlikely to be the sole problem. The differential diagnosis for widespread cognitive delay without motor involvement is similar to that for global developmental delay, discussed in the following paragraph, but a few conditions are particularly likely to affect cognition out of proportion to motor involvement. When abnormal social development and restricted activities and interests accompany language delay, autism (or, more generally, an *autistic spectrum disorder*) is the prime consideration. Uncontrolled generalized seizures may also result in learning problems, or even in intellectual deterioration (though it is often difficult to determine how much of the deterioration is due to the seizures themselves and how much is a result of the disease process that underlies the seizures). *Attention deficit hyperactivity disorder (ADHD)* is a potential cause of delayed learning. It has received a great deal of publicity in recent years, with reports of the prevalence ranging from 1–20%; this wide range probably reflects the lack of a biological marker. ADHD is characterized by inappropriate inattention, impulsivity, distractibility, and hyperactivity beyond the normal range for age. The most common treatment, methylphenidate (Ritalin), has been inappropriately prescribed for many children who do not meet specific diagnostic criteria. Psychological factors can also impede school performance; a useful clue is that the child's problems are often restricted to particular activities, with relative sparing of language skills, self-care ability, and performance in recreational activities.

Global developmental delay (affecting motor function, language, overall cognition, and social interaction) is most often a result of an infectious, toxic, or hypoxic-ischemic injury that occurred in utero or perinatally. Less often, global developmental delay may result from genetic abnormalities or the same kinds of ongoing disease processes that typically produce developmental regression. The most common inherited cause of global developmental delay is *fragile X syndrome*, caused by an expanded triplet repeat in an uncoded region of a gene on the X chromosome that codes for the "fragile X mental retardation protein" (FMRP). In normal neurons, FMRP associates with an RNA-induced silencing complex and destroys messenger RNA, preventing the synthesis of specific proteins. Most of the proteins regulated by FMRP are localized in dendrites. Neuronal activity inactivates FMRP, allowing those proteins to be synthesized. This process is probably important in neuronal plasticity. Patients with fragile X syndrome have little or no FMRP, so the FMRP's usual target mRNAs are never suppressed, and the corresponding proteins are continuously synthesized, regardless of synaptic activity. This presumably interferes with learning-dependent synaptic changes. Because the gene is on the X chromosome, the disease affects males more severely and more frequently than females. This syndrome produces features of mental retardation, autism, and ADHD. It is also associated with characteristic craniofacial features, joint abnormalities, and impaired motor skills. As discussed in Chapter 8, carriers with triplet expansions shorter than 200 repeats may develop fragile X-associated tremor ataxia syndrome (FXTAS), usually presenting after age 55 years. This condition is not due to an absence of FMRP—instead, the triplet expansion is thought to exert a neurotoxic effect by sequestering and perturbing the function of nuclear proteins.

A vast array of disease processes can cause intellectual and motor regression. These include infections, tumors, toxic exposure, vascular conditions, metabolic conditions, and endocrine disorders. Many of these conditions involve components of the nervous system and other organ systems in specific patterns that provide clues to the diagnosis. The family history is helpful in diagnosing the many metabolic conditions and malformations that are genetic. The age of onset is also helpful in narrowing the diagnosis. More detailed algorithms and tables are available in standard textbooks of pediatric neurology.

V. Paroxysmal Symptoms

As noted in Chapter 3, the most common causes of paroxysmal focal neurologic symptoms in adults are transient ischemic attacks, seizures, and migraines. Atherosclerosis is a disease of adults, and although other cerebrovascular diseases may occur in children, they are not usually associated with transient ischemic attacks. Seizures and migraines are therefore the most important causes of sudden and recurrent focal neurologic symptoms in children. Other paroxysmal conditions that can occur in childhood include breath-holding spells, night terrors, narcolepsy/cataplexy, tics, syncope, psychogenic spells, and benign paroxysmal vertigo. Most of these conditions are discussed in previous chapters, but several merit additional comment.

A. Headaches

Headaches are common in childhood, causing 10–12% of children to consult a physician. The same principles of evaluation and treatment that apply to adults (see Chapter 12) also hold for children. The abortive and prophylactic medications that are prescribed to adults are also effective in children, but the specific drugs used may differ because of different concerns about side effects. Cyclical vomiting (characterized by recurrent episodes of nausea and vomiting) and periodic abdominal pain are two variants of migraine that arise almost exclusively in childhood. These two syndromes frequently overlap. There is often no accompanying headache, but approximately 75% of these children develop typical migraine later in life, and the cyclical vomiting responds to typical migraine medications. Much less commonly, recurrent episodes of vomiting or abdominal pain may be associated with EEG changes and represent epileptic spells.

B. Seizures

Seizures in children are classified, evaluated, and managed according to the same principles that apply in adults (see Chapter 5). It is sometimes more difficult to recognize seizures in children than in adults, however. In neonates especially, the immaturity of the nervous system interferes with propagation of epileptic discharges, so classic tonic-clonic convulsions are rare. More common are brief episodes of hypertonia, atonia, or localized clonic movements. Neonatal seizures may also manifest with rhythmic or sustained eye movements, chewing, or unusual limb movements. Another unique feature of pediatric epilepsy is that certain seizure types arise only at particular ages. Infantile spasms, for example, usually present between the ages of 3 and 11 months; the first episode occurs during the first year of life in 75% of patients and before 2 years of age in 92%. Absence seizures almost always begin in childhood, with 64% of cases arising between the ages of 5 and 9 years. Benign rolandic epilepsy presents between the ages of 18 months and 13 years, usually between the ages of 5 and 10 years, and is typically outgrown by puberty. For more details regarding these conditions, see Chapter 5.

The same underlying processes that produce seizures in adults can cause seizures in children. Congenital brain defects and antenatal or perinatal injuries (especially hypoxic-ischemic and infectious) are common causes. Febrile seizures represent a separate category (see Chapter 5).

C. Breath-Holding Spells

Small children commonly hold their breath when crying, typically when fright, anger, or frustration precipitated the crying. When prolonged, breath-holding spells may result in seizures. The first attacks usually occur between the ages of 6 and 18 months, become less frequent with advancing age, and disappear by the age of 5 or 6 years. The family should be educated and reassured. No other treatment is necessary.

D. Benign Paroxysmal Vertigo

Benign paroxysmal vertigo of childhood is characterized by recurrent episodes of vertigo, vomiting, nystagmus, and diffuse pallor. The attacks usually last a few minutes, but sometimes last several hours. Children may fall during the attack, but they do not lose consciousness. Onset is usually between the ages of 1 and 4 years. The episodes eventually become less frequent and either disappear or are replaced by symptoms that are characteristic of migraine.

VI. Gait Disturbance

In both children and adults, abnormal gait can be a result of either focal lesions or diffuse processes. When the history and examination implicate a focal lesion, evaluation and treatment proceed in the same manner in children as in adults. When the symptoms are symmetric, the three most likely problems in all age groups are spasticity, weakness, and ataxia. The diagnostic considerations for each of these problems differ in children and adults.

A. Spasticity

As discussed in Part IV, conditions that produce central hypotonia in infants—notably intrauterine or perinatal damage, especially from hypoxic-ischemic events and infections—eventually result in spasticity, especially in the legs. When evaluating children with spastic gait, you should ask about intrauterine or perinatal complications and delayed motor or intellectual milestones. Structural lesions in the spinal cord or metabolic diseases (such as leukodystrophies) can also produce lower extremity spasticity, but the symptoms are usually progressive, resulting in loss of previously acquired function.

B. Weakness

The most important consideration in evaluating a diffusely weak child is whether the weakness is central or peripheral. Associated hyperreflexia and spasticity suggest a central process. As discussed in the previous paragraph, intrauterine or perinatal damage commonly results in spasticity that remains static over time, and spinal cord damage or metabolic disease typically causes progressive spasticity. Hypotonia, hyporeflexia, and muscle atrophy suggest disease at the level of the anterior horn cell, nerve root, peripheral nerve, neuromuscular junction, or muscle. The evaluation of neuromuscular disease is discussed in Chapter 6. The same principles apply in children and adults, but the particular diseases differ in the two groups. Muscular dystrophies and hereditary neuropathies are more likely to be important diagnostic considerations in children than in adults, for example, whereas conditions like inclusion body myositis (IBM) or diabetic neuropathy are common in adults but not in children.

C. Ataxia

In children, acute ataxia most commonly occurs in the setting of an infection or nonspecific febrile illness. A wide variety of organisms have been implicated, with varicella virus the most common. The condition may occur at any age, but it is most common between the ages of 1 and 5 years. It is characterized by the sudden onset of truncal ataxia, resulting in rapid deterioration of gait. Nystagmus is present in about half of the patients, and there may be prominent tremors of limbs, head, or trunk. The symptoms resolve completely in most children, usually within several months, but some children have permanent residua. The acute ataxia syndrome can also occur after children receive the varicella vaccine—which contains live, attenuated virus—but the incidence is much lower.

   Another cause of acute ataxia is toxic exposure, primarily to anti-epileptic drugs, alcohol, antihistamines, heavy metals, and mercury. Neuroblastomas are associated with a paraneoplastic syndrome consisting of ataxia, myoclonus, and opsoclonus (irregular, multidirectional involuntary eye movements). This syndrome is often the initial clinical manifestation of the tumor. The same syndrome sometimes occurs in patients with no associated tumor, and no explanation is found. Intermittent episodes of acute ataxia may occur with some metabolic diseases, such as disorders of amino acid metabolism, and also with ion channel diseases.

   Posterior fossa tumors can also cause acute ataxia, but they are much more likely to produce gradually progressive, chronic symptoms. Other causes of chronically progressive ataxia include Friedreich's ataxia and ataxia telangiectasia, both of which are discussed in Chapter 8. A number of metabolic conditions can also cause chronic, progressive ataxia.

VII. Discussion of Case Histories

Case 1. This boy has paroxysmal symptoms. They sound most like seizures; they could conceivably be tics, but tics usually occur more randomly, rather than in discrete episodes lasting up to 5 minutes. Migraine is unlikely, as the symptoms are not typical of migraine and he has no associated headache. None of the symptoms suggest any of the other paroxysmal conditions of childhood. Given the focal nature of the symptoms and the apparent preservation of consciousness, these would be classified as simple partial seizures. In particular, they are typical of the seizures that occur in the syndrome of benign rolandic epilepsy (see Chapter 5).

The history and examination should be directed at confirming this diagnostic impression and excluding any other type of seizures that might signal the need for more extensive evaluation. Thus, questions about family history are important. The patient and family should be asked about any symptoms that might suggest other kinds of seizures and about any progressive neurologic deficits. Any focal abnormality on examination should prompt further evaluation, because children with rolandic epilepsy typically have a normal neurologic examination. In the absence of any historical or examination evidence of progression, focality, or multiple seizure types, the diagnosis of rolandic epilepsy can be confirmed by finding characteristic abnormalities on EEG (epileptiform activity in the region of the Sylvian fissure). If the EEG does not show these abnormalities, an MRI would be indicated. This condition ultimately resolves, so lifelong treatment is not necessary. Anti-epileptic drugs may be used to reduce the frequency of seizures in the interim.

Case 2. This patient also has paroxysmal symptoms. They could conceivably be seizures, but the change in clinical characteristics after two months would be atypical. This would be more suggestive of a tic disorder. None of the other paroxysmal conditions of childhood are considerations in this case.

Further historical information that would be useful could be obtained by asking whether there is any impairment of awareness associated with the spells (which would favor seizures) and whether the boy can voluntarily suppress the movements, at least temporarily (which would favor tics). The boy's parents should be asked whether he has exhibited any other potential vocal tics in addition to his repetitive clearing of the throat. The patient and family should also be questioned about exposure to stimulants such as methylphenidate (Ritalin) and about weight loss, exercise tolerance, and behavioral changes to evaluate the possibility of hyperthyroidism, which can precipitate tics. A family history of similar involuntary movements, attention deficit disorder, or obsessive compulsive disorder would be consistent with Tourette's syndrome. On examination, direct observation of the involuntary movements would be particularly helpful. Unfortunately, since children can often suppress the movements transiently, they may disappear in the doctor's office even when they are reported to be very frequent at home or at school. Even so, close observation sometimes reveals subtle involuntary movements that the family may never even have noticed.

If the information gathered from the history and examination confirms that the movements are most likely tics, no further diagnostic testing is necessary. Symptoms often resolve spontaneously, so treatment is usually reserved for symptoms that have persisted and are significantly disruptive to the child. Pimozide, fluphenazine, haloperidol, clonidine, and guanfacine are helpful for treating tic disorders.

Case 3. This history is very suggestive of postinfectious ataxia, especially since varicella is the infectious agent most commonly associated with this disorder. If the history and examination confirm that the patient has ataxia rather than weakness, and if there are no other deficits, no evidence of pre-existing neurologic dysfunction, and no other potential causes of ataxia (especially toxic exposure), then additional tests may be unnecessary. It is sometimes appropriate to obtain an MRI scan of the brain (looking for hydrocephalus or a mass lesion in the posterior fossa) and a lumbar puncture (to exclude ongoing infection). If these tests are normal (or at most show a mild lymphocytic pleocytosis in the cerebrospinal fluid), only supportive therapy is required.

Case 4. This patient is also ataxic, but the several month history of associated symptoms suggests a more chronic condition. If his ataxia were intermittent, migraine would be a consideration, but this boy's gait has been growing progressively worse over the past week. The headaches and vomiting suggest increased intracranial pressure, making a posterior fossa mass lesion or hydrocephalus the two leading considerations. The history and examination should focus on any focal abnormalities that might help localize a mass lesion. In addition, increased intracranial pressure often causes papilledema, and the examiner should look carefully for eye movement abnormalities that can result from pressure on cranial nerves III, IV, or VI. In younger children, it would also be important to measure head circumference, because subacute decompensation of long-standing hydrocephalus may produce increased intracranial pressure.

If the examination confirms elevated intracranial pressure, an imaging study should be obtained urgently, because even children who look healthy may deteriorate rapidly. Either a CT scan or an MRI scan would be adequate to diagnose hydrocephalus, but an MRI scan is the optimal imaging technique in this setting because it provides much better resolution in the posterior fossa. Immediate neurosurgical evaluation is indicated if either hydrocephalus or a mass lesion is found. Temporizing treatment of increased intracranial pressure with dexamethasone, mannitol, or hyperventilation may also be necessary (see Chapter 11).

Case 5. This history suggests developmental delay rather than regression. Additional historical information about intellectual and motor milestones should be elicited to confirm or refute this impression. In a patient with gait disturbance caused by developmental delay, the examination usually reveals roughly symmetric lower extremity spasticity and hyperreflexia. If these examination findings are present in this patient, with a clear history of prematurity, consistent delays in motor development, and no regression, no additional diagnostic tests are necessary. Periventricular white matter injury is typically seen when a brain MRI scan is obtained. The cornerstone of management is physical therapy. Additional interventions for spasticity, such as tendon release procedures or botulinum toxin injections, are sometimes necessary.

Case 6. Although this patient also had delayed motor development, the history also indicates motor regression, suggesting an ongoing disease process. The main goal in the history and examination is to determine whether the prominent abnormality is ataxia, weakness, or spasticity. If there were no history of regression, and the patient had a normal neurologic examination and serum creatine kinase (CK) level (making muscular dystrophy unlikely), it would be reasonable simply to observe the child over time, because some children who toe walk have no specific neurologic deficits, but the history of recent deterioration requires prompt evaluation.

Comment: In this case, the examination was notable for prominent calf muscles and proximal weakness in all four limbs. He exhibited Gowers' sign: he marched up his legs with his hands in order to stand up from the floor. These findings suggest a primary muscle disorder, and in particular, the prominent calf muscles are typical of muscular dystrophy. Elevated CK and genetic testing confirmed the diagnosis of Duchenne's muscular dystrophy. The patient was referred to a muscular dystrophy clinic, where he was enrolled in an ongoing physical therapy program and started on prednisone.

Case 7. Although the prominent feature of this case is intellectual regression, there is also a suggestion of paroxysmal symptoms. Frequent daydreaming had been observed both in school and at home. This is often the only symptom reported for children with absence seizures, and physicians (and teachers) must be alert to this possibility. Complex partial seizures may also manifest as daydreaming spells. Absence or complex partial seizures may go unrecognized until they lead to problems at school. Further historical information about the daydreaming spells would be helpful: Can the patient respond during the spells? Are there any associated eye or face movements? Does she have any unusual feelings before, during, or after the spells? The examiner should search for focal neurologic abnormalities, which would support the diagnosis of complex partial seizures. The child should be instructed to hyperventilate for at least two minutes while the examiner watches her for absence seizures.

Comment: This girl's neurologic examination was normal, and hyperventilation provoked a typical absence attack. Her EEG showed the classic finding of 3-Hz spike-and-wave activity, and ethosuximide was started. Her daydreaming spells and school problems resolved promptly.

Case 8. In contrast to the previous case, nothing suggests that this boy has a paroxysmal condition. There has been no regression noted, and if further questioning reveals no evidence of a seizure disorder or developmental deterioration, the clear response to methylphenidate would suggest that the diagnosis of ADHD is correct. A family history of this condition would also support the diagnosis. The main goal of the examination is to exclude a structural lesion. It would not be unusual if this patient's examination revealed some "soft neurologic signs"—subtle abnormalities that do not clearly correlate with discrete, focal lesions, and that might be considered normal in a younger child. These are present in many patients with ADHD and other learning disorders, and they have uncertain significance.

If the history reveals no evidence of a paroxysmal or progressive disorder and the examination shows no significant focal abnormalities, then no diagnostic studies are indicated. The methylphenidate treatment should continue.

Case 9. Like the girl in Case 7, this boy has experienced intellectual regression, but in this case, nothing suggests paroxysmal symptoms, so the likelihood of progressive neurologic disease is greater. On the other hand, the problems began at a time of significant psychologic stress, and it was reasonable for his teachers and physicians to wonder about a connection. Historical information should be elicited regarding his behavior outside of school. If he continues to perform well at extracurricular activities he enjoys and still gets along with his friends, an underlying neurologic disease is unlikely. Historical evidence for a focal lesion (such as language disturbance or hemiparesis) and focal examination deficits should also be sought. A family history of neurologic disease would help considerably in narrowing the differential diagnosis.

If the above considerations fail to reveal a specific diagnosis, an MRI scan of the brain should be done, looking for either a focal abnormality or a diffuse process such as leukodystrophy or hydrocephalus. Depending on the age of onset, time course, family history, associated physical examination findings, and MRI findings, more specific tests for particular metabolic, chromosomal, infectious, and neoplastic diseases may be indicated.

Comment: This boy's behavior problems extended to the playground, where he had been getting in more and more fights. Even though he had not lost any motor skills, his examination revealed lower extremity spasticity. This prompted an MRI scan of the brain, which showed symmetric abnormalities in the cortical periventricular white matter bilaterally. This suggested the diagnosis of adrenoleukodystrophy. The diagnosis was confirmed by measuring very long chain fatty acids in serum. Unfortunately, the boy's clinical and MRI manifestations were sufficiently advanced that he was unlikely to respond to dietary therapy or hematopoietic stem cell transplant, so these treatments were not initiated.

Chapter 18

Geriatric Neurology

I. Case Histories

Case 1. An 82-year-old man who was diagnosed with Alzheimer's disease a year ago has had four episodes of urinary incontinence in the past 3 weeks. His family members understand that people with Alzheimer's disease are often incontinent, and they want advice on how they should deal with the problem. The patient is unable to describe the episodes of incontinence in any detail. He cannot remember whether he felt any urge to void before any of the episodes, and he is embarrassed to talk about them at all. Despite his dementia, he still converses normally, has no difficulty showering or dressing, does simple chores like dishwashing and yard work, and plays golf twice a week.

His general physical examination is unremarkable. He is alert, attentive, and jovial. He talks fluently, but he has some word-finding problems. He can follow one- and two-step commands but typically makes slight errors when given three-step commands. He has a normal digit span. He can only remember one of three items after a 5-minute delay, even with prompting. He cannot name the current president and cannot remember the ages or birth order of his children. He has eight grandchildren but cannot name any of them. He is able to perform one-digit addition and subtraction in his head, but no calculations more complicated than that.

His cranial nerve examination is normal. He walks stiffly, with no obvious asymmetry. He has marked spasticity in both lower extremities, but his strength is normal throughout all four limbs, and individual limb coordination is intact. He has diminished biceps and brachioradialis reflexes, but triceps reflexes are brisk bilaterally, and he has unsustained clonus at the knees and ankles, with bilateral Babinski signs. His mental status makes a detailed sensory examination difficult, but he seems to react much more strongly to pinprick in the upper extremities, neck, and face than in the trunk and lower extremities.

Questions:

1. Is this patient's incontinence likely to be due to Alzheimer's disease?
2. Are any other investigations necessary?
3. What interventions are indicated?

Case 2. A 78-year-old woman complains to her family physician that she has chronic pain in her elbows, hips, and knees, and it is worse at the end of the day. The woman's history, examination, and x-rays are all consistent with degenerative joint disease, but she is noted to have absent ankle jerks and markedly diminished vibration sense in her toes.

Questions:

1. Is this woman's pain likely to be caused by peripheral polyneuropathy?
2. What additional diagnostic tests are necessary?

Case 3. A 70-year-old man complains of unsteady gait since an open reduction and internal fixation procedure for a hip fracture two months ago. He received physical therapy after discharge, and it helped, but he continues to feel like "any puff of air would blow me over." He has fallen on two occasions when he got up in the middle of the night. He is afraid that he may sustain another fracture if he falls again.

His past history is notable for non–insulin-dependent diabetes. His general physical examination is normal. He has normal mental status, although he is clearly anxious. His cranial nerves are notable only for decreased visual acuity and reduced hearing bilaterally. When the examiner points this out, the patient says that he had been scheduled for cataract surgery, but it was canceled because he fractured his hip four days before the operation date. His wife has been urging him to get his hearing checked, but he has been too busy. His gait is tentative, and he limps favoring the side of the surgery, but he needs no support and has no tendency to sway to either side. He has normal coordination and strength throughout all four limbs. His upper extremity reflexes are normal, his knee reflexes are brisk, and ankle reflexes cannot be elicited. His plantar responses are flexor. Vibration sense is absent at the toes, moderately reduced at the ankles, and mildly reduced at the knees. Position sense is reduced at the toes, but normal elsewhere. He can distinguish sharp from dull throughout his body but says a pin feels less sharp in his feet and lower calves than elsewhere.

Questions:

1. What might be responsible for this patient's gait disturbance?
2. What diagnostic tests should be done?
3. What interventions are necessary?

II. Geriatric Issues

Three principles distinguish the neurologic assessment of older patients. First, and most important, people accumulate more diseases the longer they live. Second, some diseases occur primarily in the elderly. Third, even in the absence of any apparent disease, some components of the aging nervous system gradually deteriorate.

As a consequence, older patients often have numerous symptoms referable to more than one organ system. The standard approach of trying to localize all symptoms to a single lesion is untenable in many cases. Instead, the question is whether the patient has a degenerative disease affecting sites distributed diffusely throughout the nervous system or a combination of unrelated diseases. The neurologic examination provides useful information for answering this question, but accurate interpretation of the examination requires knowledge of the changes that occur during normal aging.

III. The Neurologic Examination in Normal Aging

It is harder than it might seem to characterize the changes that normally occur with aging. Because there is a wide range of variation even among normal subjects, a population study is required. The simplest kind of population study to conduct is a cross-sectional study, in which specific features are systematically observed in a random group of healthy people of a certain age and then compared to the same features in a separate group of healthy people of a different age. Cross-sectional studies can be misleading, however, because it is difficult to ensure that the groups being compared differ only in age and are identical in all other respects. For example, the elderly group might have a higher proportion of subjects with mild hypertension, cervical stenosis, or subclinical strokes than the younger group. An intended comparison of two "normal" groups then becomes a comparison of two groups with different (and often unrecognized) disease profiles.

Longitudinal studies are more reliable in this regard, but they are much more difficult to conduct. In a longitudinal study, a single group of randomly selected normal people of a certain age is observed serially over many years. Even with this kind of study it is impossible to control for the fact that a given individual might develop a disease during the period of observation, converting from "normal" to "abnormal." This would result in overestimation of the changes that occur with normal aging. Conversely, the changes could be underestimated if individuals with changes proved to be more difficult to follow over time. For example, suppose that even in the absence of any disease, 50% of normal individuals become so absent-minded as they age that they are unable to keep their appointments, whereas memory function remains completely normal in the other half of the population. A study based only on the people who were able to return for regularly scheduled memory testing would conclude that no memory problems occur in normal aging.

Even when a normal elderly subject demonstrates an abnormality on neurologic examination, its meaning may be ambiguous. It is often difficult to unravel the role played by intrinsic processes in the nervous system and the contribution of other, non-neurologic factors. For example, changes in gait can be related to fractures, sprains, and peripheral vascular disease as well as neurologic problems. Moreover, even within the nervous system there is interaction between different components. Gait changes may relate to abnormalities of sensation, strength, or coordination. Apparent changes in mental status may simply be due to primary sensory problems, especially hearing loss. Elderly people may seem to forget things just because they never heard them in the first place, and this can also cause them to ask the same question repeatedly. Speed of response is often important in interpreting the mental status examination, and this can be influenced by motor system problems. One example is parkinsonism, which sometimes causes patients to respond so slowly that examiners assume they don't know the answer and move on to another item.

Despite these limitations, some age-related changes in the "normal" neurologic examination have been consistently identified. All of these changes are of relatively low magnitude—that is, the variability between individuals of a given age is much greater than the change that occurs in any individual with aging. Even so, an awareness of these age-related changes is important when interpreting the neurologic examination in elderly patients.

A. Mental Status

The interpretation of age-related changes in the mental status examination is confounded by the deterioration that occurs in other processes (such as hearing loss and motor slowing), as discussed in the preceding paragraphs. Nonetheless, careful testing strategies that minimize these confounding factors permit the following general observations. First, older patients have difficulty thinking of words but relative sparing of vocabulary (i.e., they are still able to recognize and define words). Second, a generalized slowing of central processing occurs with aging. Third, recent memory and ability to learn new information decline, with relative sparing of remote memory. Note that the boundary between normal aging and mild cognitive impairment (see Chapter 7) is not sharply defined.

B. Cranial Nerves

The most common age-related changes noted in the cranial nerve examination relate to changes in sensory end-organs rather than intrinsic nervous system deterioration. The lens grows less clear and less elastic, the pupil becomes smaller and less elastic, rods and cones decrease in number, and the receptive fields of retinal ganglion cells change. As a result, older subjects have decreased light perception, reduced light/dark adaptation, impaired near vision (presbyopia), and changes in contrast sensitivity and color vision. Similarly, pure tone hearing declines with aging (presbyacusis), especially for high-frequency tones, and speech discrimination is diminished. Taste and smell discrimination often deteriorate slightly with aging also.

As they grow older, people often develop impairment of upward gaze. This is a supranuclear problem, so the vestibulo-ocular reflex elicits full upward excursion even though the subject cannot achieve this voluntarily. The smooth pursuit mechanisms also become less robust with aging, so "jerky" or "saccadic" pursuit is fairly common. Aging is the most common cause of ptosis; it is generally attributed to stretching of the skin and muscles of the eyelids over time, resulting in reduced elasticity.

C. Motor System

The single greatest change in station and gait that occurs with aging is a reduced ability to stand on one leg with the eyes closed. Older subjects have increased postural sway and reduced postural reflexes. They walk with a widened base, a stooped posture, shortened steps, and reduced arm swing. In short, they resemble patients with mild Parkinson's disease.

Older subjects are less coordinated when manipulating small objects. They are mildly uncoordinated without frank dysmetria when performing finger-to-nose and heel-to-shin testing. Their movements are slowed compared to younger subjects. Postural and kinetic tremors are increasingly common with advancing age.

Muscle bulk declines with age, especially in the intrinsic muscles of the hands and feet. Power is also reduced. The EMG reveals changes consistent with partial denervation and reinnervation. Paratonia is common in the elderly.

D. Reflexes

Deep tendon reflexes become less brisk as people age, with a distal-to-proximal gradient, although at least 80% of truly normal elderly subjects still have detectable ankle reflexes. Babinski signs are rare in normal subjects, regardless of age. All of the so-called primitive reflexes (grasp, snout, root, suck, and palmomental) increase in prevalence with age, but except for the grasp reflex, all of them are sometimes present in younger normal subjects, also.

E. Sensation

Ability to sense vibration declines with age, again with a distal-to-proximal gradient. Normal subjects who are more than 70 years of age are commonly unable to detect vibration at the toes. Position, light touch, and pain sensation also deteriorate, but to a lesser degree.

IV. Common Neurologic Symptoms in the Elderly

A. Dizziness

In Chapter 14, the different implications of light-headedness, vertigo, and disequilibrium were stressed. These distinctions often blur in older patients, who frequently have several coexisting problems. Arrhythmia, congestive heart failure, and orthostatic hypotension can all contribute to light-headedness, and they are all common in the geriatric population. Many of the medications that are prescribed to older patients can cause either light-headedness or vertigo. The likelihood of ischemic disease in the posterior circulation increases with advancing age. Many age-related changes in sensory function, including visual, auditory, and proprioceptive deterioration, can result in disequilibrium. When an elderly patient is able to give a clear description of a single type of symptom, the evaluation should proceed as it would in a young adult. When the history is more confusing, a careful neurologic examination should be performed with particular attention to the sensory and motor pathways that are important in maintaining balance. In many instances, dizziness is determined to be a result of many different abnormalities, each of which, in isolation, would be too mild to produce significant symptoms.

B. Gait Disturbance

The most common factors in older patients with gait difficulty are cervical stenosis, polyneuropathy, and mechanical problems such as fractures. All of the causes of dizziness and disequilibrium discussed in the preceding paragraph can also interfere with walking. Other potential causes of gait disturbance that must be considered in elderly patients include parkinsonism, strokes (causing focal weakness, spasticity, or ataxia), cerebellar deterioration (most often from chronic alcohol use), and subdural hematomas (acute or chronic). Normal pressure hydrocephalus is uncommon but should always be considered because of the potential for improvement with treatment. As with dizziness, extensive evaluation of elderly patients with gait problems often reveals a number of potential causes, each of which by itself would produce only minimal symptoms but when combined cause serious impairment.

C. Incontinence

Elderly patients who are incontinent should be evaluated according to the principles presented in Chapter 16. The evaluation can be particularly difficult in demented patients, who often have difficulty providing the historical information necessary to distinguish a spastic from a flaccid bladder. In these patients, diagnosis may depend on associated symptoms, physical examination findings, and results of urodynamic studies. Dementia can result in incontinence because of impairment of the normal cortical inhibition of the micturition reflex, but other causes of incontinence must also be considered. Incontinence may be the only symptom of prostatic hypertrophy or a urinary tract infection in demented patients. Medications frequently contribute to the problem, also. Because gait impairment is so common in the elderly, many patients have functional incontinence caused by an inability to reach the bathroom in time. Again, the problem often proves to be a combination of many slight abnormalities, none of them severe enough in isolation to cause significant symptoms. Incontinence could occur in a moderately demented patient with low-grade peripheral neuropathy and mild cervical stenosis, for example. The most important practical objective is to determine whether any of the factors contributing to the incontinence are treatable.

D. Dementia

The most common dementing illnesses occur primarily in the elderly population, so the points made in Chapter 7 do not need modification here.

E. Pain

The principles of evaluation and management of painful conditions are the same in the elderly as in younger patients, except that older patients are more likely to have more than one painful condition simultaneously. Many chronic painful conditions are incurable, and over time these may combine with accumulated injuries and mechanical stress on the musculoskeletal system to the point where some older patients complain of constant or debilitating pain. Depression may intensify pain and complicate management. Depression is common in the elderly, and chronic pain may itself lead to depression. In addition, older patients have heightened sensitivity to the side effects of drugs, and patients with several chronic conditions are often taking multiple medications. As a result, they can develop confusion or depression, further complicating pain management.

A few painful conditions occur exclusively or primarily in older patients. Polymyalgia rheumatica (with or without temporal arteritis), post herpetic neuralgia, and trigeminal neuralgia are examples.

V. Discussion of Case Histories

Case 1. Although it is true that Alzheimer's disease can cause incontinence, other possible causes should also be considered, especially in patients whose dementia is as mild as this patient's. Prostate hypertrophy and urinary tract infections should always be considered. In this case, the examination strongly suggests a spinal cord lesion. There are unambiguous upper motor neuron findings in the lower extremities, indicating a lesion above the lumbar region of the spinal cord. The brisk triceps reflexes further localize the lesion to above the C7 level, whereas the diminished brachioradialis and biceps reflexes indicate that the lesion is not above C5. In short, the reflexes alone localize the lesion to the C5 or C6 level of the spinal cord. The sensory examination cannot be performed in enough detail in this patient to provide precise localizing information, but the suggestion of a sensory level is at least consistent with a spinal cord lesion. Since the patient and his family don't even seem concerned about his gait disturbance, it probably developed gradually, but his urinary symptoms are new, indicating that the spinal cord lesion is getting worse. He needs an MRI scan of the cervical spine as soon as possible. The most likely cause of cervical myelopathy in this age group is compression from herniated discs or osteophytes. Despite his age and dementia, surgery is a realistic option. He appears to be active, productive, and happy; if he were paraplegic, his quality of life would deteriorate markedly and the cost of his maintenance and medical care would rise dramatically.

If the MRI scan shows a mass lesion unrelated to degenerative disease, the imaging characteristics will determine subsequent evaluation and management (including a search for a primary cancer if the mass looks like metastatic disease, and possible steroid treatment and radiation therapy). If no mass lesion is found, nonstructural causes of myelopathy should be considered. These include vitamin B12 deficiency, thyroid disease, and neurosyphilis. Motor neuron disease is another consideration, but it would be more likely if there were evidence of lower motor neuron dysfunction at a level below C6. The suggestion of a sensory level also reduces the likelihood of motor neuron disease. Finally, normal pressure hydrocephalus is always a consideration when the triad of incontinence, gait disturbance, and dementia is present, but this diagnosis is unlikely, given the evidence for myelopathy on examination. Similarly, multi-infarct dementia should be considered in a patient with focal neurologic signs and dementia, but multi-infarct dementia would not explain the reflex gradient or the possible sensory level.

Case 2. This patient's pain is located in her joints, not in her distal extremities, so the cause is much more likely to be degenerative joint disease than peripheral polyneuropathy. The examination findings of absent ankle jerks and decreased distal vibratory sensation are not uncommon in the elderly. Without any other examination findings or symptoms suggestive of peripheral polyneuropathy, no further diagnostic studies are necessary.

Case 3. This patient has many problems that could potentially contribute to disequilibrium. He has impaired vision, presumably caused by cataracts. He also has hearing impairment that is probably caused by end-organ degeneration, suggesting that his vestibular end-organ might be similarly affected. Note that he did not think to mention his cataracts or hearing loss when asked about his past history—most patients don't. You should get in the habit of asking elderly patients about cataracts, glaucoma, and hearing loss explicitly, not just with open-ended questions. This patient also has reduced position sense in the lower extremities, probably due to peripheral polyneuropathy in view of the other findings on his examination. All of these sensory deficits can interfere with the ability to determine the position of the body relative to the environment, so they could all be contributing to this patient's gait disturbance.

In addition, this man now has an impaired motor response because of the mechanical limitations imposed by his hip fracture (which may have resulted from a fall caused by his unsteady gait—further questioning would be necessary to determine the cause). A hint of an upper motor neuron lesion exists as well, because his knee reflexes are brisk despite evidence for a peripheral polyneuropathy. The most likely cause would be cervical myelopathy from degenerative disease. Finally, psychological factors now seem to be playing a significant role in limiting his gait. He appears to be nervous about walking even though he is not particularly unsteady.

It may prove impossible to identify which of these problems is primarily responsible for the patient's gait impairment. Indeed, each of the problems seems to be fairly mild and in isolation would be unlikely to produce significant disability. All of the problems should be addressed and treated if possible. You should urge him to follow through with the cataract surgery and also to be evaluated for a hearing aid. Although the polyneuropathy is probably due to his diabetes, other potential causes should be explored, especially thyroid disease and vitamin B12 deficiency, because these two treatable conditions can cause both polyneuropathy and myelopathy. With no evidence of myelopathy other than the brisk knee reflexes, no surgery would be indicated even if he had significant degenerative disease of the cervical spine, so an MRI scan is not necessary. He should have plain films of the cervical spine, however, to exclude more concerning causes of mild cord compression (e.g., metastatic disease). Finally, the patient should receive additional physical therapy to increase his confidence while walking and to prevent deconditioning. If the evaluation reveals no evidence of severe ongoing disease, you should make a point of reassuring the patient. Some patients restrict their walking so much because of anxiety that they ultimately develop disuse atrophy that is a more serious limitation than any of their original problems.

Chapter 19

Practice Cases

I. Case Histories

For each of the following cases, answer the following questions:

1. Is the lesion focal, multifocal, or diffuse?
2. What is the temporal profile?
3. What diagnostic category is most likely?
4. What is the most likely diagnosis?

Case 1. A 55-year-old woman came to the emergency room because of trouble speaking. She had some pain behind her left ear yesterday, but was otherwise fine until this morning, when she noted that water was leaking out of the left side of her mouth as she was brushing her teeth. Several hours later, while on the phone, she realized that her words were slurred. She looked in the mirror and saw that the left side of her face was drooping. She came immediately to the emergency department. On examination, she has weakness of eye closure, smile, and forehead wrinkling on the left side of her face. She has mild, flaccid dysarthria. The rest of her examination is normal.

Case 2. A 72-year-old right-handed man came to see his primary care physician because of trouble speaking. He is not sure exactly when it began, but notes that he gave a speech 4 months ago and neither he nor anyone else noted any problems at the time. Over the past two months or so, his speech has grown progressively more slurred, to the point where he has stopped speaking on the telephone. In the past few weeks, he has also choked while drinking water on several occasions. On examination, he has marked dysarthria, with both spastic and flaccid components. His tongue is atrophic, with prominent fasciculations. He also has some fasciculations in his quadriceps and deltoid muscles bilaterally. He has diffuse hyperreflexia, and bilateral Babinski signs.

Case 3. A 3-year-old boy was brought to the pediatrician because of trouble speaking. He attempts only single-word utterances, and his speech is loud, harsh, and imprecise. His other developmental milestones are also very delayed compared to his older sister. He has no other siblings. On examination, he has a long face, with prominent ears. He avoids eye contact, and says only a few, poorly articulated words. He does not follow directions. He has no focal abnormalities.

Case 4. A 56-year-old woman came to her physician because of trouble speaking. She first noticed the problem about two years ago, but when she mentioned it to her husband he told her she was just being neurotic. The problem has progressed slowly but steadily, to the point where her husband now acknowledges it. Her examination is notable for marked dysnomia, labored speech, and frequent paraphasic errors. Her mental status is otherwise normal, and so is the rest of her examination.

Case 5. A 58-year-old man has come to the physician because of lower extremity pain. He initially noted tingling in his toes about eight months ago, but this gradually spread to involve both feet, and over the past month it has spread above the ankles about a third of the way to the knees. The pain has a burning quality, and he has a very hard time falling asleep. He has not noticed any weakness. His examination is notable for obesity, slight weakness of ankle dorsiflexion bilaterally, reduced knee reflexes, absent ankle reflexes, and reduced sensation to all modalities from the mid-calf down, worse distally.

Case 6. A 72-year-old woman has come to the physician because of lower extremity pain. She has no problems when she is sitting or lying down, but within a minute of standing she develops severe pain in her thighs and calves bilaterally. This problem has been getting gradually worse over the past nine months. She has found that bending over a shopping cart relieves the pain to some degree. She continues to swim half a mile each day, and this does not cause her any pain. Her examination is normal.

Case 7. A 29-year-old man has come to the physician because of involuntary movements. The problem began about a year ago and has been getting gradually worse. His neck feels as if it is being pulled to the right, and although he can overcome the pulling when he tries, it requires a great deal of concentration and he finds it very painful. Superimposed on the chronic deviation to the right, he has intermittent jerking movements of the head in that direction. His examination is normal except for his head position.

Case 8. A 69-year-old woman has come to the physician because of involuntary movements. They occur during her sleep. She has had the problem for at least 15 years, but it has been getting worse, and has now reached the point where her husband will no longer sleep in the same bed. In the middle of the night, she suddenly begins thrashing wildly with her arms. She has fallen out of bed on a few occasions. During one of these episodes, her husband shook her awake, and she told him that she had been dreaming that burglars had broken into the house and were trying to tie her up. She has had no involuntary movements during the day, but she is having trouble walking for some reason. Her husband is also concerned about her memory. Her examination is notable for mild dementia, cogwheel rigidity at both wrists, a stooped posture, short steps, and slow turning.

Case 9. A 27-year-old man has come to the physician because of visual symptoms. The problem began 4 months ago, but resolved by the next morning, and since that time he has had about five episodes in all, each lasting 2 days or less. The episodes consist of double vision, which resolves if he closes either eye. He has also noticed that the two images tend to be much farther apart later in the day. His examination is notable for ptosis of the left eyelid and trouble maintaining upward gaze for more than 30 seconds.

Case 10. A 33-year-old woman has come to the physician because of visual symptoms. Her vision starts to "tunnel down" to the point where everything is momentarily black, and returns to normal within 15 seconds. These episodes can occur at any time, but she has noticed that they are particularly likely to happen when she first stands up from a chair. She has had this problem for 5 months, and during that time she has also had a dull, constant headache. Her examination is notable for obesity and bilateral papilledema.

Case 11. A 52-year-old man has come to the emergency department because of trouble using his left hand. He has had intermittent tingling in the fourth and fifth fingers of his left hand for more than a year, and for the past month the tingling has been continuous. His left hand has been getting gradually weaker over the past month, and over the past 2 weeks he has noticed that the hand is shrinking. He has no neck pain. His examination is notable for atrophy and weakness of the intrinsic muscles of his left hand, with reduced sensation to all modalities in the fourth and fifth digits of that hand. Percussion at the left elbow exacerbates the tingling in his fourth and fifth fingers (Tinel's sign).

Case 12. A 22-year-old woman has come to the emergency department because of trouble using her left hand. She had experienced some neck pain for the past few weeks, but it had responded to chiropractic manipulation, and she was otherwise fine until about 10 a.m. today, when she suddenly dropped her coffee cup. When she tried to clean up the mess, she discovered that she could not control her left hand. She came immediately to the emergency department, where her examination reveals marked ataxia of the left upper extremity, and mild ataxia of the left lower extremity. Her strength, reflexes, and sensation are normal, as are her mental status and cranial nerves. She has no history of previous medical problems, takes no medications (including contraceptive medications), and does not smoke.

II. Answers

Case 1.

1. focal (left facial nerve)

2. acute

3. vascular

4. Bell's palsy

Comment: This is a situation in which the principles of Chapter 3 lead to the wrong diagnostic category—Bell's palsy is thought to be an inflammatory condition, not a vascular one. The principles lead to the correct diagnostic approach, however, because vascular disease must always be considered in a patient with acute facial weakness. Patients must be examined carefully for additional neurologic findings (especially weakness or numbness of the ipsilateral face and leg) before diagnosing Bell's palsy. This patient had a completely normal examination except for her left facial weakness. She received prescriptions for prednisolone and acyclovir, and instructions for eye care to prevent corneal injury. Her face continued to get weaker for a day, then reached a plateau. It started to improve three weeks later, and returned to baseline over the subsequent four weeks.

Case 2.

1. diffuse (upper motor neurons and lower motor neurons)

2. chronic

3. degenerative

4. ALS

Comment: This patient was started on riluzole and BiPAP, but developed aspiration pneumonia about a month after his disease was diagnosed. In accordance with his advance directives, he was treated with antibiotics but not intubated, and when his respiratory function continued to deteriorate he was given opiates to minimize his discomfort. He died shortly thereafter.

Case 3.

1. diffuse (supratentorial)
2. chronic
3. congenital-developmental
4. fragile X syndrome

Comment: Although the craniofacial abnormalities suggested fragile X syndrome, this boy had careful testing for hearing impairment and other potentially treatable causes of developmental delay. Genetic testing eventually confirmed the presumptive diagnosis of fragile X syndrome, and he was enrolled in a therapy program directed at speech, language, and behavioral problems. His parents were also provided with extensive counseling, including genetic counseling.

Case 4.

1. focal (left frontal lobe)
2. chronic
3. neoplasm
4. frontotemporal dementia

Comment: This is another situation in which the principles of Chapter 3 lead to the wrong diagnostic category, but the correct diagnostic approach, because neoplasm must be considered in any patient with a progressive focal lesion. In this patient, an MRI scan was normal except for mild left frontal atrophy. A PET scan showed prominent abnormalities in the left frontal and temporal lobes. This patient and her husband were counseled regarding the diagnosis, prognosis, and techniques for facilitating her communication.

Case 5.

1. diffuse (sensory and motor peripheral nerves)
2. chronic

3. toxic-metabolic

4. polyneuropathy

Comment: This patient had a normal fasting glucose, but an abnormal 2-hour glucose tolerance test. The results of all other tests for common causes of polyneuropathy were normal. He was given the diagnosis of impaired glucose tolerance and counseled regarding exercise and diet. Studies have shown that patients with impaired glucose tolerance who comply with dietary modification and a regular exercise program are less likely to progress to overt diabetes during the follow-up period; these measures also produce a short-term improvement in small fiber nerve function and a more sustained benefit with respect to pain.

Case 6.

1. focal (cauda equina/lumbosacral nerve roots)

2. chronic

3. neoplasm

4. lumbar spinal stenosis

Comment: As discussed in Chapter 3, structural disease of the spine is another situation in which the diagnostic principles lead to the wrong diagnosis but the right approach. This patient's lumbar MRI scan showed no neoplasm, but significant lumbar spinal stenosis. She responded well to surgery.

Case 7.

1. focal (though specific site unknown – left basal ganglia?)

2. chronic

3. neoplasm

4. spasmodic torticollis

Comment: The failure to reach the correct diagnostic category in this case is hardly an indictment of the principles of Chapter 3, because the etiology of torticollis remains unknown. This patient had an excellent response to botulinum toxin injections, and said that only after he started "to feel normal again" did he appreciate how much his symptoms had been limiting his activity.

Case 8.

1. diffuse (basal ganglia and cerebral cortex bilaterally)

2. chronic

3. degenerative

4. REM sleep behavior disorder as a component of DLB (dementia with Lewy bodies)

Comment: Her history was classic for REM sleep behavior disorder, and a polysomnogram confirmed the diagnosis. This syndrome often precedes other manifestations of degenerative disease by years or decades, as it did in this case. Her sleep disorder responded to a low dose of clonazepam at bedtime. Her examination also revealed dementia and parkinsonism, consistent with DLB. She was given a prescription for donepezil; she and her husband thought that it made her thinking a little sharper, but the effect was not dramatic.

Case 9.

1. multifocal (neuromuscular junction)

2. intermittent

3. inflammatory

4. myasthenia gravis

Comment: Because this patient's symptoms are intermittent, the principles summarized in Table 3.1 do not apply. The purely motor manifestations, the predilection for ocular muscles, the intermittent time course, and the worsening at the end of the day all suggest myasthenia gravis. His symptoms responded to pyridostigmine. A thymectomy was considered, but deferred.

Case 10.

1. focal (increased intracranial pressure)

2. chronic

3. neoplasm

4. idiopathic intracranial hypertension (IIH, pseudotumor cerebri)

Comment: It may seem strange to think of this case as focal, because the symptoms and signs were symmetric, but it is probably best to consider increased intracranial pressure focal until proven otherwise, with the assumption that a focal lesion has interrupted the flow of CSF or the brain's venous outflow. In fact, that is the basis for the name pseudotumor – this condition mimics a tumor. An MRI scan was normal, and a lumbar puncture revealed an opening pressure of 300 mm of water (normal opening pressure is 180 mm or less). This patient's symptoms responded to acetazolamide. She managed to lose 55 pounds over the next two years, at which point the medication was successfully tapered.

Case 11.

1. focal (left ulnar nerve)

2. chronic

3. neoplasm

4. compression neuropathy of ulnar nerve at the elbow (cubital tunnel syndrome)

Comment: This patient's sensory and motor symptoms could be consistent with a lesion either of the ulnar nerve or of the C8 nerve root, but the fact that the symptoms could be reproduced by percussion at the elbow is strong evidence for an ulnar nerve lesion, because the elbow is the most common site of ulnar nerve compression. This is another situation in which "neoplasm" must be understood in its most general sense ("new growth"). Although cancer is certainly in the differential, connective tissue is responsible for the compression in most cases. Conservative therapy with protective elbow padding is usually adequate, but the rapid progression of weakness in this patient prompted his physician to recommend surgical decompression. His sensory symptoms resolved soon after the surgery, and his strength gradually returned to baseline.

Case 12.

1. focal (left cerebellar hemisphere)

2. acute

3. vascular (ischemic)

4. stroke, likely due to vertebral artery dissection

Comment: A stroke in a young person with no cardiovascular risk factors raises the possibility of less common causes. In this case, the recent chiropractic manipulation suggested the possibility of arterial dissection, which was confirmed with MRI/MRA scanning. This patient was treated with warfarin. Repeat MRI/MRA scanning six months later showed that the vertebral artery had recanalized normally, and the warfarin was stopped.

Index

Note: Page references followed by "*f*" and "*t*" denote figures and tables, respectively.